D0777010

Treating People in Families

TREATING PEOPLE IN FAMILIES
An Integrative Framework

WILLIAM C. NICHOLS

Foreword by Augustus Y. Napier

RC
488.5
.N5353
1996

Indiana University
Library
Northwest

THE GUILFORD PRESS
New York London

© 1996 The Guilford Press
A Division of Guilford Publications, Inc.
72 Spring Street, New York, NY 10012

All rights reserved

No part of this book may be reproduced, stored in a retrieval system, or transmitted, in any form or by any means, electronic, mechanical, photocopying, mi-
crofilming, recording, or otherwise, without written permission from the Pub-
lisher.

Printed in the United States of America

This book is printed on acid-free paper.

Last digit is print number: 9 8 7 6 5 4 3 2 1

Library of Congress Cataloging-in-Publication Data
Nichols, William C.
  Treating people in familes : an integrative framework /
William C. Nichols : foreword by Augustus Y. Napier.
  p. cm. — (The Guilford family therapy series)
  Includes bibliographical references and index.
  ISBN 1-57230-036-1
  1. Family psychotherapy. I. Title. II. Series.
RC488.5.N5353 1996
616.89'156—dc20   95-25437
                                             CIP

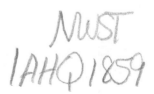

To Mary Anne

FOREWORD

In reading this important book, I am reminded of how far the field of family therapy has traveled from its beginnings. The movement I entered as a graduate student in the 1960s was dominated by a few bold pioneers. The people who influenced me then were Nathan Ackerman, Murray Bowen, Carl Whitaker, Don Jackson, Virginia Satir, Lyman Wynne, Salvador Minuchin, and Jay Haley. Inevitably, family therapy was caught up in those tumultuous years. Family therapy was going to overthrow the entrenched bastions of psychoanalytic tradition; and it might save the world. In order to accomplish its aims, family therapy had to embrace a wide net of social systems and influences, and it needed to cut loose from psychoanalytic thinking that grounded psychotherapy in the intrapsychic processes of individuals. Systems theory helped send us to the moon, and it provided conceptual reassurance to those of us who were defining the "patient" in more and more ambitious (some would say grandiose) terms: the nuclear family, the extended family, the friendship and "helping network," the community. The writings and conferences of those years were full of argument and bravura, and, because we were dealing with so much conceptual complexity, we fell into camps around the most charismatic leaders. Was one a structuralist follower of Minuchin? A Whitakerite? A Bowenian? It was an exciting, anxious, and largely feudal world where new lands were being explored and fought over.

The family therapy presented in this book represents a far different world from the social experiments of the 1960s and 1970s. While William Nichols also casts a wide conceptual net, this work is grounded in the more modest world of the *practice of family therapy*, and of several intervening decades of that activity. Written for the student of family therapy and for the practitioner, it is an impressive compilation, a winnowing of the experiences of many others' work, and an integration of diverse approaches and concepts. The common ground is a kind of sensible pragmatism: It is a wise and very experienced therapist's summation of *what works*. I find it accessible, logical, helpful; and I trust that others will also find in it valuable assistance in their efforts to help couples and families.

The book is divided into two sections. Section I, entitled, "Personality, Context, and Integration," is general and theoretical. Chapter 1 presents the field of family therapy, its popularity, its power, its efficacy, and its social context. Nichols reminds us of the force of the individual human personality and makes the call for an integrative approach, particularly one that "reincludes" the individual.

Chapter 2 outlines Nichols's own integrative mix. Of particular note here is the prominent reappearance of principles of psychodynamic psychotherapy, especially the work of Harry Stack Sullivan and W. R. D. Fairbairn and object relations theory. The spirit of Nathan Ackerman is alive in this emphasis; and as one who cut his psychological teeth on Sigmund Freud, I am delighted to be reminded of these pioneering thinkers who are the real link between the intrapsychic world of Freudian theory and the abstract realms of systems thought. The other planks in Nichols's platform are a highly pragmatic behavioral approach, which he explores in both marital and family contexts, and systems concepts. The latter he explores thoroughly but cautiously, reminding the reader that although one needs to think about systems dynamics, one always works with people. In fact, throughout this book one has the sense of Bill Nichols the person, who is engaged intelligently, sometimes firmly, always warmly— with other people.

Chapter 3 lays out the other main emphasis in this book: an embrace of the development over time of the family life cycle. The challenges and opportunities of these predictable cycles provide a health-seeking, normative context for "pathology," one that grounds the author in the conviction that if one can remove the often temporary impediments to a family's mastery of a difficult transition, the flow of life can resume. Several times in later chapters Nichols refers to "midwiving a relationship," and one develops a sense of the author's belief that the therapist needs mainly to lend an informed push or pull to the client system, freeing the family to move through its present dilemma into new territory. It is a hopeful, confidence-building point of view.

Section II is about therapy, and it follows two broad "developmental" scenarios: first are the challenges the therapist faces in working with various stages in the development of the family system, from marriages in formation to the "postparental couple," with of course much emphasis on families with children of various ages and dilemmas. Two final chapters deal with the noteworthy "detours" of divorce and remarriage. The second "developmental" focus is on the emerging therapy relationship, from initial assumptions about therapy, to techniques of engagement, to eventual termination. The author follows these two "stories" more or less in parallel, now picking up one strand, now another; but the evolution over time of family life is the guiding metaphor.

In Chapter 4 we are treated to a careful and thoughtful perspective on the family therapy process by a mature and wise therapist. We think carefully about the therapist–client relationship: who is responsible for what; the need for a respectful approach by the therapist; the principle of least pathology; the education of clients; issues of motivation, gender, ethnicity; ethical considerations. We look at the family's structure and decide how to begin an intervention. Throughout this chapter we are impressed by the author's flexibility and by his reluctance to prescribe formulas; we are sobered by the demand that the therapist think carefully about the possibilities of intervention.

Chapter 5 is about the evaluation of the client system and the beginning stages of treatment. Here Nichols presents the reader with a variety of tools, from the use of the genogram to various observational and interview strategies, as well as more formal assessment devices such as the Family Assessment Device and the Beavers Family Systems Model. We learn history taking, helping clients set goals, giving feedback, and planning treatment.

Chapter 6, "Therapy with Families in Formation," is vintage Bill Nichols. We begin with the formation of families through a review of the mate selection process, then proceed to the development of the therapy relationship with the marrying or newly married couple. After a tour of the initial interview, we "settle in" to the therapy process, exploring the dimensions of marriage through Nichols's "five C's": commitment, caring, communication, conflict and compromise, contracts and complementarity. We learn what he means by "midwiving the relationship" and how to deal with confidentiality issues and secrets. We even take an early look at termination! One gets the sense that the author is juggling many balls here, but we admire the performance.

Chapter 7, "Therapy with Expanding Families," and 8, "Therapy with Contracting Families," deal with the bread and butter issues of family therapy: the problems kids have raising their unhappily married parents. Nichols presents a variety of problems and calmly and sensibly offers an array of approaches to them. In each of these chapters we are treated to the author's own cases, and these illustrations—both here and in other chapters—are the richest aspects of the book. I like Nichols's clear, lively, compassionate approach to therapy.

Chapter 9, "Therapy with Postparental Couples," is poignantly and powerfully presented. It is about grief and loss and the other issues that

aging couples face. I found it richly meaningful as, of course, my eye would
be drawn to the phase of life in which Margaret and I find ourselves. (By
the way, marital satisfaction *does* take a great leap upward for many
postparental couples, a fact that Nichols neglects, perhaps because those
couples do not often seek therapy.)

I think I learned the most from Chapters 10 and 11, which deal,
respectively, with divorce and remarriage. These most difficult of treatment dilemmas for family therapists are often dealt with superficially in
texts, and I am glad to say that such is not the case here. In addition to
summarizing the work of others, Nichols guides us in his unflappable style
through these turbulent situations. His belief in the power of a kind of
"compassionate education" of clients shines through.

The family therapy I learned early in my career was full of the dogma
born of uncertainty; Nichols's approach to the therapy process is full of
the flexibility inspired by confidence. The field has come a long way, and
the rich lode of material that Nichols incorporates from the work of others
is ample testimony to that growth. Nichols's freedom in mixing diverse
elements in a unique way that reflects the person of the therapist is yet
another result of the evolution of the field. This is the true benefit from
an integrative approach: a challenge and model for today's family therapist
whose personhood shapes profession.

AUGUSTUS Y. NAPIER, PH.D.

PREFACE

My intention in writing this book was to try to advance the emphasis on integration in psychotherapy that has marked my endeavors in this field. Specifically, I have tried to go beyond what I have offered in two previous books in The Guilford Family Therapy Series, one coauthored with Craig A. Everett and one written alone. Most of all, I have tried to offer a framework for treating people in families that can be useful to practitioners who favor several different kinds of therapeutic interventions and techniques.

There is some material in this book that appeared previously, although virtually all of that material has been edited and rewritten specifically for this book. I appreciate the gracious agreement of Craig A. Everett, Ph.D., to the use of material from our 1986 book.

Augustus Y. Napier, Ph.D., now my colleague at the Family Workshop in Atlanta, merits a tremendous expression of gratitude for his perceptive criticisms and sharp editorial pencil. Gus not only read the manuscript as the superb clinician he is but also with the skill of an English teacher. The increased clarity and greater illustration in the present form of the manuscript are due largely to Gus's comments and suggestions. He not only went "above and beyond" any expectations one could have in critiquing the manuscript but also graciously consented to write a foreword to the book.

To Alan S. Gurman, Ph.D., founding Series Editor, and Seymour Weingarten, Editor-in-Chief of The Guilford Press, once again I say "Thank you" for your guidance and the pleasant working relationship in our third effort together.

Most of all, I express loving appreciation to my wife, Mary Anne Pace-Nichols, Ph.D., for being herself and for being there, for coming into my life and bringing great happiness and renewed meaning after I had been through a period of major pain and loss, and for her support while I snatched time from our overcrowded schedule to write.

WILLIAM C. NICHOLS
Oconee County Georgia

xi

CONTENTS

Treating People in Families

Personality, Context, and Integration

FAMILY THERAPY: REVOLUTION AND EVOLUTION

> *. . . the boundaries between the intrapersonal and the*
> *interpersonal are subtle. . . .*
> —ALAN S. GURMAN AND DAVID P. KNISKERN,
> *Handbook of Family Therapy*

There is little doubt that family therapy represents one of the major revolutions in the mental health field. When this vigorous new approach began to appear on the scene in the 1950s, it brought to psychotherapy a novel and powerful emphasis on the context in which a client develops and lives.

Traditionally, psychotherapists had focused on the individual and ignored the context. Generally, the problems presented to therapists were viewed as stemming from disturbances in the client's intrapsychic functioning. Hence, therapeutic interventions were aimed at dealing with the internal dynamics of the individual. Practitioners and teachers of orthodox psychoanalysis strongly cautioned against contact between the therapist and members of the client's family because of fear that any such association would contaminate the transference relationship between therapist and client. What was considered important was to treat what emerged from within the client. This was done essentially in isolation, in a special two-person relationship consisting of therapist and client in which the client's transference to the therapist provided the occasion and vehicle for achieving therapeutic change.

During the late 19th and early 20th centuries psychoanalytic theory and practice evolved and staked out a preeminent position in psychotherapy. At the same time, venerable nature–nurture arguments continued regarding the development of human personality. An either/or atmosphere prevailed in which explanations of personality development favored the influence either of human biology or of the environment. With some risk of oversimplification, this can be described as an emphasis on either "inside" or "outside" dimensions. Following the lead of the pioneering genius Sigmund Freud, early Western psychotherapy traditionally focused on the "inside" dimension of human personality, that is, on intrapsychic processes and conflicts.

Given that western culture had produced a romanticized and highly inaccurate view of "rugged individualism," it is understandable that the pioneering and dominant psychotherapy approach with its 19th-century roots embraced an "isolated individual" conception of personality and focused on treating individuals. Add to this the fact that Freud and his contemporaries were guided by a premodern physics that permitted a conceptualization of a human being as a "closed system," and it becomes even more clear how the idea could readily be accepted in Europe and North America that a person could be treated as if he or she stood alone.

Even group therapy, when it developed, focused on treating individuals who were unrelated to one another. One of the major controversies at one phase in group therapy, for example, was whether the group was to be heterogeneous (comprised of individuals with different symptoms and problems) or homogeneous (made up of individuals with similar symptoms and problems). Whatever the preference of the therapist for group composition, the focus in treatment typically was on the individual and his or her internalized conflicts and problems. With the exception of the marital therapy movement (Broderick & Schrader, 1981, 1991; Nichols & Everett, 1986) and elements of the child guidance techniques (Nichols & Everett, 1986) that were forerunners of family therapy, psychotherapy consisted largely of the treatment of individuals as individuals until the family therapy revolution erupted.

Such extreme emphasis on one aspect of human personality and human functioning virtually begged for corrective reactions. These were not long in coming. There were movements toward treatment of persons in marital settings and other forms of "relationship counseling." In addition, important developments began to arise within psychiatric theory and practice.

Harry Stack Sullivan's interpersonal theory of psychiatry, for example—which strongly influenced some early family therapists such as Don D. Jackson—was well under way during the 1920s. Focusing on communications and the patterns of interaction between people, Sullivan made it clear that the therapist does not deal with a patient/client as an "isolated and self-contained entity" but as a participant in an interpersonal situation

(Sullivan, 1953a, 1953b, 1954). Manifesting an animus against the excesses of the "rugged individual" and isolated individual concept (Mullahy, 1955), Sullivan went so far as to define personality as "the relatively enduring pattern of recurrent interpersonal situations which characterize a human life" (Sullivan, 1953b, pp. 110–111).

Family therapy threw down the gauntlet, taking the point of view opposite to an isolated individual approach. It insisted that the "outside" dimension was important. Adapting principles from a 20th-century scientific paradigm, General System Theory, to living systems, family therapists focused on the family system and functioning within that system rather than on the individual's internal processes. In a family systems approach, the individual is conceptualized "as an interdependent, contributing part of the systems that control his or her behaviors" (P. Minuchin, 1985, p. 291). More than anything else, this emphasis on a systems approach has characterized the family therapy perspective.

Generally, the early adherents of family therapy were correct in affirming the values of the new approach. But were they accurate in denying the values of other approaches? While emphasizing the significance of family systems, some highly visible and vocal early family therapists disavowed the necessity and importance of attending to the client's internal processes. Claiming that it was impossible to view individuals' mental processes at work, they adopted a "black box" concept from telecommunications—that is, comprehending the complexity of processes inside an electronic device is neither possible nor necessary in order to understand its use in a larger system. Adapting this approach to human beings, they put the emphasis in therapy on input–output relations (communication) rather than on the internal functioning of the person. They indicated that one can infer what goes on inside the person from the input–output relations. Knowing what "really" occurs internally is not essential for studying "the function of the device in the greater system of which it is a part," they insisted. The symptoms of an individual thus were conceptualized not as an indication of intrapsychic conflict but as a kind of input into the family system (Watzlawick, Beavin, & Jackson, 1967, pp. 43–44).

This kind of approach can dismiss not only the individual's internal processes but the individual as well. A significant portion of family therapists continue to concentrate almost entirely on the system. They view historical factors in the client's life and intrapsychic phenomena as irrelevant to therapy and proclaim a concern only with "horizontal" relationships in the here-and-now. Such family therapy purists tend to focus entirely on intervening with the family system. They emphasize discontinuity between family therapy and other therapeutic orientations that developed both before the emergence of family therapy in the 1950s and subsequently.

The adamant and sometimes dogmatic stance of early family therapists who emphasized "outside" factors in one side of an "either/or" approach to therapy is understandable in the context of the 1940s and 1950s. They were up against an entrenched, one-sided approach that emphasized the "inside" dimension. Without the strong statements and claims of their often dramatic fight, it is unlikely that they would have been able to establish the efficacy and legitimacy of their theory and practice against the hegemony and dogmatism of what can rightly be called "the [psychoanalytically dominated] psychotherapy establishment."

Today, it is unnecessary for family therapists to wage war against 19th century views of physics or personality. Neither is it necessary to seek to obliterate the values of psychodynamics or to go to extremes in order to establish appropriate claims regarding the effectiveness and place of family therapy in the psychotherapy field. An old adage holds that we frequently are right in what we affirm and wrong in what we deny or dispute. Family therapy and systems approaches are here to stay.

THE POPULARITY OF FAMILY THERAPY

Family therapy has had an impressive impact on the field of psychotherapy. Currently, it boasts the fastest growth rate of any modality in the mental health arena (Pinsof, 1990). Not only is it used with a large number of problems formerly treated only with individual psychotherapy, but also new meanings continue to be given to the notion that problems arise "between" persons and in the system itself. Other systems in the society that affect the family and its members, such as the educational, mental health, medical, and occupational systems in particular (Friedman, 1985; Imber-Black, 1988, 1991; Wynne, McDaniel, & Weber, 1986), increasingly are being studied and worked with by family therapists.

Some view the substantial and continuing popularity of family therapy as problematic, noting that a kind of "technolatry" exists among many who have embraced techniques of family therapy without a comprehension of the theory and substantive content on which the approach is based (Pinsof, 1990).

THE POWER OF FAMILY THERAPY

Family therapy is not only popular but also powerful. For example, having members of a family present for the psychotherapy session brings an immediacy to therapy that is not present in individual treatment. Rather than have a therapist and client discuss the client's relationships with absent family members, the client and his or her family members interact directly in the therapy setting. Family therapists have expended a considerable amount of ink in extolling the advantages that directly seeing and experiencing family relationships and interaction give the clinician in understanding pathology and assessing and treating various therapeutic issues.

Similarly, dealing with family issues "live" in a family therapy session can have dramatic and potent outcomes for clients as well as for therapists. For example, Ted, a young adult male, sought assistance individually because of hindering anxiety and fears that were interfering with his vocational and personal adjustment. He related how he was often "paralyzed" by reactions to his hard-driving, highly successful father. Exploration of his families of origin brought out the fact that his paternal grandfather was a powerful man but that Ted was not afraid of him. After careful preparation, Ted's parents were invited to join him for two sessions.

In the midst of one meeting, Ted's father described how frightened he had been early in his career and how he had driven himself to achieve success by deliberately doing what he was afraid to do.

TED: I never knew that you were afraid.

FATHER: Whew! I was scared spitless!

TED: Of what?

FATHER: That I would fail. I was scared all the time. [He then described how he had joined a public speaking group and "sweated blood" to learn how to speak, taken courses on assertiveness training, earned a master's degree in business administration, etc.]

TED: I always saw you as a powerhouse who could do anything. You were so self-confident . . . and angry.

FATHER: Scared. I was scared.

THERAPIST: (to Father) When did you stop being scared?

FATHER: Last year, when I merged my business with [another corporation] and cut a good deal for myself [that assured his financial future and an early retirement].

The most dramatic episode in the sessions took place when the therapist asked Ted's father about his own father.

THERAPIST: (to Father) What was your father like?

FATHER: (virtually rising out of his chair) He was a dictator! He was a tyrant!

TED: (quietly) Grandpa?

FATHER: Hell, yes! I was scared to death of him! Everything had to be his way. You had to do what he said. You couldn't fail.

For the moment, the highly successful executive was a frightened little boy once again, and his son could see the picture in living color and action. While Ted could understand his father's fear, he was personally not nearly so fearful of his grandfather as was his father. Hence, seeing his father as the frightened, fearful person that he was, the "scared son of a tyrant," rather than as an ogre in his own right, released Ted directly and dramatically from some of his own fear and anxiety. Whether or not the therapist's statement, "Those two sessions—and particularly that incident—saved us a year or so of work in individual therapy," was totally accurate, he was correct that they produced an immediate and powerful impact that would have been difficult to attain without the presence and direct therapeutic involvement of Ted's parents.

A considerable amount of what is generally regarded as individual psychotherapy can be facilitated and conducted much more rapidly and effectively by working with the identified patient or client in a family context. Bringing in the client's family of origin or parts of it can be done in order to deal with specific issues, as in the case of Ted, and for general therapeutic purposes as well. For example, a 38-year-old, single dentist being treated for depression (*Diagnostic and Statistical Manual of Mental Disorders*, revised third edition [DSM-III-R], 296.3; American Psychiatric Association, 1987) was boosted significantly when his elderly parents accepted the therapist's invitation to meet with him and their son and flew halfway across the country for the therapy session. The son's fervent statement, "Yeah, I know they care, because they really hate to fly, and they came anyway," was only a symbolic reflection of the positive impact of the parental actions.

THE PRAGMATISM OF FAMILY THERAPY

Family therapy is also pragmatic: It works. At least, it works for many kinds of problems, and it works very well. Gurman, Kniskern, and Pinsof (1986), for instance, found that improvement could be expected in nearly three-fourths (71%) of cases of childhood and/or adolescent behavioral problems treated by any of a number of clearly defined family therapy or eclectic psychotherapy methods. Additionally, the same researchers also found that family therapy methods also are successfully used with marital problems.

Family therapy, including marital therapy, is used effectively with selected psychiatric disorders. Clinicians and researchers have described its successful use in the treatment of a number of conditions from DSM-III-R and DSM-IV (American Psychiatric Association, 1987, 1994). These include agoraphobia (Hafner, 1986), alcoholism (O'Farrell, 1986; Steinglass, Bennett, Wolin, & Reiss, 1987), depression (Coyne, 1986,

1988; Dobson, Jacobson, & Victor, 1988), drug abuse (Kaufman & Kaufmann, 1979), eating disorders (Foster, 1986; Minuchin, 1974), narcissistic disorders (Lansky, 1986), schizophrenia (Anderson, Reiss, & Cahalane, 1986; McFarlane, 1983), and other individually diagnosed psychiatric conditions.

CONTINUING EVOLUTION: THE SCHOOLS PHASE

The growth of the family therapy field has paralleled that of other fields in that "schools" of theory and treatment have emerged. This development seems to be an inevitable stage in the evolution of an academic and practical field. Early, sometimes tentative discoveries tend to be elevated and hardened into dogma, then staunchly defended and propagated as "the truth," "the right way."

Salvador Minuchin (1982), one of family therapy's pioneering figures, has decried the development of these rigid positions. Describing how many of the early explorers "each selected a piece of territory, using the reality of this segment to reach families in pain" (p. 662), Minuchin notes that those in the forefront knew and privately acknowledged that their "private truths" were only part of the picture. As they acquired students, Minuchin points out, "larger buildings" were needed in order to accommodate the growing number of followers. Those buildings became "castles" with turrets, drawbridges, and watchmen to protect the "truth" presumably lodged behind the castle walls. Expensive and needing to justify their existence, the castles demand ownership of the total truth, declares Minuchin. Observing that those who seek him in his castle will not find him there, he implies that this period of multiple castles, each claiming and strenuously defending "the total truth," will end.

In the general field of psychotherapy, the proliferation of schools seems to have provided an overabundance of choices along with an awareness that no single theory has a monopoly on clinical effectiveness and adequacy for all cases. Over the past two decades, these and other factors have fueled a movement toward integration (Norcross & Newman, 1992). Family therapy trails the general field of psychotherapy in that the process of proliferating schools of family therapy may not yet have crested. Nevertheless, there are some signs that the eventual diminishing of the crowds flocking to the family therapy castles of "truth" is beginning, as Minuchin hinted would happen.

Currently, there are several classifications of schools of family therapy, but change is under way. Gurman and Kniskern (1981, 1991) in their highly regarded and widely used handbooks have indicated that some of the rigidity and purity of approach are undergoing mutation. Their original *Handbook of Family Therapy*, published in 1981, classified approaches to family therapy under four broad headings: psychoanalytic and object relations; intergenerational (contextual, symbolic–experiential, Murray Bowen–family systems); systems theory (Mental Research Institute [MRI] interactional, structural, strategic, functional, problem-centered, integrative); and behavioral (marital).

A decade later, Gurman and Kniskern (1991) expressed the view that most schools of family therapy were less "pure" than when they produced the first handbook and that there was an "increasing synthesis in clinical theory in the field, especially at the technical level" (p. xvi). Accordingly, rather than grouping the models into categories as in the 1981 handbook, they listed them in alphabetical order. These included behavioral (behavioral family therapy, behavioral marital therapy), Bowen theory and therapy, brief therapy (MRI approach), contextual, Ericksonian family therapy, focal family therapy, Milan systemic approach, family psychoeducational treatment, strategic, structural, and symbolic–experiential.

Individuals who take the examination in marital and family therapy that is used as part of qualifying for licensure as marital and family therapists in a majority of the states of the United States are expected to be familiar with 13 major models of family therapy: behavioral, cognitive-behavioral, contextual (Boszormenyi-Nagy), experiential, integrative, intergenerational (Bowen), network, psychodynamic/object relations, psychoeducational, strategic (Haley et al.), strategic (Watzlawick et al.), structural, and systemic (Milan) (Association of Marital and Family Therapy Regulatory Boards, 1989, p. 10).

All of these approaches are successful in some instances and with some cases, or they would not continue to be used, as Alan S. Gurman has appropriately noted (personal communication, February 14, 1994). Similarly, these approaches are not likely to be successful with all problems and all kinds of cases (Papp, 1983).

Family therapy continues to evolve. Essentially, the point has long since been made by family therapists that context is important. It is to be hoped that the field will move steadily and without delay beyond the schools stage into an atmosphere of openness toward various viewpoints and a welcoming attitude toward integration of theory and practice. Anyone who has visited a castle should be thoroughly aware that castles are often damp and gloomy and that they certainly are relics of a bygone era.

PERSONALITY IS HERE TO STAY

Just as family therapy and systems approaches are here to stay, so also are human personality and psychotherapy with the individual. Personality is a major focus of therapy. The therapist always works with human behavior, and that means dealing with persons, that is, living, feeling, anxious, fearing, desiring human beings.

Human Personality

There are nearly as many definitions of personality as there are students of personality. When the various definitions are drawn together and analyzed, however, two emphases emerge. That is, personality definitions tend to stress the "internal" or the "external" aspects of personality, depending largely on the orientation of the person making the definition. Psychologists have tended to focus on the internal aspects, the psychological and psychophysiological factors in personality. Sociologists and cultural anthropologists understandably have emphasized the external aspects, which can be related more directly to cultural and social forces.

Some theorists combine both the internal and the external aspects in their definition and understanding of the meaning of personality. The psychiatrist-family therapist Nathan Ackerman (1958), for example, proposed a biopsychosocial model of personality in which attention was given to intrapsychic events and interpersonal events, the real and the unreal, the unconscious and conscious organization of experience, related modes of social adaptation, and a person's view of both the future and the past. As mentioned above, the assumption here is that understanding personality is impossible without comprehending the context in which it is formed and sustained as a system and subsystem in a hierarchy of systems.

Traditionally, discussions of personality development have involved arguments over "heredity versus environment" or "heredity and environment," or some related attempt to grapple with the recognition that a biologically endowed human organism functions in a physical and sociocultural setting. At this point in history, we assume that most serious students of human personality acknowledge the fact that both heredity and environment, as well as their complex interplay, must be considered in dealing with personality. As the psychologist Gordon Allport (1961) put it, "The most important point of scientific agreement is that no feature or quality is exclusively hereditary and none exclusively environmental in origin" (p. 67). The old arguments concerning heredity versus environment are essentially meaningless, because the two sets of forces cannot be separated in any meaningful way. Both genetics and environment provide potential, and both set limits for human development and functioning. The question of what determinants shape and sustain human personality has to be refocused and framed in other ways.

Framework of Personality Formation

Kluckhohn and Murray (1956) have provided one of the most comprehensive frameworks for understanding the factors that determine personality formation. They discussed four classes of determinants: constitutional, group membership, role, and situational. These, along with the interaction of the four, further our understanding of the ways in which every person is like all, some, and no other members of the species. I have borrowed their list, changing the last category from situational to idiosyncratic experiences. The discussion that follows was influenced by the Kluckhohn and Murray material but essentially reflects my views and understandings, not theirs (cf. Nichols & Everett, 1986, pp. 93–99, for a more comprehensive discussion).

Constitutional Determinants

Age, sex, and physical traits, such as stature and physiognomy, influence not only a person's needs and expectations but also how that individual is treated by other people. Temperament is sometimes included as a significant constitutional factor. Temperament refers to the individual's mode and intensity of emotional response (e.g., whether one is lethargic and phlegmatic, "laid back," or intense and highly active, "hyper"); quality of prevailing mood (e.g., whether one tends to be optimistic and lighthearted or pessimistic and gloomy); and susceptibility to emotional stimulation (i.e., whether one is quickly or slowly emotionally aroused). Although there is a lack of consensus about the role that temperament plays in human behavior and precisely how to define temperament, the more solidly a personality disposition is rooted in one's constitution, the more likely it is to be referred to as temperament (Allport, 1961).

A major implication for family therapy, in addition to the differences in behavior and reaction related to age and sex, is that temperamental differences among children often affect in significant ways the reactions of parents to their offspring. A compliant, "good" baby may be handled differently than a colicky, "difficult" baby, for example, and a "responsive" child may be rewarded differently than a youngster labeled "hyperactive."

Group Membership Determinants

This refers to any lasting, organized group from the family through to entities at the national, or even international, level. Membership tends to expose individuals to both general and specific influences and to shape them in both general and specific ways. That is, there are general cultural patterns and social dimensions that impinge on individuals, as well as things that are mediated to the individual through agents of the society or groups such as parents or teachers.

A society is composed of people and the ways in which they are organized and linked together in a system. Their system of relatedness is partly ideational; that is, they behave and think in ways that are normative for their group. Culture, simply defined, is the shared, learned behavior that forms a characteristic way of life for the society. Culture includes, of course, material aspects and artifacts as well as nonmaterial components such as ideas, values, and concepts. Individuals learn about or absorb a culture from other individuals and through participation in small groups, as well as from general exposure to the culture. The subsystems of the society such as the family, school, peer groups, and work groups provide filters through which important aspects of the culture and social order are mediated to the individual. Socioeconomic class, or social class, also serves as a highly significant filtering and shaping factor in one's development and living. There are many possibilities of deviation from the norms of a culture, and there are many important subcultures within the confines of a large and complex nation.

Despite the existence of filtering factors and the possibilities for idiosyncratic learning as a private individual, some things can be predicted with a fair degree of accuracy on the basis of group membership. For example, one can make some informed guesses about Mr. Smith's values and behaviors by knowing that he is American, Protestant, and upper-middle-class in origin, as well as being a lawyer, a Southerner, and a lifelong resident of Nashville, Tennessee. Similarly, some predictions about Ms. Jones's values and behaviors could be made from the knowledge that she is an Irish-American, Roman Catholic pediatrician from a blue-collar background and a resident of Boston, Massachusetts. Add race to the equation and the possibilities of making informed guesses or accurate predictions about attitudes and behaviors of individuals are increased still further. One can also make reasonably informed guesses about families on the basis of social class, occupational level, ethnicity, and other factors related to culture and value considerations.

Instinct is not as important for human beings as it is for the lower portions of the animal world because in the process of evolutionary development Homo sapiens attained the capacity for symbolic functioning and use of language that permitted the development and transmission of culture. Man became a "symboling" creature par excellence who could think abstractly and communicate with other members of the species verbally. Human functioning and interaction were greatly facilitated by the accomplishment of language.

Planning, self-observation, introspection, and other ego functions became possible. It was no longer necessary to pass along what had been learned through direct training or observation. Ideas and descriptions could be expressed through words. Nor was it necessary to act solely on the basis of instinct. It was no longer necessary, in order for the species to survive, for all members of the species to carry within their nervous systems the means for instinctive patterning to emerge at crucial points (e.g., mating). What was required for survival and what was valued could be learned and stored through symbolization and thus transmitted to succeeding generations.

Parenthetically, one of the interesting and important contributions of family therapy has been a renewed emphasis on communication, including nonverbal communication, in human interaction. The use of words and language to obscure communication, rather than to facilitate direct and clear understanding, in schizophrenic behavior was one of the early focal points of interest among those who found themselves becoming family therapists.

Role Determinants

Playing a particular role for a long period of time leaves a distinct impact on an individual and roles become the basis for differentiating or distinguishing personalities within a group.

Roles have been defined in many ways, including the expectations (rights and obligations) that accompany a given status in a social group. Role playing is different from role taking, another important behavioral science concept. Role playing involves organizing one's conduct in conformity to the norms of the group. Role taking has to do with placing oneself in the position of the other, imagining how a situation looks from the standpoint of another person. Role taking is much closer to empathic functioning and empathic relating to another person or persons. Role playing is expected to be fairly standard for all players (persons) who occupy a given position in a social system.

Roles may also be characterized in several other ways. "Conventional" roles are learned through participation in the life of an organized group and involve fulfilling modes of conduct appropriate to that group. Roles also may be described as "situational" or "interpersonal." Situational roles are peculiar to given social circumstances and situations and, again, would be considered standard for all role players encountering such situations. Interpersonal roles are defined by the personal characteristics of individuals participating in reciprocal relationships.

There is overlap, of course, in that there are conventional ways of being a husband and special interpersonal ways of being a husband in relation to the particular other person who is one's wife. John Jones is expected to behave in certain general, conventional ways as a middle-class husband, but he also is called upon to be a husband in certain specific ways in relating to Mary Jones. In almost all group transactions, persons act as both conventional role players and as unique human beings at the same time, although the mixture of conventional and individual interpersonal behaviors will vary widely from situation to situation. Therapists must attend to both the conventional and the unique aspects of the situation and behavior and make their interventions in terms of both dimensions.

Within families there are role determinants of both varied natures and varied functions. One may have the role of older child, family pet, family scapegoat, decision maker, as well as parent, child, sibling, and many others. Playing any one of these for an extended period of time generally makes a distinct impression upon the personality of the person playing the role.

Idiosyncratic Experiential Determinants

These refer to experiences that are not normative for the group in which the individuals live. That is, the other members of the group do not undergo such experiences as a result of being a member of the group. The events or experiences may occur on a single occasion or on many occasions and can be regarded as idiosyncratic experiential determinants so long as they are not common to the experiences of the other group members.

Examples would include having a physical accident, being physically handicapped, being adopted, and a long list of other possibilities, all of which could be expected to have a strong impact on the formation of personality.

Not only the four classes of determinants but also the interaction or interrelatedness of the determinants has to be taken into account in understanding the foundations out of which personality is shaped and sustained. Personalities of males and females differ because of physical differences and because of different cultural expectations and demands at various points of the life cycle. There is an interactive or interrelatedness component among all four determinants throughout the life cycle of the individual. Those who undergo similar experiences and who have similar constitutional makeups will tend to exhibit some common characteristics. Culture, as well as society (including its organizations and groups), tends to play a significant integrating, shaping role in the formation of personality in continuing and complex ways.

All four of these determinants need to be taken into account in addressing the needs of human beings for help with their pain and difficulties. Intervention may be aimed at elements of any one of the four or at all of them in a given case.

None of what is written here should be construed as implying that standardization prevails in personality formation. The human organism—male or female—should never be considered merely as something being acted upon by the environment in which it develops. Neither should it be regarded as developing inexorably in some predetermined fashion, regardless of the setting. Allport's (1955) idea of a proactive organism that interacts with its environment, instead of being merely reactive or a passive recipient of environmental impress and pressures, has considerable explanatory merit. The outcome of the interrelatedness of organism and setting in dynamic interplay is what determines the personality that emerges and that appears in situation after situation. It is the integration, the gestalt, of components that defines the person.

TIME TO EMPHASIZE INTEGRATION, NOT SEPARATENESS

With both systems and personality here to stay, it is time, and past time, to strive for integration of both emphases into therapy. It is better that their advocates be on speaking terms than either spewing pejoratives or playing ostrich and attempting to ignore each other.

The family therapy revolution, with its introduction of a systems perspective, interjected into the broader field of psychotherapy not only a new way of looking at human problems but also a division among psychotherapists that continues today. Once again, family therapists were correct when they proclaimed the importance of the context in which persons develop and function. For a considerable portion of the psychotherapy field—although, admittedly, not for all of it—the point has been made that context is so significant that it can be ignored only at the peril of missing something vital. Making interventions only with systems and ignoring the individual's internal states has limitations, just as treating individuals in isolation has definite drawbacks. As Karpel and Strauss put it, "We can no more remove the person from the system than we can the system from the person" (1983, p. xvii).

Fortunately, a purist family systems view has scarcely been the only orientation in family therapy. Other family therapists also deal with the present and consider systems perspectives to be vitally important. In addition, however, they give attention to "vertical" relationships involving the client's family of origin and, in some instances, to intrapsychic processes. Increasingly, efforts are being made to combine "outside" and "inside" perspectives in various types of integrative approaches to family therapy (e.g., Duhl & Duhl, 1981; Feldman, 1992; Kirschner & Kirschner, 1986; Nichols, 1988; Nichols & Everett, 1986; Pinsof, 1983; Sander, 1979; E. F. Wachtel & Wachtel, 1986).

Today, therefore, although it may be tempting and appear easier for family therapists to be systems purists and to ignore the individual, it is unnecessary and exceedingly shortsighted. We are not doomed to ignore history and thus compelled to repeat it. Family therapy does not have to repeat the error of traditional psychotherapy (which implied that the person could be understood solely in terms of what went on inside them) with an error of its own by assuming that an individual's dynamics are unimportant. "No systems theory has ever adequately explained the dynamics of a relational system without some reference to individual dynamics" (Karpel & Strauss, 1983, p. 14). Systems and individuals need to be considered together.

Treatment of persons in context does not mean that all interviews and all interventions are conducted with the family system present. Sometimes, the method of choice is individual interviewing and treatment of the individual without other family members being present.

In sum, treatment does not have to be "either/or," that is, either treatment of the individual or treatment of the system. Therapy can, and typically needs to be "both/and," that is, focused on both the individual and the system. Neither the systemic forces and processes nor the individual's intrapsychic processes needs to be dealt with as if they are unrelated to the other. Neither the family nor the individual is a closed system; they interact—their processes are in transaction. They are not hermetically sealed and thus prevented from being in transaction with one another; it is the sealing of minds rather than the sealing of those systems that hinders considering them together.

The time certainly has arrived for a new phase in the psychotherapy dialectic. If the family therapy revolution with its emphasis on systems was the antithesis to the psychoanalytic revolution's focus on the individual, it is surely time now to work toward a synthesis of those major approaches in helping people who are in pain.

This book is intended as another contribution to the process of integration in family therapy. It will be concerned primarily with three major foci of therapy: the individual system, family subsystems including specifically the marital subsystem, and the family system. Family therapy at its best treats the person in context, the family subsystems, and the total family system, emphasizing the various aspects as indicated by the nature and extent of the problems presented to the therapist.

AN INTEGRATIVE FAMILY THERAPY APPROACH

The integrative approach presented in this book is not aimed at constructing a grand theory for psychotherapy. Rather than an attempt to devise a totally new approach from scratch, it involves synthesizing what is known already and putting it together in the most useful ways possible at this time. The result is expected to produce something that is different from the sum of existing parts, something new and better. More changes and additions will be made as new findings become available from clinical experience, empirical research, and fresh ideas from theoretical advances. The model presented here is both theoretically driven (cf. Wachtel & McKinney, 1992) and empirically driven, in other words cutting across theoretical grounds (cf. Prochaska & DiClemente, 1992).

Prochaska and DiClemente (1992) indicate that there are five distinct but interrelated levels of psychological problems that can be addressed in psychotherapy: symptoms/situational problems, maladaptive cognitions, current interpersonal conflicts, family systems conflicts, and intrapersonal conflicts. These are interrelated in that (1) the symptoms frequently reflect interpersonal conflicts, and maladaptive cognitions often stem from family system rules or beliefs; and (2) change at one level of problem is likely to result in change at another level.

Prochaska and DiClemente (1992) describe five basic stages of change: precontemplation, contemplation, preparation, action, and maintenance. They sketch the particular processes of change (consciousness raising, self-liberation, social liberation, counterconditioning, stimulus control, self-reevaluation, environmental reevaluation, contingency management, dramatic relief, and helping relationships) to be emphasized during particular stages of change (pp. 302–307). They also suggest where to fit what they term the major systems of psychotherapy into an integrative framework. With family systems conflicts, for example, strategic therapy is used during the precontemplation stage, Bowen therapy during the contemplation and preparation stages, and structural therapy during the action and maintenance stages (p. 309).

In theoretical integration, a synthesis is formed in which both the underlying theories of various therapies and the therapeutic techniques from each are integrated. London (1986) calls these mergers "theory smushing" and "technique melding," respectively. Examples of such approaches include Feldman and Pinsof (1982), Gurman (1981), Seagraves (1982), Wachtel (1977b, 1987; Wachtel & McKinney, 1992; E. F. Wachtel & Wachtel, 1986), and others (Norcross & Newman, 1992, p. 11).

Theoretical schools may not be as different as their proponents assume and claim. Norcross has suggested that theoretical schools may not be contradictory but complementary. He points out that such complementarity is the basis of Pinsof's (1983) Integrative Problem-Centered Therapy (Norcross, 1991; Norcross & Newman, 1992). It is not always easy or even possible to demonstrate such complementarity and to find a ready "fit" between different theoretical and empirical components. Elsewhere I have referred to the necessity of a therapist being able to tolerate some apparent contradictions when it is known that there is validity in two or more divergent "truths"; a therapist must develop a tolerance of "lumps in the oatmeal" (Nichols & Everett, 1986). Blending is the goal, but all parts cannot always be whipped into a smooth concoction.

Although my avid general and theoretical interest in human personality formation and functioning, now in its fourth decade of my professional life, will continue to claim a considerable amount of time, my purpose in presenting the material set forth here is primarily practical in nature, as it has been in some earlier writings (Nichols & Everett, 1986; Nichols, 1988). That purpose is consistent with the objective of the integration movement in general psychotherapy—to improve the efficacy of treatment (Norcross & Newman, 1992)—although in this instance family therapy integration rather than general psychotherapy integration is the focus. The goal, in brief, is to continue working toward the development and presentation of a family therapy model that brings to bear appropriate knowledge from whatever sources will help therapists to work with clients and help clients to deal with their difficulties. The aim here also is broadly compatible with Wachtel's stated integrative goal of seeking "to provide an internally consistent approach to personality functioning, as well as a way of proceeding clinically within the therapy hour" (Wachtel & McKinney, 1992, p. 335).

Integration is different from eclecticism. As compared with integration, for example, eclecticism is concerned much more with technical (as opposed to theoretical) blending, with differences in therapies (rather than with similarities), with applying the parts of therapies (instead of unifying the parts), with applying what is (vs. creating something new), with focusing on the sum of parts (as contrasted with an entity that is more than the sum of parts from different therapies), and is atheoretical but empirical (as compared with being more theoretical than empirical) as is the case with integration (Norcross & Newman, 1992).

Integration, as used in this book, includes the combination of therapy formats—individual, marital, family (e.g., Nichols, 1988). Most clinicians also consider the combination of formats and the combination of medication and psychotherapy to be appropriate in integration (Norcross & Napolitano, 1986). There is complete agreement with Pinsof (1990) that family therapy needs to be informed by findings and theory from a wide range of sciences—physical, biological, behavioral. My longtime claim that "I have learned far more about the plasticity of human personality from cultural anthropology than I ever have from dynamic psychology" is only a slight exaggeration at best.

My notion that family therapy is the treatment of the "individual in context," primarily in his or her family setting, implies a set of priorities.

With the family serving as the crucible for personality formation, the primary need of the family therapist is to comprehend how families develop, how they function, and what role they play in the normal and abnormal development of personality and human behavior. Although the study of family merits priority over psychotherapy as such and certainly over techniques, an integrative approach does not end with the study of family and with what has been discovered and demonstrated by family therapists.

As powerful as it has been, family therapy represents only one of the major revolutions in psychotherapy. The other two, of course, are psychodynamic psychology (starting with Sigmund Freud and psychoanalysis) and behavior therapy. Each has made its contributions to understanding and aiding human beings who are in pain and distress. Psychodynamic psychology and behavior therapy have vitally important theoretical and practical offerings to make to a family systems approach.

It is time to reconnect with our roots. This needs to be done consciously and knowledgeably, blending together ways of understanding from the old and the new so that we work in the most effective ways that we can.

We turn in Chapter 2 to a brief description of systems theory/family therapy, psychodynamic psychology, and social learning theory and to the issues involved in integrating them into family therapy.

2

AN INTEGRATIVE APPROACH
TO FAMILY THERAPY

*Integrative family therapy selects from systems, behavioral, and
psychodynamic perspectives "those aspects of each that can be
put together in a new system."*
      —PAUL L. WACHTEL AND M. K. McKINNEY,
        Handbook of Psychotherapy Integration

What are the aspects from existing major theoretical perspectives that
need to be included and integrated in order to assemble a new system of
therapy? Which theoretical contributions are useful, if not essential, from
each of those approaches? What needs to be brought together in order to
establish a useful and reasonably comprehensive theoretical synthesis?

The point was made in Chapter 1 that therapy need not be restricted
to an "either/or" approach in which the focus is either on the individual
or on the system. Rather, it can be, and in order to be comprehensive and
integrative must be, "both/and," focusing on both the individual person
and the key systems in which he or she is involved. The fact that the five
problem levels described by Prochaska and DiClemente (1992) (symp-
toms/situational problems, maladaptive cognitions, current interpersonal
conflicts, family systems conflicts, and intrapersonal conflicts) tend to be
interrelated increases the importance of establishing a theoretical base
from which to address them flexibly as indicated by the needs of the client
system.

An integrative family therapy approach needs to be one that takes into account the following:

- Individuals and their intrapsychic processes as part of their development and functioning; how they are attracted to and relate to other persons, including their entry into and continuation in voluntary relationships of intimacy such as mate selection and marriage; and how they learn and how their behavior is changed.
- Systems and subsystems in which individuals participate, including the development and functioning of family systems and their subsystems—marital, parental, sibling, and individual.

While intervening at one level, a therapist using an integrative approach will be thinking about and attempting to keep up with what is occurring on multiple levels. At times, when it seems clinically appropriate, the therapist is likely to make those concerns about other levels explicit in interventions with the clients. While dealing with marital interaction, for example, the therapist may ask one of the clients, "Can you share your feelings about your father's illness? How do you suppose that is affecting you?" At other times, the therapist may note similarities in several systems or subsystems in which a client is involved but say nothing. Eventually, when a pattern emerges, connections between those patterns and the thinking and feeling of the client may be made explicit.

This chapter begins with a brief introduction to the three theories of psychotherapy—psychodynamic, behavioral, and family systems—that contribute to the integrative approach to family therapy presented in this book and closes with a brief depiction of what is extracted from each of them.

The reason for starting this discussion with psychodynamic therapy is essentially historical. That is, I am starting with the approach to psychotherapy that developed first, moving next to behavioral therapy, and then to the family systems approach. I regard systems theory as the umbrella under which the other two approaches fit. It is the broadest level, the context in which individuals exist and function. For my purposes, psychodynamic theory is, of the three approaches, the most closely tied to individual personality and the raw materials out of which it develops. Social learning theory occupies an intermediate place between the other two.

PSYCHODYNAMIC PSYCHOTHERAPY

Psychodynamic theory and therapy arose out of the tradition of psychoanalytic theory and techniques established by Sigmund Freud (1856–

1939), beginning a century ago. Freud first used the term "psychoanalysis" in 1896 (Jones, 1953). As Mishne notes (1993, pp. 4, 20), over four decades Freud "independently and alone" conceptualized the basic idea and techniques of psychoanalytic theory and therapy: transference, resistance, repression, the significance of the unconscious, and the Oedipus complex.

Freud saw the human organism, the human infant, as driven by a need to alleviate somatic (bodily) tensions and to seek pleasure. For Freud, both libido (love impulses) and aggression were aimless. He saw the impulses as having a life of their own. The "ego" (the personality's executive functions and structure) was conceptualized as arising on top of a sea of seething impulses (the "id") as a result of those impulses coming into contact with the realities of the world.

Freud did not invent intrapsychic processes. Presumably, they have been around since the time in the hazy past when our ancestors moved beyond instinct and combined thinking with feeling. Freud did, however, demonstrate the ubiquitous and significant role that unconscious motivations play in human behavior. Nevertheless, some of his theories have not withstood the test of time and the methods of psychoanalytic treatment are open to criticism on several fronts. Psychoanalysis has been in a state of flux and controversy almost since the beginning. Today, it is "neither a monolithic nor a homogeneous entity" but "a heterogeneous hodgepodge" (Eagle, 1984, p. 184).

My focus here is on psychodynamic theory and not on psychoanalysis as such. Psychodynamic theory in its various permutations and clinical adaptations provides a legacy for understanding and treating individuals that seems unlikely to fade from the scene. New interest in psychodynamic psychotherapy approaches in family therapy has emerged in recent years. Slipp has produced two works on object relations, one on object relations as a bridge between individual and family therapy (1984) and one on the technique and practice of object relations family therapy (1988). The Scharffs have published three volumes, one on object relations family therapy (Scharff & Scharff, 1987), one on foundations of object relations family therapy (J. S. Scharff, 1989), and one on object relations couples therapy (Scharff & Scharff, 1991). Willi (1982, 1984, 1992) has provided several works applying a psychodynamic approach to couples and couples therapy.

The contributions regarded here as sufficiently durable and appropriate for integration into family therapy come from diverse sources within the broad rubric of dynamic psychotherapy. Those materials stem from among those theorists who have abandoned Freud's drive (instinct) theory and have struggled with comprehending personality in relation to social and cultural forces. These contributors have been labeled "relational/structure theorists" (Greenberg & Mitchell, 1983) because they conceptualize personality structure as coming from interactions with other persons rather than being derived from transformations of drive energy as conceived in the original drive/structure model of Freud.

Although the ideas adopted here come from psychodynamic clinicians who are considered as relational/structure theorists, the concepts from two different relational/structure sources cannot always be integrated easily.On the one hand are Harry Stack Sullivan's (1953a, 1953b, 1954, 1962, 1964) interpersonal theory and Erik H. Erikson's (1950) psychosocial theory of development which place emphasis on the contributions of the social and cultural context to personality. On the other are constructs taken from the British school of object relations, particularly from the theory of W. R. D. Fairbairn (1952, 1954, 1963) and from Henry V. Dicks's (1963, 1967) applications to marital therapy.

Sullivan's interpersonal theory and the British object relations theory as exemplified by Fairbairn offer a "two-person psychological model," rather than the one-person intrapsychic approach provided by classical psychoanalysis. The interpersonal theories they provide emphasize relationships and represent an open system in which interaction between the child and the environment is viewed as "responsible for personality development and psychopathology" (Slipp, 1988, p. 13). Sullivan provides an important "outside" and Fairbairn an important "inside" psychodynamic perspective. Sullivan emphasizes the cultural content and the critical role of communication processes in human development and interaction. Fairbairn, drawing significantly from Melanie Klein (1932, 1948; Segal, 1964), provides more specificity regarding the internal organization of the person and the interaction processes themselves. The major clinical import of their work is the emphasis on taking other persons and the environment into account in working with a troubled client.

Harry Stack Sullivan's Contributions

Sullivan's focus was not on the individual psyche as in classical psychoanalysis, but on the relationship field and the relational patterns that emerge from it. Personality cannot be separated from its network of interpersonal relationships; we are born, develop, and exist in relation to other persons (Sullivan, 1962, 1964). He emphasized also the organization of one's experience, which deals with the patterning of those relations and is thus interpersonal and relational (Greenberg & Mitchell, 1983).

Sullivan abandoned the earlier psychoanalytic emphasis on drives and forbidden strivings as the source of psychopathology and the organization of the self. Instead, he viewed anxiety, interpersonally generated between parent and child, as the source of those matters (Mishne, 1993). The self, or self system as Sullivan called it, was a process, not a static, structural entity isolated within the individual. It was a reflection of interpersonal relations, a product of the individual's interaction with the family, society, and culture (Slipp, 1984). The self system, in Sullivan's theory, protects the remainder of personality from the threat of anxiety and maintains a sense of security in which satisfactions are possible (Greenberg & Mitchell, 1983).

Perhaps more than any other psychodynamic theorist, Sullivan was concerned with what persons do with each other, with their actions and relationships. In this, as well as in other areas, his theory and practice reflected a concern with one's behaviors in relation to and in interaction with others rather than a focus on one's intrapsychic functioning. For example, Sullivan described a case in which a patient came in complaining that he had a homosexual problem. At the end of what Sullivan termed the "reconnaissance" phase of intake, he told the man that he had no psychiatric time for the patient's interest in homosexual problems and did not know anybody who did have. However, Sullivan added, if the man wished to discover why he continually got into collisions with his bosses and could not hold a job for more than 6 months despite initial rapid progress, he could find him some psychiatric help. Sullivan notes that during the exploration of the job difficulties, concerns with homosexuality "caved in" (Sullivan, 1954, pp. 91–92).

Extrapolations and adaptations of his theory have given Sullivan a tremendous influence over psychiatry and psychotherapy in the United States (Mitchell & Greenberg, 1983). His influence undoubtedly can be seen in the "black box" approach of some early family therapists, particularly Don D. Jackson, who eschewed a concern with intrapsychic functioning. Jackson, during his psychiatric residency at Chestnut Lodge in Maryland, was greatly impressed by the interpersonal theory and the empirical approach taken by Sullivan. Abandoning the exploration of the development of the individual as a self, Jackson viewed pathology as residing only in the relationship and emotional dysfunction as essentially the product of family interaction (Slipp, 1984).

It is Sullivan's emphasis on cultural contributions to personality that most clearly distinguishes his theory from the British object relations theorists. Cultural conditioning shapes one's desires and pursuit of security as an end state, according to Sullivan (1953b, 1954). He stated emphatically (1954) the great importance of signs, symbols, vocalization, and other cultural factors in the formation and functioning of human personality and emphasized how the person's personal environment is expanded by other channels of communication, including the telephone, radio, and printed word. (Today, of course, television would be included.)

It is that emphasis and the stress on the interpersonal context, as well as the synthesizing of information about human development and functioning from a variety of social science fields, that makes his theory so intriguing and useful in the pursuit of integration in family therapy. As Slipp (1984) has noted, some of the theoretical underpinnings of Sullivan's interpersonal theory can be seen in general system theory, communications theory, game theory, field theories, cybernetics, and in behavioral science generally.

Fairbairn's and British Object Relations Theory's Contributions

Object relations theory has been described as the bridge between individual systems and the family system (Scharff & Scharff, 1987; Slipp, 1984). The Scharffs (1987, p. 52) described it as providing a bridge between the internal world of the child and the reality of life within the family. Object relations connect the intrapsychic with the interpersonal and, in family theory and therapy, with the family-as-a-whole levels of functioning. In broad terms, object relations theory attempts to deal with certain aspects of human relatedness, development, and motivation from infancy onward.

Object relations theory as it developed in Great Britain includes several important theorists, some of whom attempted to remain in the Freudian mainstream and others who split off rather radically. Melanie Klein (1932, 1948) made significant and controversial contributions to the development of object relations theory at the same time that Sullivan was departing from Freud's instinct theory. Klein, however, retained the drive theory, continuing to regard instinct as the source for object relations. My concern is not with Klein but primarily with the tradition of object relations launched by Fairbairn.

Fairbairn's theory, along with Sullivan's, "provides the purest and clearest example of the shift from the drive/structure model to the relational/structure model" (Greenberg & Mitchell, 1983, p. 151). He explicitly developed a "theory of the personality conceived in terms of object relations, in contrast to one conceived in terms of instincts and their vicissitudes," noting that "there is no such thing as an 'id' " (Fairbairn, 1963, p. 224). Fairbairn conceptualized the human organism as primarily object seeking, as driven by a need to be involved in social interaction and relationships, rather than being propelled by instinctual urges.

Some of Fairbairn's basic theoretical points, as he summarized them (Fairbairn, 1963, p. 224), were as follows:

An ego is present from birth, and libido is a function of the ego.
The ego, and hence libido, is fundamentally object seeking.
Aggression is a reaction to frustration or depression.
The earlier and original form of anxiety, as experienced by the child, is separation anxiety.

The child, concerned with relating to objects (persons) in outer reality, does not internalize an object as the result of a fantasy of incorporating the object orally (as in classical psychoanalytic theory). Rather, the internalization occurs as "a distinct psychological process" (Fairbairn, 1963, p. 224), that is, in reaction to unsatisfying relations with real persons. Children emotionally identify with a person, or persons, whom they need and internalize that person as an object, constructing an inner psychic world that replicates the original frustrating and unhappy situation. "Bad" object situations are handled differently from "good" object situations. A person needed by an infant becomes a bad object by, for example, (1) ceasing to love the infant, (2) disappearing, (3) dying, or (4) doing something else that is experienced as frustration or rejection. Linked to the bad object and continuing to feel deprived and unhappy, the child subsequently has a temptation to project the bad object back onto someone in the real world.

Clinically, this process may be seen frequently in collusive marital interaction. Each partner, for example, unconsciously functions as a split-off negative parent for the other. They thus complement or complete each other's personality needs. The wife, for instance, may be regarded by her husband as an internalized bad object (representing his internalized bad parents who rejected and exploited him) and treated as a scapegoat. The husband serves the wife as an internalized bad object (representing a parent who did not adequately fulfill her emotional needs) whom she punishes. They quarrel, but at the same time they need and seek each other emotionally. In Fairbairn's terms, the antilibidinal object and ego attack the libidinal (exciting) object (Scharff & Scharff, 1987; Slipp, 1988). It may be easier for them to quarrel incessantly than to acknowledge their hurt and longing to be loved (Scharff & Scharff, 1987).

As Fairbairn conceptualized the internalization process, the child retains satisfying parts of the relationship with significant objects as conscious memory, but internalizes unsatisfying aspects in an effort to deal with them internally. As the bad object is internalized, splitting occurs and exciting and frustrating aspects are split off from the main core of the object and repressed by the ego. In other words, the infant/child takes into itself the bad object that it cannot handle in the real world. It does not take the good object into itself, because there is no need to do so.

Good, or satisfying, objects and experiences are retained as memories in a routine and rather straightforward manner. For example, when outer experiences of pleasure, such as tactile stroking and holding and the provision of emotional, physical, and feeding satisfaction, meet one's inner needs, there is no conflict. Therefore, there can be confidence in the ability to possess the real object, both in the present and in the future. Confidence in the present and predictability for the future are possible when an infant's needs have been met satisfactorily, as theorized in Erikson's (1950) basic need for trust in the earliest stage of life.

Clinically, this may present in the form of persons who exhibit high amounts of trust and optimism. Sometimes, the person is overly optimistic and expects to achieve and to be gratified too easily in a current environment that is not as rewarding and gratifying as was the early environment that he or she remembers. This puzzling experience may result in anger toward the desired person who fails to gratify the person's wishes. In some instances, it leads to disappointment and confusion that result in reactive depression.

Details of the splitting process and more explicit implications for personality development and therapy can be ascertained from Fairbairn (1952, 1954, 1963), Guntrip (1969), and, in relation to marital choice and interaction in particular, from Dicks (1963, 1967).

Another way of stating Fairbairn's ideas is to say that because of our nature and condition in the world we are dependent upon objects (persons) from the beginning and that the origins of psychopathology have their roots in early life, in the stage of infantile dependency. Fairbairn viewed normal development as consisting of three stages: the stage of infantile dependence, the transitional stage, and the stage of mature dependence (1952). These stages represent the maturation of different ways of relating with others. Rather than following Freud's idea of an instinct-driven oedipal situation, Fairbairn held that the child attempts to keep good relations with his or her parents throughout life (Mishne, 1993, p. 227).

Simply put, "the development of object-relationships is essentially a process whereby infantile dependence upon the object gradually gives place to mature dependence upon the object" (Fairbairn, 1952, p. 34). The process starts with a situation in which the infant does not distinguish itself from the object. In a normal process, things move to a situation in which there is dependence based upon a clear differentiation of the object from the subject.

This process occurs gradually. The infant starts out with its libidinal aims being oral, sucking, incorporating, and predominantly "taking" in nature. If adequate maturation and development occur, this basically "taking" aim is replaced by a "mature, non-incorporating, and predominantly 'giving' " aim (Fairbairn, 1952, p. 35).

The basis for good functioning later is the satisfaction of the child's "greatest need." This is the need to "obtain conclusive assurance (a) that he is genuinely loved as a person by his parents, and (b) that his parents genuinely accept his love" (Fairbairn, 1952, p. 39). If this happens, the child is able to be assured that he or she can depend on real objects and can gradually give up infantile dependence. If such assurance does not exist, the child's relationship with his or her objects is loaded with too much anxiety over separation. A child turns to relationships with internalized objects "in default of a satisfactory relationship with objects in the outer world" (Fairbairn, 1952, p. 40).

Object relations theorists generally agree that the patterns of relating and the internalized residues of the early experiences, as developed subsequently, provide the basis for later intimate relationships. What negatively affects later relationships is the anticipation that they will not be satisfactory. Guntrip (1969) has described object relations in terms of the person's need to maintain a continuity with the past and thus to have a basis for present functioning and relating. What would it be like if every new interpersonal experience were novel and unique and there were no guidelines for reacting to it and deciding how to deal with it? According to Guntrip, persons form some guidelines or bases for reacting and dealing with the present by carrying experiences in their minds, either as memories or as internal objects.

Fairbairn's theory, which views internalization of objects as stemming from reactions to actual situations and relationships rather than from fantasy, should be particularly appropriate to family therapy and its focus on actual relationships and their significance in an individual's development and functioning. For example, in family therapy one may meet with the client and his or her family of origin to elucidate and deal with issues that turn out to be residues from actual events and relationships in the past rather than being constructed from the client's imagination. This applies especially to questions of childhood physical and/or sexual abuse. Fairbairn's theory should also be compatible with Sullivan's emphasis on interaction and relationships. The most useful theoretical ideas of object relations for integration into family therapy are discussed below.

Splitting

Splitting in object relations theory refers to a primitive defense maneuver in which one splits the good from the bad in an external object and internalizes the split perception. The construct has been used in family therapy to describe an interactional style in which positive and negative thoughts and feelings are split and experienced in isolation from each other (American Association for Marriage and Family Therapy, 1992).

Splitting presumably occurs in all human beings. Human experiences are not uniformly positive. All persons have limitations to their ability to trust and to love another object or person. They have not always received the love or emotional support that was needed. When they have put out feelers or emotionally given to another significant person (object), the object has not always reciprocated. Therapy is concerned with both the normal, garden variety splitting of human experience and with the problematic versions and their aftermath.

Projective Identification

Projective identification refers to externalizing a feeling, attitude, or other aspect of one's psychic processes onto another person or external object. The identification reference pertains to a person's identification with his or her projected part as perceived and experienced in the object. We relate to the projected part of ourself in the other person as we would to the self part, as if it were within ourself. We then attempt to involve the other person in collusively behaving in the way in which we perceive him or her (Zinner, 1976). An example is provided by a father who unconsciously projects his own unacceptable aggressive feelings onto his adolescent son and covertly encourages or provokes aggression on the part of the youngster. When the adolescent "accepts" or "owns" the projection and acts aggressively, the father then can reprimand him without having to acknowledge what is occurring or to accept the aggression as part of himself (Everett, Halperin, Volgy, & Wissler, 1989).

Dicks (1967) described spouses' attributions to each other of unconsciously shared feelings as constituting a "symbiotic" or collusive process in marriage. It is as if an unconscious agreement exists, for example, that "I will regard you as not sexual, if you will regard me as not aggressive," and conversely. Dicks also illustrated the unconscious work that couples often do to keep "bad feelings" out of the marriage, to conceal inner realities, and to maintain a smooth facade of happiness (Dicks, 1967, p. 73). An implicit, conscious level collusion to maintain a marital myth is illustrated in George and Martha's marriage in *Who's Afraid of Virginia Woolf?*, which has been analyzed in family therapy terms by Don Jackson (Watzlawick et al., 1967).

Projective identification is first of all a primitive defensive mechanism and probably the earliest form of empathy (ability to put oneself in the place of the other). It also is, as illustrated above, an interactional style within marital and/or family relationships. Projective identification involves projecting onto another person a rejected part of oneself. Also, it may involve making projections onto the ideal object in an attempt to avoid separation from it or in order to gain control of the source of perceived danger (Segal, 1964). Projective identification may produce anxiety in the author of the projection by activating the fear that the object of our projections will respond with projections of his or her own or that parts of us will be grasped and controlled by the object (Segal, 1964).

Projective identification is not always problematic or pathological. It occurs along a continuum (Zinner, 1976). At one end of the line it operates in such a way that there are distorted and perhaps even delusional objects. On the other end of the continuum, there may be a healthy empathic connection with the subjective world of the object. Whether one's projective identifications are pathological or healthy depends in large measure on the ability to use the mechanism for approximating shared experience in an empathic fashion instead of as a means of externalizing conflict (Zinner, 1976).

Other terms have been used by clinicians and researchers to refer to essentially the same phenomena that are included under the heading of projective identification. Zinner and Shapiro (1989) suggest that a number of relationships in which one interacts with others as if they were not themselves but someone else may all be variants of projective identification. These include the family projection process (Bowen, 1978), trading of dissociations (Wynne, 1965), merging (Boszormenyi-Nagy, 1967), scapegoating (Vogel & Bell, 1960), and others.

Dicks (1967) says that the partners in such a marriage treat each other "as if" the other were the original frustrating object. In this mechanism a deeply unconscious "deal" is struck by which the fixed view that one member has of another family member is unconsciously swapped for a fixed view that that person has of him or her (e.g., "I will regard you as nonaggressive if you will perceive me as nonsexual"). Each person is dealing with a part of the other that the other cannot acknowledge is present. Such reciprocal interaction in the family of origin would, of course, be powerful "basic training" for similar patterning of interaction in marriage. (Mechanisms of defense and adaptation referred to as "externalization" also may take the form of projective identification.)

Introjection

Introjection has been described by Fairbairn as the process by which "a mental structure representing the external object becomes established within the psyche" (1954, p. 107). One incorporates the picture of a person as one conceives him or her to be and then transfers affect from the actual person in a real-life environment to the mental picture in one's psyche. This process is, like projection, unconscious; one is not aware of doing it. Introjection is also different from identification, which is based on a desire to model after the object and in effect to be the object.

An illustration of introjection can be found when a person internalizes and invests affect in the image of a person rather than in the real person. Henry, for example, falls in love with the idealized image of Mary and, consequently, is unable to love the real person. Or, Betty, who is depressed because of the loss of her husband in combat, redirects her feelings to the mental image she has of that person and acts toward the image as if it were in reality the lost loved one (Hinsie & Campbell, 1960).

Projection

In projection, one "casts out" undesirable parts or qualities of oneself and places them onto another person, or persons, in the external world. Meissner (1980) distinguished between projective identification and projection as follows: What is projected is experienced as belonging to or coming from the object, whereas what is projected in projective identification is "simultaneously identified with and is experienced as part of the self" (p. 55).

In Fairbairnian terms, where there is continuing rejection on the part of the parental figure(s), the unsatisfactory parts of the objects are internalized and invested with a significant amount of strong feeling. Such objects, loaded with a large amount of hate and accompanying guilt feelings, are felt by the person to be outside one's self. The person comes to feel that such negative and undesirable feelings are also held by the object toward him or her. These patterns of reactivity last over the years as the person deals with external real persons as if they were the same as his or her internal bad objects (Guntrip, 1969). Thus, a cycle of introjection–projection that begins early is carried into later life by many individuals as a prototype for intimate interpersonal relationships. A clinical example is found in the man who carries within himself denied anger but attributes anger to his wife.

When transference—distortions based on earlier relationships, treating present objects (persons) as if they were figures from the past—is present, the transference reactions in such transactions do not emanate from only one of the participants. There must be an interlocking of perceptions and needs of both participants based on transference.

Collusion

Projective identification requires a reciprocal action on the part of one's object. The other must accept the projection and act in accordance with it if projective identification is to be part of an ongoing interaction. This is part of what occurs when projective identification becomes involved in the process of mate selection and ongoing marital interaction. Such a relationship does not begin and continue unless each spouse colludes by agreeing at an unconscious level to accommodate by accepting and identifying with the projective identification from the other.

Participants in projective identification are involved in a collusive process and relationship in ways that are not present in simple projection.

That is, it is not simply a one-way process in which one person projects something onto another. Instead, in this kind of collusion, each partner "carries" something for the other in a collusive process of splitting and projective identification. For example, a man who is "kind, sweetly reasonable, and somewhat dependent" may be married to a woman who is "angry, excitable, and bossy." She does not have to be kind or reasonable as long as he will bear those feelings for her, and he does not have to be angry or assertive as long as she will carry those attitudes for him. The denied, split-off, "bad" parts of one's self are carried by the other so long as the unconscious agreement prevails. While the collusion lasts, one does not have to try to become comfortable with the denied and projected parts of oneself.

As a marriage continues, there is a continual shaping of the mate through the collusive process (Slipp, 1984). Greater degrees of predictability emerge for the partners as the relationship evolves. They begin to feel more comfortable and trusting as the responses of the other confirm their object-seeking efforts. Similarly, the spouse's efforts to induce one to play a particular role increase the predictability of the relationship (Boszormenyi-Nagy, 1966).

Dicks (1967) has extensively illustrated how the process of unconscious marital collusion operates in many marriages. In some pathological relationships, there is an unconscious "bargain" in which each partner sees in the other the promise that old problems will be worked through, old hurts redressed, and the even stronger reassurance that nothing will change. Mate selection in such situations is based on a mutual signaling system. Unconscious signals or cues convey the dual message that the other (1) has the capability for engaging in joint working through for unresolved conflicts or splits in one's personality, while (2) simultaneously guaranteeing the paradoxical message that they will not be worked through with that person. This latent interaction is initially concealed by idealization, much of which is conscious. To the extent that both continue to play their roles, a kind of rigid and pathological relationship continues.

Through case materials Dicks (1967) has specifically demonstrated how "cat and dog" marriages (in which couples "can't live with and can't live without" the other) work. At a conscious level the partners' expectations for an ideal union attempt to keep "bad" feelings out of the marriage. Unconsciously, they collude to deny that there are any troublesome inner realities. Together, they thus maintain a shared resistance to change. Reality testing in the marriage often exposes the unreality of their idealization and permits frustration and regressive demands to surface. If the repression holds and there are other inner resources and adequate living conditions, such marriages frequently last. There are genuine needs for growth and integration (e.g., the mental health truism that the basic thrust of the organism is onward) that keep the marriage going. There may be tensions, however, that show up in depression, psychosomatic difficulties, or problems with the children.

Dreams

Fairbairn (and Melanie Klein) rejected Freud's idea that dreams constitute only wish fulfillment. Fairbairn saw dreams as representing the current state of affairs, as dramatizations of situations existing in the person's inner reality, the situations thus being relationships between the self and its internalized objects. Dream content today often is viewed not as containing unconscious wishes but as reflecting the dreamer's current life problems and dealing with incomplete emotional business from day-to-day life (Mishne, 1993). In brief, the emphasis on the meaning of dreams is shifting to a model that focuses more on their "integrating, organizing, problem-solving function" (Glucksman, 1987).

Significance of the Unconscious

The issues with regard to unconscious motivation today do not concern whether mental activity takes place outside one's awareness. Rather, the questions are how significant is the unconscious mental activity and how is it dealt with in therapy? A psychodynamic perspective sensitizes the clinician to conflict and the widespread presence and nature of self-deception. It also provides guidelines regarding where and how to look for experiences and tendencies that are being disavowed (Wachtel & McKinney, 1992). For example, the chances are very good that probing for potential anniversary reactions to past losses or trauma that occurred at approximately the same time on the calendar as the present will locate sources of unexplained current depression.

Psychodynamics and Integrative Family Therapy

Psychodynamics offers integrative family therapy an emphasis on an intrapsychic perspective. Although it continues to be ignored by some segments of today's family therapy field, attention to intrapsychic perspectives serves as a partial corrective to the tendency toward the impersonal and mechanical "technolatry" (Pinsof, 1990) that often is evidenced by family therapists. An integrative approach regards psychodynamic theory (which emphasizes the person) and family systems theory (which stresses the social setting) as complementary rather than as conflicting or having no relevance for one another.

The interpersonal conceptions of Sullivan and object relations from the Fairbairnian tradition focus not only on the internal structures of internal personality but, importantly, on the interactive nature of personality processes. Mallouk (1982) notes that object relations theory identifies relatedness as "the most fundamental of all psychic phenomena" (p. 429). He cites Dicks (1967), Framo (1976), Feldman (1979), Gurman (1981), and Sager (1981)—all of whom can be identified as bridging figures between psychodynamics and marital and family therapy—as examples of "depth-psychology advocates who have become convinced of the necessity of an interactional viewpoint" (p. 429).

The Fairbairnian approach, as noted above, views the quest for relatedness (or object relations) as being present in the human organism from birth. Seeking relatedness continues into adulthood but does not have to be driven solely by what happened in infancy and early childhood. It is significantly affected by the nature of current interaction with other persons and the systems in which they live. It is as important to comprehend what persons are reacting to in the present as to understand why, on the basis of their past history, they react to the present situation in they way they do (Wachtel & McKinney, 1992).

Object relations provides a theoretical explanation for the psychological choice of mate and, in many instances, the continuation of a marriage. Although pathology is generally more spectacular and receives the lion's share of attention, object relations theory helps in explaining more than just pathological choices; healthy choices also can be described in object relations terms.

On the pathological side, object relations can be useful in describing and treating specific family transactional patterns. Slipp (1988), for example, has developed a typology in which specific family transactional patterns are related to specific forms of psychopathology in a family member.

Although Heinz Kohut's (1971, 1977) self psychology is not used here as part of the psychodynamic base for integrative family therapy, there are at least three interesting theoretical parallels and points of agreement between Kohut's theory and the psychodynamic theory used here. First, Kohut's theory holds that we continue to need objects. Normal development is marked by the changing nature of what he terms "selfobject" relationships in which we move away from early, archaic selfobject relationships. Second, his interpersonal emphasis appears to be generally agreeable with Sullivanian and Fairbairnian emphases on interpersonal relations. Third, Kohut views actual traumatic events, particularly deficiencies in the interaction with parental figures, as the main etiological factors in engendering pathology (Eagle, 1984). That emphasis is compatible with Sullivanian and Fairbairnian theory regarding actual noxious encounters with significant figures in the person's life, rather than fantasied situations, as sources of pathology.

BEHAVIORISM

Behaviorism may be described as the second major paradigm to develop in psychotherapy, joining psychoanalysis in the 1950s as another way of doing therapy with individuals. Based on learning theory and emerging from the experimental laboratory rather than from the clinic, behaviorism introduced quite different emphases from those of the dominating psychoanalytic model. The emphasis in behaviorism, of course, is placed on behaviors and not on the internal processes of the individual (R. L. Weiss, 1978). The cognitive-behavioral version of the behavioral approach (Baucom & Epstein, 1990) does have a specific concern with the mental processes of the individual, but with cognition rather than with unconscious processes and personality dynamics.

In behaviorism, symptoms are seen neither as symbolic and meaning something other than their obvious meaning nor as indicative of unconscious conflict, as in psychodynamic theory. Instead, they are viewed as learned responses that are not adaptive. Behaviorism shares with psychodynamic theory an emphasis on the individual and also holds in common the fact that much of its theory deals with reciprocity, with individuals in reciprocal interaction with other persons.

The core assumptions in behaviorism are that behavior is learned, that social reinforcement (receiving attention and recognition) is the most important source of human motivation, and that intermittent reinforcement produces very durable, continuing behavior (Liberman, 1970).

Therapeutic applications of learning theory began to receive attention with the work of B. F. Skinner (1953) and his operant conditioning theory and research. Operant or "instrumental" conditioning and learning focus primarily on the conditions that follow the behavior, that is, the consequences and the absence or presence of rewards. Social learning theory holds that "behavior is controlled by its consequences (operant conditioning) and antecedent discriminative stimuli that signal to the individual that particular reinforcement contingencies are operating" (Baucom & Epstein, 1990, p. 18). In the operant learning perspective, "changes in behavior follow the laws of learning, including primary and secondary reinforcement contingencies, generalization, and extinction" (H. A. Klein, 1974, p. 353).

Another contribution to behaviorism came from the classical conditioning approach advocated by Joseph Wolpe (1958), whose work on systematic desensitization was applied to a number of individual human difficulties. At the risk of oversimplifying the two approaches, they may be described as follows: Classical (also called "respondent") conditioning basically is concerned with behaviors that are elicited by preceding stimuli, instrumental (also called "operant") conditioning focuses primarily on the conditions that follow the behavior (i.e., on the consequences and the absence or presence of rewards). There is a considerable amount of overlap between the two approaches. Both were used originally in devising treatment methods for individual problems.

From a behavioral viewpoint, both individual and family interactional problems result primarily from interpersonal problem stimulation and problem reinforcement processes. That is, behaviors by one or more individuals result in the arousal of dysfunctional emotions, cognitions, and behaviors in another or other persons. Responses by another or others to the dysfunctional behavior that result in increased probability of recurrence of the dysfunctional behavior constitute interpersonal problem reinforcers (Feldman, 1992, pp. 11–12).

Behavioral Approaches to Family Therapy

Social learning theory has been applied to family problems, particularly parent–child situations, very effectively for several decades. Gerald Patterson and his colleagues at the University of Oregon, for example, have provided many descriptions of and research reports on their work (Patterson, 1974, 1982; Wills, Weiss, & Patterson, 1974). Their application of social learning theory to the treatment of disturbed children emphasizes altering the social environment in which the children live. Skills training work is conducted with parents in an effort to teach them to diminish the rates of deviant and undesired behavior by the child and to increase the rates of adaptive and more desirable behaviors and social interaction. Typically, observation procedures are used and the parent's efforts are supervised by the therapist. Behavioral family therapists typically report good success rates. For example, in one study with families in which at least one male child was aggressive, a 60% reduction in observed target behaviors was noted at the time of termination (Patterson, 1974).

Patterson and the Oregon group have succeeded in depicting reciprocal coercive patterns in family interactions in which an individual's behavior elicits and reinforces other members' aversive acts (Baucom & Epstein, 1990). They have found many parents using ineffective norms of punishment in their attempts to alter their children's undesired behavior. For example, the parents threaten but do not back up their threats with serious punishment such as consistent suspension of privileges, or the parents use physical force that results only in a temporary suppression of the youngster's behavior (Patterson, 1982).

Behavioral Approaches to Marital Therapy

Applications of learning theory to marital interaction have come from two major sources, operant conditioning theory and social exchange theory (Thibaut & Kelley, 1959). Operant conditioning theory contributes the idea that the external environment provides significant determinants of behavior. Social exchange theory offers a perspective in which a marriage is viewed in quasi-economic terms. It holds that a relationship is satisfying if the benefits that are derived from being in the relationship exceed the costs; that is, it is concerned with costs and benefits (R. L. Weiss, 1978). The degree of satisfaction gained by a marital partner thus stems from the reward–cost ratio. Clinicians using a behavioral approach, therefore, would be concerned with the variables that maintain positive and negative behaviors.

Social exchange theory appears to be deficient in its ability to explain the choice of a mate. Similarly, it does not explain why one continues in a marital relationship when examination appears to demonstrate that the costs significantly outweigh the benefits. That is, from all indications, it would not be worth it for a person to enter or continue in such a voluntary relationship, but he or she does so anyway. Object relations theory appears more likely to explain the person's actions in such situations than social exchange theory's quasi-economic rationale.

The central emphasis of a behavioral approach to marital therapy has been described (O'Leary & Turkewitz, 1978) as helping spouses to learn more productive and positive ways of causing behavioral changes in one another through such techniques as contingency contracting, problem solving, and communications skills training. Useful definitions as well as a sketch of the history of behavioral marital therapy may be found in a review of the literature by Jacobson and Martin (1976).

The concept of reciprocity (Thibaut & Kelley, 1959) may be applied by some persons in a quid pro quo (literally "something for something") manner (Lederer & Jackson, 1968; and others). That is, one partner agrees to do something in exchange for a different behavior of an equal weight from his or her partner. For example, a wife may agree to be pleasant and enter into sexual relations once a week, provided the husband manifests certain kinds of attention and offers affection in certain ways. Reciprocity in a general sense refers to the tendency for couples to reward each other at approximately equal rates (Jacobson & Margolin, 1979; Patterson & Reid, 1970). The quid pro quo approach, which has not proven to be as effective as early behavioral marital therapists supposed it would be, is only one of two kinds of contracts used. Another is the "good faith" contract introduced by Weiss and colleagues (R. L. Weiss, Hops, & Patterson, 1973). Stuart (1980) later introduced a third type, the "holistic" contract.

Patterson and colleagues (Wills et al., 1974) not only have researched the concept of reciprocity and found evidence supporting it, but also have made several other contributions to behavioral marital therapy. These include the development of several ways of assessing marital relationships, such as the Willingness to Change Scale, the Marital Activities Inventory, the Spouse Observation Checklist, and others (L'Abate & McHenry, 1983).

Behavioral marital therapy continues to be a complex matter, involving several different approaches to dealing with marital discord. As long ago as 1980, Gurman noted that as a treatment model, behavioral marital therapy was in a state of transition and change. One of its major strengths has been its successful focus on the outcome of therapy; like nonbehavioral approaches, it has been effective approximately two-thirds of the time (J. P. Vincent, 1980). Some of its limitations include a lack of emphasis on therapist–client relationships, the assumption that changing behaviors will result in increased marital satisfaction, and a lack of applicability for severe marital disorders such as those involving alcoholic and psychotic spouses (Gurman & Kniskern, 1978; L'Abate & McHenry, 1983).

By the early 1980s, much of the early animosity between practitioners of behavioral and nonbehavioral marital therapy approaches appeared to have diminished. Efforts were being made to integrate social learning perspectives with other points of view. Behavioral marital therapy had won its place as a significant approach to dealing with marital (and family) difficulties. Paolino and McCrady (1978), for example, attempted to deal with marriage and marital therapy from psychoanalytic, behavioral, and systems perspectives. Seagraves (1982) tried to combine psychodynamics and behaviorism into a general approach to marital problems and marital therapy.

Behaviorism and Integrative Family Therapy

Behavioral therapists have a considerable amount to contribute to integrative marital and family therapy in terms of both theory and technique. Human existence is as much a learning process as it is anything else. Behavioral approaches emphasize that family therapy should be a learning experience for all the family members who are involved in the therapy. As Liberman (1970) notes, instead of rewarding maladaptive behavior with attention and expressions of concern, family members learn to provide recognition and approval for desired behavior. It can be useful in therapy to help family members understand the practical implications of the social learning theory discovery that any response to a behavior is a reward, and that undesirable behavior tends to be extinguished not by negative responses but by being ignored.

Psychoanalysis and even much of psychodynamic theory and practice do not give sufficient attention to the role of social skills in human behavior and therapy (Wachtel & McKinney, 1992). By contrast, behaviorists in their emphasis on social reinforcement help family members to learn new behaviors by means of modeling, including imitative learning through observation of other family members, and by "shaping" of behavior through role playing and role rehearsal (Liberman, 1970). Other techniques that are used include providing guidelines for problem solving, communication training, and behavioral contracting methods (good faith contracting), as well as focusing on the learning and relearning involved in certain problems such as jealousy and anxiety (Baucom & Epstein, 1990).

Behaviorists share with family therapists "an attempt to focus upon observable behavior, a lack of enthusiasm for insight, and a stronger emphasis on bringing about change than exploring pathology," according to Haley (1986, p. 44). Other observers see evidences of affinity to behaviorism in Haley's own work. His communication analysis, for example, has been used to interpret the techniques of behavior modification (H. A. Klein, 1974).

Similarities between therapy techniques used by psychodynamically oriented family therapists Framo (1965) and Zuk (1967) and behavioral therapists have also been noted. Liberman (1970) points to Framo's stated preference for techniques that prompt family interaction, concentrate on here-and-now feelings, and involve taking active, forceful positions in order to loosen a family from its rigid positions; and he highlights Framo's illustration of clinical work in which the therapist provides differential reinforcement for approved, desired behavior. Liberman describes Zuk's techniques as fitting into a reinforcement pattern.

Behaviorism also emphasizes the variability of human behavior and experience in different contexts. Although the behavioral focus here is on the individual, its "outside-in" emphasis regarding the direction of causality fits well with systemic perspectives.

Behaviorism's emphasis on change is highly consistent with family therapy's focus on change. This is opposed, of course, to the traditional accent in psychoanalysis, and in much of continuing psychodynamic psychotherapy, on insight as being essential to behavioral and personality alteration. As Wachtel and McKinney (1992) put it, new behaviors provide change and new insights which in turn generate increased motivation to attempt new behaviors. This, of course, stands in contrast to the classical psychoanalytic idea that insight is a necessary prerequisite to personality change. They also emphasize that providing opportunities for clients to experience corrective emotional experience is very much at the heart of what good behavior therapists do (Wachtel & McKinney, 1992, p. 338).

Another point relating to change is the fact that separation of affect (feeling), cognition (knowing), and action (behavior) is more easily done for purposes of analysis than can be accomplished in reality. Human beings cannot be conveniently split precisely into feeling, thinking, and acting creatures. As cognitive behaviorists Baucom and Epstein (1990) point out, the person's affect is "complexly interrelated with cognitions and behavior patterns" (p. 124). Emotions can have positive or negative effects on cognitive and behavioral processes in a relationship. Conversely, behaviors or cognitions cannot be altered without "some impact on the emotional quality of the relationship" (p. 124). Hence, there is more kinship in practice between behaviorism and psychodynamic and systems approaches in this respect than adherents of any of the three models generally have acknowledged.

Gurman (1980) described the major challenge of behavioral marital therapy in the 1980s as integration with alternative models of marital treatment. In order to integrate successfully, he noted, the treatment would have to attend to the fact that family members require reintegration as individuals in order for the family as a system to function effectively (p. 88). This means, as Gurman is interpreted here, that individual, intrapsychic elements give significance to interpersonal events and, along with systems conceptions, must be taken into consideration in the integration of behavioral marital therapy and behavioral theory generally with alternative models.

The key to reconciling behavioral and psychodynamic perspectives, according to Wachtel and McKinney (1992), is the recognition that causality in human behavior is largely circular in nature. They indicate that the events that have a causal role in human behavior are very often themselves a function of human behavior as well (p. 344). Thus, the "outside-in" and "inside-out" emphases must be considered together in order to include the entire picture instead of simply a partial representation.

SYSTEMS AND GENERAL SYSTEM THEORY

The emergence of General System Theory (GST) represents one of the major conceptual and practical changes in the scientific and clinical worlds in the 20th century. Although named by the eminent biologist Ludwig von Bertalanffy, who made significant contributions to the concepts, GST emanated from long-term evolutionary developments. Many persons in several different scientific fields were working on similar conceptions when von Bertalanffy published his concept of GST in 1945. Consequently, his ideas found widespread acceptance in the scientific world, where the major research orientation previously had been that of mechanism/reductionism.

A brief sketch of the background out of which GST emerged is helpful in understanding the significance of this new approach to scientific work, which soon became accepted as a major new orientation to clinical work as well. For some 1,900 years, Western thought tended to be dominated by Aristotelian teleology. "Teleology" is variously defined as the study of final causes, as the fact or quality of being directed toward a definite end, and as a belief that natural phenomena are determined by an overall purpose in nature. When Aristotle's view of nature was combined with medieval theology and ethics, the basis for the scientific outlook of the Middle Ages was established. Founded on both reason and faith, this organic world view had as its major goal understanding the meaning and significance of things, rather than prediction and control as in later scientific approaches. The Aristotelian/medieval outlook generally discouraged the empirical study of natural phenomena and the formulation of explanations other than those of a teleological nature.

Beginning approximately with the 17th century, a new scientific approach developed. Variously referred to as Galilean, Cartesian, and Newtonian, this mechanistic outlook ruled Western scientific thought and explanation for the next 300 years. According to mechanical theory, everything in the physical world is governed by the inexorable laws of mechanical or linear causality. Galileo's (1564–1642) major contributions included his emphasis on an empirical approach to nature and his use of quantification, that is, studying nature mathematically. Descartes (1596–1650) made significant contributions to the general framework of science with his view of nature as a machine governed by exact mathematical laws and with his analytic method of reasoning in which ideas and problems are broken into pieces and arranged in logical order. Newton (1642–1727) effectively synthesized the work of Galileo, Descartes, and others and provided the mathematics for the mechanistic view of nature. Newton's invention of differential calculus gave physics a mathematical basis for measuring natural phenomena and behavior and completed the Scientific Revolution, and Newtonian physics provided the model to be followed. As the mechanistic viewpoint became solidly established, physics became the basis of all the sciences (Capra, 1983).

Mechanistic/analytic thinking became the scientific approach. The scientist's goal was to reduce reality into ever smaller units in order to determine the causes of individual events or units. Scientists attempted to discern the rules or laws governing the parts and then to understand the complex phenomena as a result of understanding the elementary parts. That approach has been characterized briefly as "the whole is nothing more than the sum of its parts" (Beavers, 1977, p. 11). The best-known example of the resultant linear thinking probably is the stimulus–response explanation in psychology. A leads to B, B leads to C, C leads to D in a chain of linear causality. Reductive analysis thus became the operational procedure used in the physical sciences. Eventually, it became evident that reductive analysis is not appropriate for use in certain instances. Analytic procedures, for example, are not applicable to situations in which the actions or behaviors are not linear in nature. Some parts of reality are not explained as a result of efforts to reduce them to ever smaller units.

The breakdown of what can be called the classic mechanistic/reductionist outlook began in the 19th century with the discovery of evolution in biology and with other developments that pointed to the inadequacies and shortcomings of the Cartesian/Newtonian views of the universe. The major blow came, however, early in the 20th century, with the introduction of two theories that focused on the nature, function, and relationship of objects. Einstein's revolutionary theory of relativity and further developments in physics that resulted in quantum theory became a major part of scientific explanation. These developments—the emergence of relativity theory and quantum theory—spelled the end of the reign of the mechanistic view of the universe as the only way of explaining and dealing with nature. Newtonian physics was joined by a new physics embodying a world view using holistic, organic, and ecological concepts. This systemic approach set the stage for the development of GST (Capra, 1983).

While these scientific developments were occurring, another factor was evolving. This was the emergence of organismic theories in several different fields. Organismic theory calls for the study of the organizing principles or relationships that result when the entire entity is taken into consideration. This approach obviously is very different from a reductionistic perspective in which isolated parts of processes are studied. Reductionism deals with parts in isolation. Organismic approaches focus on the entire entity and on the relationships that result from the dynamic interaction of the parts of the whole. Any organism is considered as a living system. Goal-directed behavior, including growth and creativity, can be considered and accounted for by the dynamic interaction among the components of the living system.

The early work of von Bertalanffy in biology led him to adopt the organismic principle, which means that organisms are organized things and must be regarded as such by scientists. Subsequently, he began to lecture and write about GST in an attempt to provide a theory that would account for systems and organization in general. By the time he made a published presentation of GST following World War II, von Bertalanffy found that parallel developments were appearing in cybernetics, information theory, game theory, decision theory, typology or relational mathematics, and factor analysis (von Bertalanffy, 1968). To some extent, the phenomenon of independent invention was functioning in the area of scientific explanation as systems approaches were emerging in several different areas simultaneously. Nevertheless, it was von Bertalanffy who developed GST and led the way in introducing its concepts to the psychiatric and psychological world in particular. At the same time, he noted that there were many organismic developments in psychiatry that could be traced back to Adolph Meyer and that, in American psychiatry and psychology, organismic/systemic approaches could be found in the work of Kurt Goldstein, Karl Menninger, Roy Grinker, Carl Rogers, Silvano Arieti, Gordon Allport, Abraham Maslow, and J. S. Bruner (von Bertalanffy, 1968). Similarly, Gregory Bateson (1979) was dealing with human life in terms of a systems approach when he emphasized "the pattern which connects" (p. 8). Sullivan (1953b), the interpersonal psychiatrist, was using a kind of systems approach when he defined personality as "the relatively enduring pattern of recurrent interpersonal situations which characterize a human life" (pp. 110–111).

GST arose in the biological sciences as a result of attempts to provide better and more appropriate explanations of natural phenomena. Linear thinking had some definite and demonstrable effects and advantages. By relying on a series of linear cause-and-effect occurrences, one could predict outcomes by linking such sequences, or one could start with an event and work backward until a basic cause was discovered. However, such an approach left many things unexplained. Frequently, many of the phenomena being studied had to be left out of consideration in order to predict outcomes or find beginning causes (Steinglass, 1978). Life phenomena, or living things, do not yield easily to study under the analytic methods of the physical sciences (A. Rapoport, 1968).

As GST theory developed, organization rather than reductionism came to be regarded as the unifying principle in science. Briefly, "the whole is different from the sum of its parts" is a systems approach. That is, when parts or components are examined separately, the results or findings cannot simply be added together in order to determine what the whole will look like. The whole must be examined as a whole, as a system, rather than as the sum of a number of parts.

As significant as it was, the emergence of GST did not render previous scientific work invalid. There are still uses for reductionistic work in modern technology. The point is that neither reductionistic thinking nor systems thinking should be accepted as the only possible way of regarding the world.

Concepts for Family Therapy

The new organismic world view introduced such relevant concepts for family therapy as systems, organization, ecology, open systems, complexity, positive feedback, negative feedback, and negative entropy. The following definitions of GST concepts serve both to introduce the reader to their salient meanings and to provide an in-context glossary of terms used throughout this book.

System

A "system" was defined by von Bertalanffy as a set of elements standing in interaction. Others have referred to a system as something that is put together in such a way that whatever affects one part of it affects other parts. GST involves a search for "general structural isomorphisms" (Gray & Rizzo, 1969, p. 7).

A family may be viewed as a system whose various members and subsystems interact much like the organism of the human body, with its ongoing interaction of organs, blood flow, and nerve endings. An injury to a portion of the body summons the resources of the entire organism to combat the danger and ensure survival, just as stress experienced by a member or subsystem of the family requires adjustment and accommodation of the remainder of the system. For example, when a member of the family is injured, the entire family system may flock to the hospital, change their schedules, and otherwise help and give indications that they are affected by that member's difficulty.

Organization

This is to be considered the first concept among the concepts of living systems. Steinglass (1978) describes it as follows:

> If a *system* is defined as a set of units or elements standing in some consistent relationship or interactional stance with each other, then the first concept is the notion that any system is composed of elements that are *organized* by the consistent nature of the relationship between the elements. (p. 305)

The organization of the family defines its basic structure, that is, how the various members and subsystems are arranged in an interactive field. A family may be organized, for example, around a rigid, dominant male head, his compliant and passive wife, and a group of either rebellious or compliant children.

Subsystem

This is part of a system that carries out a particular process in that system (J. G. Miller & J. I. Miller, 1980). The major subsystems identified within the nuclear family, for example, are spousal, parent–child, and sibling. The individual also may be considered a subsystem within a family system.

Subsystems have their own organization, boundaries, and interactive patterns. The marital subsystem—which can be regarded as both a system in its own right and as a subsystem of a family—is composed of husband and wife; the parent–child subsystem, of the parents and children; and the sibling subsystem, of the children in the family. The children will have their own patterns of relating, their own rituals, and their own difficulties and competencies as a sibling subsystem.

Wholeness, Boundaries, and Hierarchies

These are key notions within the concept of organization (Gurman & Kniskern, 1981). "Wholeness" has to do with seeing patterns rather than with reducing entities to their parts in a reductive fashion. For example, the family system may be described as "depressive" as a result of observations of the enmeshing characteristics of the system, rather than of observations made only of an individual member's reactive depression or of other individual characteristics.

The concept of "boundaries" describes who is to be included within a certain system and the quality of the interactive process and feedback that occurs with other related systems. Boundaries serve to regulate the flow of information and feedback to the systems so that a family with "closed" boundaries would allow limited information to come in and would restrict the outward flow of information. An isolated family that had little to do with outside systems would be described as one with relatively closed boundaries. Clinically, such a family might provide little helpful descriptive information.

The concept of "hierarchy" refers to the fact that living systems have several different levels in which the simpler, more basic system levels compose the more advanced and complicated higher level systems. J. G. Miller and J. I. Miller (1980) have indicated that seven such levels may be conceptualized easily in living systems: cells, organs, organisms, groups, organizations, societies, and supranational systems. In the family, the "simpler" individual, spousal, parental, and sibling subsystems compose the more complex nuclear family system that is part of the even more complex intergenerational system.

Open Systems

A living system is relatively open. That is, it exchanges information and other material with the environment and with other systems in the environment. The relatively open family system not only processes information freely but also allows its members to come and go with a balance of both protecting and engaging mechanisms. The school, the community, the church, and various other groups influence and are influenced by a relatively open family system.

Closed Systems

A "closed system" is one in which there is no exchange with the environment and the system components are not influenced by the environment. Families are relatively open or relatively closed. A family that maintains a very low interchange of information and interaction with the schools, the workplace, or other parts of the community would be described as a relatively closed family system.

Living systems exist in a "steady state" rather than in a state or condition of equilibrium or homeostasis. In a steady state, there is a combination of homeostatic and viable or adaptive mechanisms operating. Viability, which refers to spontaneity, growth, creativity, and general capability of living, is necessary for the system's survival. The concept of a steady state is difficult to illustrate clearly, but a clinical example would be a family in which the fluctuations between behaviors that would maintain the status quo and actions that would deal with new challenges in the environment keep the family system going in a kind of dynamic tension. A family, for example, struggles to maintain desired family participation and behaviors on the part of its teenage members at the same time that it permits them to leave the family unit to be with their friends and to adopt behaviors that are different from those of the family elders and even from those of the younger children. The steady state also is the means by which the organism maintains the disequilibrium that produces growth and development while continuing as a viable organism.

Equifinality

This is an important characteristic of the steady state. "Equifinality" refers to the fact that the same results can be obtained by different means and by starting from different beginning points. The nature of the system's organization determines the outcome. For example, there is no single kind of "good parent" subsystem that will produce healthy children. Westley and Epstein (1970) found that healthy offspring come from families with disturbed parents as well as from families with healthy parents.

Equifinality is related to "circular causality" and to the fact that feedback may cause changes in a process and provide corrective mechanisms that make it unnecessary to proceed from a beginning point to a predetermined outcome in a mechanistic fashion. "Linear causality," by contrast, results in the ability to reach only a particular given conclusion as a result of starting from a particular beginning point (e.g., *A* leads to *B*).

The concept of equifinality has immense practical value for clinicians in that one may start from any one of several different points in many cases or use any one of a variety of different methods, techniques, or approaches in order to obtain a desired result. It obviously is quite different from a mechanistic, reductionist approach in which, for example, a given symptom would be considered to be derived from a particular earlier condition or cause and treatable only by dealing with that presumed prior cause.

Feedback

"Feedback" refers to a situation in which there are two channels carrying information in such a fashion that one loops back from the output to the input, feeding back into the system information that affects succeeding outputs from the system. The understanding and use of feedback loops has provided an alternative to the old deterministic/teleological debate in which there had to be predetermined outcomes. Systems may have both deterministic and goal-seeking characteristics that can be explained in terms of self-correcting behavior on the part of the system through the use of feedback (information). In a family, the children's socialization experiences in school provide new incoming data that the total system must process and to which it must attempt to accommodate and adjust adequately. In a relatively closed system, of course, the feedback from the school may be perceived as threatening and potentially dangerous in that it threatens to pull the children away from the family system.

Feedback may be either negative or positive. "Positive feedback" makes things change. The positive feedback loop may even set up a runaway situation in which the system moves beyond its limits of functioning and self-destructs. Positive is not to be interpreted here as desirable but merely as descriptive of a feedback loop that increases deviation in a system and causes change. Clinicians sometimes encourage the use of positive feedback in ways that are intended to break up the existing system or patterns of relating and behaving. "Negative feedback," in contrast to positive, provides information that decreases the output deviations and helps to achieve and maintain stability in relationships (Watzlawick et al., 1967). Negative feedback, in short, cancels errors and helps to maintain a steady state in systems. This, also, is a concept frequently used by family therapists in their interventions that are aimed at stabilizing systems. The study of methods of feedback control, "cybernetics," is a significant part of GST.

Negative Entropy (Negentropy)

This concept is the opposite of the idea of "entropy," a major concept in thermodynamics, which states that, over time, there will be a gradual loss of energy. The degradation of energy occurs because over time, heat energy cannot be converted into an equivalent amount of work. As such change occurs, the system becomes disorganized and even chaotic. In contrast to entropy in a closed system, an open, living system secures energy through an exchange with the environment. This leads to an increased degree of organization and more complex patterning. The concept of negentropy is essentially the same as that of "information." The influx of information into a system provides a kind of "energy" that leads to the reduction of uncertainty within the system, and thus helps the system to become increasingly organized and complexly patterned, rather than becoming disorganized and perhaps chaotic (Steinglass, 1978). For example, a family that is isolated from its context and has very little interaction and communication with its community may become suspicious, fearful, and disorganized.

Nonsummativity

The family system cannot be understood merely by summing up the attributes or characteristics of the individual members, although characteristics partially determine the nature of the family. As noted, the family as a whole is different from the sum of its parts and one must attend to the pattern, not merely to the parts. A clinician who separately interviewed five members of a family, for example, would not get the same picture—the same understanding and comprehension of the family—as would the clinician who brought the five members together and observed them in interaction.

Communication

All behavior is considered to be communication. One "cannot not communicate" because one "cannot not behave," and communication is behavior. Communication defines relationships and establishes roles in the family system through the setting of rules. The transactional nature of the family system, including verbal and nonverbal communication, shapes the behavior of members of the family. Patterns of communication among family members and with external sources are indicative of the relative openness of both internal and external boundaries. For example, the manner in which family members organize themselves around a dinner table or seat themselves in a therapist's office defines boundaries, hierarchies, coalitions, and triangles. The look of a parent toward a child or the tone of a wife's voice in addressing her husband are indicative of roles, rules, and moods.

Stability and Change

Feedback loops that bring information and other forms of input into the system operate so as to promote both stability and change in the system. Families are thus self-regulating in that any input that affects a member is modified during the process of feedback. In the most simple explanation of stability and change, family stability is maintained by means of negative feedback mechanisms, and family change is brought about through positive feedback mechanisms. In most cases, change in a system is a result of accommodation to new input. The change may at times be dramatic but is usually gradual, often with a step forward followed by a step sideways or backward.

Structure

"Structure" can be defined in several different ways, for example, as in the common dictionary meaning of the "arrangement or interrelationship of all the parts of the whole" or "the manner of organization." The Millers's (1980) emphasis on the structure of a living system as "the arrangement of its parts in space at a given moment in time" is important, as is their assertion that structure refers to the arrangement of both subsystems and components, and that a structure may be either fixed or changing.

Process

As defined by J. G. Miller and J. I. Miller (1980), "process" refers to change over time and includes the ongoing functions and history of a system. Again, as with the structures of a system, process may involve one or more subsystems. Process describes a quasi-organic quality that undergoes movement, growth, and change. Erikson's (1950) description of an epigenetic principle in individual developmental theory provides one example of a process, although it is much more narrow than what we think of when we talk about family process. Similarly, I am not using process to refer simply to the movement through various life cycle stages or substages, as the concept is employed in some textbooks.

The processes or functions in a living group such as a family may be subject to change; that is, they may be reversible. A living system carries its history with it in the altered structures of the system and the consequently altered functions (J. G. Miller, 1969). In human groups, communication or information exchange and processing is an exceedingly important process, contributing, as noted above, to change in either positive or negative directions. "Process," of course, is a neutral term and may refer to desirable or undesirable change, depending on the values of the viewer.

Steinglass (1978) distinguished between process and structure as follows: "Organization or patterning observed along a spatial dimension is called structure. Patterning along a temporal dimension, on the other hand, is referred to as process or function" (p. 317).

A Caution Regarding Systems Theory

It needs to be recognized that GST differs from family therapy systems today. GST has much more kinship with thought from the days of "rugged individualism" than with ideas developed since the introduction of Sullivan's interpersonal theory and contemporary family therapy. Thinking systemically in family therapy does not mean that one needs to or can follow GST closely. GST, after all, is oriented toward matter and is essentially mechanistic in nature. Human beings are not balls on a billiard table that follow presumably inexorable laws of physics. Bateson (1979) pointed out that structures in the human, living world are not closed, mechanical systems. Rather, they tend to be open, so that energy in the form of information may enter, thus permitting the system to become more organized rather than to run down. Some early family therapy adaptations, including the family homeostasis concept, have been questioned and their abandonment urged (Dell, 1982, 1986; Slipp, 1984, 1988).

GST, as Slipp (1988) notes, is honored by therapists only at a highly abstract level. At a practical level, a linear approach is used. Recently, correctives have been issued to the uncritical acceptance of a "circular" epistemology in family therapy. One of its pioneering figures, Lyman C. Wynne (1986), calls for family therapy to drop its pretense that therapy follows a circular epistemology and recognize that not all causality involves feedback and circularity. Wynne argues that the effectiveness of most family therapists stems significantly from the use of powerful lineal techniques. Two therapeutically crucial lineal processes operate: the time line that prevents genuinely circular processes from occurring, and family therapists' linearly directional orientations toward goals of relieving symptoms (Haley, 1976), producing growth (Whitaker & Keith, 1981), or balancing the ledger of merit and obligation (Boszormenyi-Nagy & Ulrich, 1981). Family therapy involves spiral transactions rather than circular transactions.

TOWARD A SYNTHESIS

This section will offer a brief introduction to the parts of the three theories that are being synthesized into an integrative family therapy approach (Table 2.1). The synthesis is still in a comparatively early stage and is far from being complete. Additional illustration of the points offered in this

TABLE 2.1. Selected Emphases of Therapeutic Models

Psychodynamic

"Inside-out" dimension (individual, intrapsychic)
Unconscious processes
  Dream processes
Interpersonal (Sullivanian) emphasis
Object relations (dyadic and choice emphasis)
  Projective identification
  Introjection
  Projection
  Collusion

Behavioral

"Outside-in" dimension (individual, observable behavior)
Learning processes
  Cognitive emphasis
  Teaching–learning emphasis
  Techniques for change
Emphasis on change

Systems

Contextual dimension (interactive, systemic)
New epistemology
Systems perspective
  Organization
  Subsystems
  Wholeness, boundaries, hierarchy
  Open systems
  Closed systems
  Equifinality
  Feedback
  Nonsummativity
  Communication
  Stability and change
  Structure
  Process
Emphasis on change

section will be made in subsequent chapters, which focus on assessment and treatment.

Viewed from a broad perspective, psychodynamic psychotherapy provides theoretical constructs useful not only for explaining the individual's intrapsychic functioning but also for comprehending important interactive processes that contribute to both healthy development and pathology.

Sullivan's theory, with its interpersonal emphasis, offers assistance in explaining the role of anxiety in human experience, for example. His theory also lends itself to the explanation of tensions in large groups and systems as well as in units as small and restricted as the mother–infant dyad. At the time of his death in 1949, Sullivan was involved in efforts to apply interpersonal theory to international tensions. Similarly, his description of the induction of noxious feelings in the infant during contacts with the mothering one has implications not only for understanding and intervening in early parent–child interaction but also for expanding explanations into interaction in later life and other intimate relationships.

Sullivan's emphasis on communication, including work in integrating linguistics into his theory, has contributed far more to psychodynamic and systems thinking in the United States than is generally recognized. Many of his emphases fit neatly into a family systems perspective.

Fairbairnian object relations theory offers a basis for understanding, in particular, one's attachment and interaction with parents and the initial attraction to another person for purposes of marriage. It is helpful in answering such questions as the following:

- How does the infant relate to the primary nurturer (the mothering one)?
- How does it discover that it is separate from that person (or that object)?
- What are the consequences of that discovery?
- What are the processes involved in making that discovery and in reacting to the discovery?
- What are the implications of the early experiences with the nurturing one and other close figures for other and later intimate relationships, particularly the relationships of mating and marriage?

Therefore, Fairbairnian theory has significant implications for comprehending infant and child development and for working with parent–child relationships and interaction, as well as for crucial aspects of choices of objects in intimate relationships such as marriage. It helps to explain continuation in unhealthy relationships. As noted earlier, Dicks (1967) has extensively illustrated how persons continue in certain kinds of unsatisfying and painful relationships because of splitting, projective identification, and collusion. Fairbairnian theory is somewhat less effective in explaining healthy attachment with its trust and dependency aspects. It does not, as such, provide an adequate basis for understanding and interpreting continued growth and "risk" in healthy adult relationships, but it is not alone in that deficiency.

In brief, psychodynamic theory as used here deals not only with unconscious processes and implications of interpersonal theory and object relations for human development but also pertains to the kind and degree of attraction and attachment that prevail in later intimate relationships and to the kind and degree of intrapsychic conflict that exists within the client–client system.

Behaviorism concentrates primarily on individuals but does have some implications for explaining as well as altering human interaction. Social learning theory provides explanations of how learning (adaptive and maladaptive) occurs and how behaviors are sustained by reward systems. In addition to its theoretical contributions, behaviorism offers extensive practical assistance in terms of techniques for affecting and helping to change behavior. As noted, its stress on change is highly compatible with a similar emphasis in a family systems approach.

The systems perspective has brought a new epistemological emphasis to psychotherapy. Once the systems paradigm found its way into the therapy field, it was no longer possible to treat clients as if they were isolated atoms. Combining a systems perspective with interpersonal theory and object relations, one reaches the conclusion that the individual is not simply acted upon by outside forces, but is proactive, as Allport (1955) and others insisted. The developing person is not merely acted upon by the family system or any other external entity, but is proactive from the beginning of his or her existence. The importance of the systems approach is that it provides some of the best constructs and explanations found thus far for explaining how the individual functions in his or her context and the roles that the context plays in the interaction shaping process.

Sullivan's description of personality as consisting of the recurrent patterns of interaction is an overstatement, but the emphasis on the interpersonal and interactive nature of life is a helpful contribution to therapy.

The integrative approach that is described here is one in which treatment is tailored to the needs of the client system. Devising a treatment approach to a particular client system does not imply that other approaches would not work, because it is possible that they would, but it does imply that the approach selected is one that the therapist thinks would be effective. Additionally, the approach selected is likely to be one with which the therapist feels reasonably comfortable.

What are the factors that determine the form and nature of the therapeutic intervention?

• The presenting problem(s) of the client system, including the nature and severity of the problems and symptoms, and the problems that are manifested subsequently during the course of therapy.
• The strengths and current functioning abilities of the client system. The latter includes the current functioning and difficulties as well as the historical elements that are affecting the current functioning.
• The stage or stages of development of the client system and the effectiveness or lack of effectiveness of the client system in discharging the essential developmental tasks of the relevant stages.
• The orientation and abilities of the therapist, including the kind of alliance that the therapist is able to form and maintain with the client system.

A METAPHOR FOR SYNTHESIS

What are the key elements in the three models of therapy that I attempt to synthesize? Perhaps the use of a simple visual metaphor will provide some indications. If I am in the room with a married couple, for example, and am trying to understand what their marriage looks like and how it functions, I try to think integratively. I take my visual and cognitive "photographs" and try to put them together so that I can determine how best to proceed with therapeutic interventions.

One "photograph" will focus on the kinds of systemic patterns that are present to sustain the problems. What kinds of structures prevail? What kinds of boundaries surround the marital subsystem? Are the boundaries too loose and too permeable? Are they overly rigid? Do they shut out too much of the external world, including the extended family systems of each spouse's family of origin? Is there an adequate hierarchy in the married couple's nuclear family? Is the marriage negatively affected by the parentification of a child? Are there family triangles that are maintaining the problem(s)?

A second "photograph" will focus on the dynamics that maintain the problem(s). What kinds of projective processes, what kind of Fairbairnian processes, maintain the problem(s)? What is the nature of the mutual projection process? the collusion between the partners? What kinds of (Sullivanian) transactional processes communicate anxiety from one person to the other?

A third "photograph" will focus on the clients' defensive behaviors.

When I examine this third "photograph," how are the first two reflected in it? What can I infer about the dynamics of the relationship and about the subsystem structure and processes from the picture of the defenses presented in the clients' behavior? Also, what kinds of cognitive processes are being used by the clients? What kinds of belief systems are operating? How can the beliefs be changed? How do the clients learn?

Similar processes are used in synthesizing the different models in therapeutic intervention. For example, the usual starting point is with the obvious behaviors. Can the clients respond positively and productively to a cognitive approach, to a teaching–learning emphasis (in the context of a respectful and accepting relationship)? Can efforts at helping them to change their behaviors and learn new skills provide the basis for altering pathological dynamics? Similarly, can the therapist's efforts to effect change in the family system help to alter the clients' defenses and their nonproductive dynamics?

3

THE FAMILY SYSTEM
AND DEVELOPMENT

It is often very important to distinguish between the merely very difficult and the actually impossible.
—Attributed to MARY E. WOOLLEY,
Former President of Mount Holyoke College

Integrative family therapy is developmental in its orientation and outlook. Family development is used here in a broad sense to refer to the responsibilities generally assigned to families in meeting the needs of adults and children. Within that framework are included the concepts of a family life cycle, a marital life cycle, and an individual life cycle. The family life cycle is concerned with the developmental tasks of the family itself as it deals with the needs of the adult members and the development needs of the offspring. The marital life cycle pertains to the needs and developmental tasks of marital partners as marital partners. The tasks of those married persons who are parents are part of the broader family life cycle.

It is recognized that nontraditional family forms abound and that diversity and plurality in relationship configurations continue to grow in the United States and the western world generally. Attention is given to divorce, single parent living, and remarriage, as well as to the role of family-of-origin factors in the life of differentiating single adults.

I have not made an attempt to define developmental life cycles for other types of relationships. With respect to adoption, Rosenberg (1992) has

57

constructed "the adoption life cycle." She has established the developmental tasks of birth parents, adoptive parents, and adoptees. Each of the charts she presents describes phases, with goals/tasks and emotional issues for each phase. Although a life cycle perspective does not appear to be available for other "sexually based primary relationships" such as homosexual or lesbian partnership statuses, readers will find some guidance for understanding those issues in Baber and Allen's recent work on feminist reconstructions of women and families (Baber & Allen, 1992, p. 6).

Developmental tasks and life cycle constructs, whatever their limitations, provide significant benchmarks for assessment and treatment. Symptoms manifested by an individual or by the functioning system may be reflections of failures/deficits in discharging developmental tasks effectively. Beavers (Beavers & Hampson, 1990), for example, uses "competence" and "family style" as major assessment factors in dealing with families.

Family therapy in a general sense is most directly concerned with family development, the dynamics of authority in the family system, the maintenance of structure and discharge of functions within the system, and appropriately assessing and treating subsystems (parent–child, marital, sibling, and individual) while recognizing the specific characteristics and needs of each subsystem. For example, although marital therapy is a part of the larger domain of family therapy, it is significantly different from total family treatment and has some dynamics, emphases, and techniques of its own (Nichols, 1988). Among the differences are a concern with choice and attachment, the dynamics of peer relationship choices of an opposite sex partner including the motivations for entering and leaving or remaining in the relationship, and emotional and sexual intimacy. Thus, the focus in the integrative approach described in this book is on acknowledging the differences among individual, marital, and family therapy and putting the three emphases together in a larger (family therapy) treatment framework.

Family therapy is developmental in that it is concerned with a family as it moves through the processes of formation, expansion, contraction, and continuing changes, as well as being concerned with its individual members as they navigate the passages of their own life span. Families go through stages of development that follow a broadly predictable course. The mainstream family development conception holds that the family's predictable stages of development can be understood in terms of the development of the individual family members and of the family as a whole (Duvall, 1971). This chapter not only will broaden the traditional view of family development and stages, but also will go beyond the perspective generally espoused by family therapists. Before moving to a description of the new offerings, however, we will take a look at the origins and meanings of the family development approach.

THE FAMILY DEVELOPMENT PERSPECTIVE

Historically, the family development perspective emerged from collaboration beginning in 1943 between Evelyn M. Duvall, from the human development program at the University of Chicago, and sociologist Reuben Hill. The work was refined in the preparation of background papers they developed for the National Conference on Family Life held in Washington, D.C., in 1948. As noted by Duvall (1977), their efforts involved bringing together the life cycle approach that was already well known among sociologists and the developmental task concept that was emerging in (individual) human development research and theory.

The life cycle began to be conceptualized as involving a series of developmental tasks throughout its span. Formulation of the concept of family developmental tasks was accomplished by a work group in family development research at a workshop on marriage and family research assembled and led by Duvall in 1950 (Duvall, 1977). Students and professionals alike became familiar with the family development approach through the writings of Duvall (1957, 1971, 1977), Hill (1970, 1971), Hill and Rodgers (1964), Rodgers (1973), and others. Unfortunately, family therapists have tended to view the family life cycle as being the only part of the developmental framework that is pertinent to their work (Breunlin, Schwartz, & MacKune-Karrer, 1992).

The Family Life Cycle

Various divisions have been made of the family life cycle. Duvall (1977) divided it into eight stages. Childrearing is the stackpole around which family life is organized in Duvall's schema. She viewed each family as going through the stages with the oldest child and essentially repeating the process with subsequent children. Acknowledging the conceptual problems involved in establishing the family life stages in connection with the progress of the first child, she noted that there is no simple way to deal with the conceptual difficulties posed by families with more than one child (p. 145).

The eight stages delineated by Duvall (1977) are as follows: married couples (without children), childbearing families (oldest child, birth to 30 months), families with preschool children (oldest child, 2½–6 years), families with school age children (oldest child, 6–13 years), families with teenagers (oldest child, 13–20 years), families as launching centers (first child gone to last child's leaving home), middle-aged parents (empty nest to retirement), and aging family members (retirement to death of both spouses).

Duvall also pointed out that some persons do not fit into the family life cycle typology. These include individuals who do not marry and who, theoretically at least, remain part of their family of origin; couples who never bear, adopt, or rear children; and others such as homosexual pairs, communes, and other family-like households (Duvall, 1977, pp. 145–146). It should also be noted that Duvall's framework has a significant middle-class flavor and must be adapted in order to address family differences based on race, ethnicity, and culture. Similarly, it can be criticized for failure to recognize and deal with some important gender issues such as some of the inequities featured in contemporary feminist literature.

Family Developmental Tasks

Each stage of the family life cycle has stage-appropriate developmental tasks. A family developmental task has been described as a growth responsibility that appears at a certain stage of a family's life, emerging from biological needs, cultural imperatives, and family goals. These tasks must be successfully completed in order to secure present satisfaction, social approval, and future success. Failure to deal with a task adequately leads to dissatisfaction, social disapproval, and difficulty with later tasks (Duvall, 1977).

The concept of developmental tasks has been made even more useful to family therapists by those who have freed it from its strong ties to biological roots and have related it more closely to role theory and systems theory. Rodgers (1973), for example, redefined a developmental task as a set of norms or role expectations arising "at a particular point in the career of a position in a social system" (p. 51).

Developmental tasks for a family range from those that are critical to a particular stage to those that are less significant and certainly not crucial to that stage. A stage-critical task for a family with a teenage child, for example, would involve balancing freedom with responsibilities for teenagers as they mature and emancipate themselves. For the adult, a stage-critical task would be that of establishing postparental interests and careers (Duvall, 1977).

THE FAMILY DEVELOPMENT PERSPECTIVE
AND FAMILY THERAPY

Publication of a 1971 posthumous article by social worker Frances Scherz marked one of the first introductions of a family development perspective into the family therapy literature. Scherz relied heavily on the work of Theodore Lidz (1963), who appreciated the fact that adults continue to develop and stressed the interactional nature of development in which each family member affects the course of the others' development. Noting the interrelationship and mutual influence of individual and family tasks, Scherz characterized family tasks as "universal in the sense that, despite differences in social and family cultures and rapid changes in family lifestyles, every family apparently needs to live through the same tasks" (Scherz, 1971, p. 363). She regarded conflict as being inherent in family development "because of the needs for the family to regulate interaction in order to accomplish its tasks and from the needs of the individual to assert his [or her] own developmental wishes" (p. 363).

The family development perspective, particularly the family life cycle aspect, subsequently has been accepted by many mainstream family therapists (e.g., Carter & McGoldrick, 1980, 1988; Glick & Kessler, 1974; Haley, 1973).

FAMILY LIFE CYCLE CLINICAL ADAPTATIONS

Several modifications of the number of stages of the family life cycle have been made for clinical purposes. M. A. Solomon (1973), for example, constructed a five-stage clinically oriented framework that included a developmental task conception. Each of the developmental family stages that he proposed poses a life crisis situation that must be resolved if adaptive growth is to be continued by the family. Solomon's five stages of the family life cycle are the marriage, the birth of the first child and subsequent childbearing, individuation of family members, departure of the children, and integration of loss.

Howells (1975, p. 94) described the family in terms of seven stages or phases. Each of these involves changing structure and functions.

Barnhill and Longo (1978) divided the family life cycle into nine stages and emphasized the transitions from one stage to the next. They attempted to set forth a key issue in the transitions of each of the nine stages, as follows: committing, developing new parent roles, accepting the new personality (in the family), introducing the child to institutions, accepting adolescence, experimenting with independence, preparing to launch, (the spouses) letting go and facing each other again, and accepting retirement and/or old age.

The appearance of symptoms in one or more family members—for example, depression or delinquent behavior—during a transition often indicates to Barnhill and Longo (1978) that the appropriate life cycle tasks are not being mastered. In other words, disruptions or failures in the achievement of family developmental tasks may result in the appearance of symptoms and symptomatic behavior in a family member. Changes in family size, for example, frequently are accompanied by the appearance of symptoms. That is, losses from the family or additions to it may produce symptomatic reactions in one or more family members. Although this is far from universal, it occurs often enough to warrant careful attention by the clinician at both the original assessment and the ongoing assessment–treatment stages. These correlations have obvious implications for both clinical assessment and intervention.

Carter and McGoldrick (1980) established a family life cycle of six stages. They emphasize the central importance of transitions and the disturbance of the family homeostasis at the points at which members enter and depart from the family system. They used a variation of a Barnhill and Longo (1978) idea to suggest that "the central underlying process" that has to be negotiated "is the expansion, contraction, and realignment of the relationship system to support the entry, exit, and development of family members in a functional way" (Carter & McGoldrick, 1980, p. 16). The life cycle transitions require second-order change (change of the system itself), according to Carter and McGoldrick (1988).

Changes within a stage appear to be relegated to a comparatively minor position by Carter and McGoldrick. Problems inside a stage are viewed as frequently being amenable to solution through rearrangement of the system and incremental change. Therapists are cautioned not to become "bogged down with a family in first-order details" when the family has not negotiated the prescribed second-order changes (Carter & McGoldrick, 1988). Carter and McGoldrick (1988) do not appear to recognize the possibility that successful therapeutic intervention with the problems of family members within a stage can lead to or be a prerequisite to the eventual successful achievement of "the key principle of the emotional process of transition" and accomplishment of the "second-order changes in family status required to proceed developmentally" (Carter & McGoldrick, 1988, p. 15).

The six stages described in the latest version of Carter and McGoldrick's (1988) schema are leaving home (single young adults), the joining of families through marriage (the new couple), families with young children, families with adolescents, launching children and moving on, and families in later life. They also conceptualize useful frameworks for major variations in the family life cycle (divorce, postdivorce, and remarried family). The first two of these involve tasks associated with the "emotional process of transition: prerequisite attitude" and "developmental issues" and the last (the remarried family) with prerequisite attitudes and developmental issues (Carter & McGoldrick 1988).

Nichols and Everett (1986) conceived a four-stage, developmental-clinical framework for intact families: formation (mating and marriage), expansion (parental beginnings and subsequent years), contraction (individuation and eventual separation of youth), and postparental. A fifth stage deals with marital breakup and family reorganization with the major stages of divorce, single parent living, and remarried families.

The Nichols and Everett approach differs from the path followed by McGoldrick and Carter in that they treat the entry into marriage more explicitly as part of an ongoing process of detachment–reattachment (detachment from one's family of origin and reattachment to an opposite-sex peer for the purpose of forming new marriage and family relationships) rather than as a more separate and discrete stage. Acknowledging the validity of Carter and McGoldrick's conceptualization, we note that a considerable amount of overlap exists between differentiating from one's family of origin and forming a marriage and new nuclear family of one's own. Leaving the old family is less a stage than a process in which realignment of relationships with one's own family of origin usually begins with an increasing differentiation of self in late adolescence and is advanced by one's entry into marriage.

IMPLICATIONS FOR THE CLINICIAN

Comprehension of the processes and issues involved in family development is useful, if not crucial, to all family therapists. Some family therapists take a synchronic or cross-sectional approach, it is true, dealing primarily with the problem(s) of the moment and claiming that their approach is ahistorical. Even they, however, tend to adapt their interventions to the stage of development the family and its members are in at the time of the therapy intervention. On the other hand, a considerable segment of the family therapy field focuses mainly on dealing with the family and its members explicitly in terms of development, a life cycle perspective, and a three-generational outlook. Among the major implications of taking a family development approach are the following:

1. The developmental perspective embodies the recognition that family members may carry within themselves and in their relationships unresolved tasks from an earlier period of their life. A major difference between this understanding and that of classic psychoanalytic explanations is that the family system approach recognizes that unresolved tasks are not simply contained within the psyche of the individual and, hence, can be dealt with effectively by working with the system as well as with the person.

2. Recent research and theory in child development have highlighted the emphasis that parent–child interaction is reciprocal. There is an ongoing mutual influence process operating with the child and its envi-

ronment. More than two decades ago, Lewis and Rosenblum (1990) showed, and others have supported the finding, that even small infants have the power to influence the response of their caretakers. As Patricia Minuchin (1985) has noted, a "relational, bidirectional framework has become increasingly prevalent in developmental research" (p. 292).

3. Use of a developmental stage concept for the classification of families has some definite implications for the consideration of family pathology. As noted by L. Fisher (1977), there are two fundamental views regarding the nature of family pathology. One, illustrated in the work of Duvall (1957, 1971, 1977), Haley (1973), and others, is that family pathology is based on a combination of life-stage events and external circumstances. The other view suggests that pathology stems from the family system itself, with the developmental stage simply defining the nature of the symptoms or coloring the particular expression that the pathology takes.

Fisher also notes that the two views lead to somewhat different emphases in clinical intervention. The first focuses on environmental manipulation in conjunction with working with specific family members. The second, which embodies a stronger emphasis on a systems conceptualization, involves intervention that includes all family members and deals with the family structure, according to Fisher (1977).

4. The existence of various stages and tasks of the life cycles makes it possible to predict accurately that certain problems may arise at specified times. Examples are the transitional periods in the family life cycle when a member leaves the family or is lost from it and transitions in the marital and individual life cycles. Unexpected disruptions also may arise, such as those resulting from losses due to accidents, occurrence of chronic illness in a child, discovery of extramarital affairs, and other incidents that are not standard for all families.

An intervention strategy called "previewing," developed by Trad (1990, 1992, 1993) for individual development, can be adapted for use with family stages and tasks as well. In previewing, forthcoming developmental changes are envisioned and enacted in order to rehearse forthcoming skills (Trad, 1993, p. 225).

5. The existence of various stages and tasks of the life cycles also provides the therapist with guidelines for determining some of the tasks that must be accomplished in order to establish adequate functioning in the system. Failure to accomplish the ordinary developmental tasks because of lack of knowledge of what is needed, inability to discharge responsibilities, and other reasons may cause major problems in the family and its members.

6. Transacting with families from a developmental perspective is a complex business in that the constituent units of the family go through

their respective and different stages and transitions simultaneously. It is essential that the therapist be able to conduct his or her assessments of the client system by recognizing the different life cycles and developmental tasks in which the client system is involved—family, marital, individual— as well as to comprehend the sociocultural factors impinging on the family and its members. The different problems and strengths in each cycle and component and how they may contribute to the client system's problems and to problem resolutions need to be taken into consideration in determining interventions.

7. Changes are underway in the use of the family life cycle approach. Some family therapists have abandoned their earlier attention to and use of the family life cycle. Fisch (1983), for example, has written that the family life cycle is no longer central to the brief therapy model of the Mental Research Institute (MRI) group. Breunlin (1988) suggests that one possibility for the abandonment may be the fact that the family life cycle lacks the complexity to deal with the major models of family therapy. It has stagnated in the form of an underdeveloped stage-transition model, in his terms (p. 153). Breunlin (1988; Breunlin et al., 1992) has offered a broader family development "metaframework" that gives attention to development at five levels: biological, individual, subsystemic, familial, and societal. Rather than definite, discrete stages, Breunlin and associates (1992) emphasize microtransitions and the negotiation of these changes through an oscillation.

Although I find Breunlin's theory interesting and helpful in several respects, my own speculation is that one reason some family therapists lost their interest in the family life cycle may have been an overemphasis on the transitions between stages and on the production of pathology in relation to failures or difficulties in effecting those between-stage transitions. The other side of the overemphasis on transitions and the related spawning of pathology appears to have been an underemphasis on the significance of normal "inside-the-stages" developmental tasks. Family therapists do not seem to have recognized and adequately used a comprehension of the family life cycle during less overtly eventful periods—that is, when significant transitions between stages are not in process—for understanding (a) how the failure to successfully discharge the phase-specific developmental tasks within a stage results in difficulties and (b) how knowledge of the pertinent tasks and the use of support and education of family members in order to help them succeed in accomplishing the requisite tasks can help both to solve problems and, less dramatically, to prevent problems.

8. There are other uses and adaptations of the family life cycle concept. Among them are the advent of the women's movement and changes in the roles of females that have resulted in corresponding changes

in marital relationships and a need to revise traditional views of marital developmental tasks. Conceptualizations beyond those made earlier are required, such as the "floating marital task" described by Zemon-Gass and Nichols (1981) which is concerned with obtaining an equitable balance between the marital partners.

INTEGRATION OF CYCLES

The view in this book is that the therapist needs to be wary of oversimplifying the concept of the family life cycle in at least two ways. One possible oversimplification is to view the family life cycle as if it were useful only with regard to understanding and dealing with potentially negative disruptions of the transitions between stages. The other is to overlook the rich complexity and interlocking nature of the various life cycles that affect individuals and families at any one time and throughout the spans of those cycles.

The developmental perspective described here is more inclusive than the typical approach of family therapists and gives attention to the family system, the marital subsystem, and the individual subsystems as they unfold over time. The stage concept is retained, although the notion of distinct lines between stages that have to be crossed in a step-like or "leaping" fashion is modified. The system and each of its subsystems is concerned with developmental tasks that need to be mastered at each stage in order for the system or subsystem to proceed successfully to the next stage.

Hill (1970) emphasized the three-generational properties of the family life cycle. The marital pair in the nuclear family form a "linkage bridge" between their own parents and their children's generation. Therefore, a linking and mutual interdependence exists among the generations as they move through the life cycle. Like interlinking cogwheels, each individual's life cycle meshes with and affects the movement of the life cycles of other individuals and of the various systems themselves. This linking and cogwheeling is an important emphasis of this book. I shall refer to the linkages in a description of stages of the marital life cycle and various individual life cycles in connection with various stages of the family life cycle.

The Marital Life Cycle

Materials for formulating marital developmental tasks and constructing a marital life cycle have long been available. Eight tasks in the couples' interpersonal preparation for marriage and three for a honeymoon phase were described by R. Rapoport and R. N. Rapoport (1964) three decades ago. Nevertheless, family therapists typically have not appeared to be concerned with the construction of a marital life cycle.

Writers who have given some attention to marital development and life cycle issues include Scherz (1971; she was primarily concerned with the parent–child relationship), Haley (1963), M. A. Solomon (1973), Berman and Lief (1975), Barnhill and Longo (1978), Carter and McGoldrick (1980, 1988), Nichols and Everett (1986), Nichols (1988), and others. Some of these approaches have dealt with marital developmental tasks under the rubric of either individual or family life cycles. Even Carter and McGoldrick (1980, 1988) in their widely used work, despite naming some marital tasks in their stages of the family life cycle under the heading of second-order changes in family status, provide no separate, systematic schema of marital developmental tasks. Berman and Lief (1975) combined their marital life cycle materials with an adult individual life cycle. I did not separate the marital cycle adequately from the family life cycle (Nichols, 1988), including several parental tasks under the marital rubric.

The marital life cycle presented below is taken from Nichols and Pace-Nichols's (1993) recent attempt to devise a specific marital life cycle with appropriate developmental tasks. We intended to provide clinicians with a marital life cycle that included the following criteria:

- Based explicitly on the marital relationship and developmental tasks of marriage.
- Based on mutual responsibility and privilege between mates, embodying gender equity.
- Focused both on couples who have children and on couples who do not have children, with most features applying to all marriages, but some being limited to those with children.
- Focused both on intact marriages and on marriages that are ended by divorce (although only the parts dealing with intact marriages will be presented in this chapter).
- Based on major Western values and behaviors and thus culture specific. (Although applicable in some instances to non-Western marriages, the tasks and perhaps the stages themselves need to be adapted for non-Western marriages.)
- Essentially applicable to marriages in all social classes.
- General and illustrative rather than exhaustive in its coverage of marital tasks. (Some core tasks possibly could be placed elsewhere and interpreted differently, and additional tasks could be added.)
- Clinically useful.

It was derived primarily from clinical experience with married couples and a broad comprehension of marriage and marital interaction formulated from studying pertinent research across several decades (Nichols & Pace-Nichols, 1993).

Rather than focusing on either individual tasks or family tasks, the marital life cycle and marital therapy are concerned with the levels of development achieved by the partners together and on the tasks they need to achieve jointly in order for the marriage to function adequately. The associated parental tasks are included because of the importance of parental roles and because the spouses need to master parental tasks as a couple in order to function satisfactorily in their marital and family roles. It should be recognized that each couple will seek to fulfill their marital tasks in their own distinctive way but within a broad framework established by the culture and their family heritages.

The joint tasks of the married couple may be grouped into two broad categories, internal relationship tasks and external relationship tasks. The central, or core, internal relationship tasks described here are as follows:

Commitment: How and to what extent the partners value the relationship and their intentions with regard to its maintenance and continuation. (Attention to this task is exceedingly important because marriage is the only voluntary family relationship and, hence, the most fragile.)

Caring: The kind of emotional attachment that ties the partners to one another. (This term is used instead of the ambiguous term "love." Caring, like commitment, is highly significant because of the nature of mate selection—largely on the basis of personal choice and sentiments—and the fragility of marriage.)

Communication: The ability to communicate verbally and symbolically, to share meanings.

Conflict/compromise: The ability to recognize and deal with the disagreements that are inevitable in any intimate relationship.

Contract: The set of expectations and explicit, implied, or presumed agreements held by the partners. (These may be conscious and verbalized, conscious but not verbalized, or outside awareness levels, as described by Sager, 1976.)

External relationship tasks are concerned with forming and maintaining appropriate associations and affiliations with other subsystems within the family, with other systems, and with other individuals. The ability of the spouses to sustain a satisfactory balance of power, balance of roles, and degree of intimacy is crucial to good marital functioning (Nichols, 1988).

A developmental model of what Kovacs (1988) has called "couplehood" provides the therapist with a kind of map for interventions with problematic couples and marriages. Kovacs regards lasting intimate relationships such as marriage as an arena following adolescence for adults to complete unfinished developmental business and attain additional individual differentiation and development as a couple.

The Individual Life Cycle

Family therapists may fall into the trap of ignoring the individual while accentuating the system. There is a strong need for the therapist to develop an adequate knowledge of individual development and how it fits into and links with the family life cycle and the marital life cycle. The individual has developmental tasks to perform at given stages in life. As described by Havighurst (1953), successful completion of them leads to happiness and subsequent success with later tasks, and failure results in individual unhappiness, social disapproval, and problems with subsequent tasks. These tasks have been described in various ways and grouped into stages.

Duvall (1977) listed developmental tasks for individuals in 10 categories of behavior: achieving an appropriate dependence–independence pattern, achieving an appropriate giving–receiving pattern of affection, relating to changing social groups, developing a conscience, learning one's psychosociobiological sex role, accepting and adjusting to a changing body, managing a changing body and learning new motor patterns, learning to understand and control the physical world, developing an appropriate symbol system and conceptual abilities, and relating oneself to the cosmos. Each of the seven stages in the individual's life—infancy, early childhood, late childhood, early adolescence, late adolescence, maturity, and aging—contains its version of the task for each category of behavior (Duvall, 1977, pp. 172–175).

Achieving an appropriate dependence–independence pattern is described as one such developmental task. In Duvall's (1977, pp. 172–173, adapted) framework, this task in three of the stages would be as follows:

- In *late childhood*, the task is to free oneself from primary identification with adults.
- In *late adolescence*, the task is to establish oneself as an independent individual in an adult manner.
- In *aging*, the task is accepting graciously and comfortably the help needed from others as powers fail and dependence becomes necessary (Nichols & Everett, 1986).

This kind of individual developmental task approach leaves adequate room for incorporation of human development materials and psychosocial concepts from many sources, from Piaget to object relations and numerous other stations in between.

PUTTING THE CYCLES TOGETHER

What follows is an attempt to list and relate the various cycles and their respective developmental tasks for each of the four stages of the intact family life cycle used in this book. The stages are expanded from the framework erected by Nichols and Everett (1986).

The Family Life Cycle, Stage 1–Formation: Mating and Marriage

This stage is concerned with three life cycles: the marital life cycle, which at this time is synonymous with the family life cycle of what typically will become a new family unit; the individual life cycle—young adulthood (for the two persons who separate out from their families of origin and enter into the mating and marriage process, and the family life cycle for each of the families of origin of the mating partners. (The postparental tasks of the parents of the young couple are given in Stage 4 of the family life cycle.)

The Family Life Cycle, Stage 2–Expansion: Parental Beginnings and Subsequent Years

This stage is concerned with the introduction of a new member(s) into the life of the couple, thereby creating a family and significantly increasing the complexity of life in the home. Five types of life cycles are involved: the family life cycle, the marital life cycle, the individual life cycle—adulthood (for each of the adults), the child individual life cycle—child (for the new infant/child), and the family life cycle of the families of origin of each of the marital partners in this family (the older generation's life cycle). Each time an additional child becomes part of the new family, another life cycle adds to the mix and its complexity.

   Although an argument can be made for conceptualizing expansion-stage families as comprising three different stages—childbearing, preschool years, and school-age years—a different pattern is followed here. The family life cycle during the expanding years is viewed in a broader and more inclusive sense. A major guideline is the child's, or children's, status, involving the movement from initial total dependency to a period, usually in adolescence, when the child begins manifesting increased independence and sharing with the parents a growing degree of responsibility for him- or herself in preparation for getting launched.

The Family Life Cycle, Stage 3—Contraction: Individuation and Eventual Separation of Youth

This stage is concerned with the departure of the children from home and the contraction of the nuclear family so that eventually it becomes a couple once again. In a very genuine sense, this stage "starts before it starts" in that there is a fairly lengthy preparation process before the adolescent member(s) finally departs from the home. As with Stage 2, five types of life cycles typically are involved, including the individual life cycle—middle adulthood for the original couple. (See the older generation's life cycle for the tasks of the grandparents [family of origin].)

The Family Life Cycle, Stage 4—Postparental Years

This stage begins when the children have left home and ends when both of the original marital partners have died. Between those two markers, the family life cycle rolls forward so that the children in the family typically become parents; their parents (the original marital partners) become grandparents; their own parents, if still living, move into the role of great-grandparents to the youngest members of the family. The life cycles involved here are the marital life cycles (of the original marital couple and of their married children); the individual life cycle—aging, the individual life cycle—adult and/or middle adulthood (for the children of the original marital couple), and the child individual life cycle—child, adolescent, and/or young adulthood.

Evaluation and Treatment

4

PERSPECTIVES ON THERAPY

Working directly with the totality of the forces that influence the
individual is such a logical idea that it is hard to deny its validity.
—AUGUSTUS Y. NAPIER,
The Family Crucible

Every therapist should be as aware as possible of his or her assumptions regarding therapy. This is an evolving process; our perceptions and conclusions are continually changing. We may not be readily aware of the ideas and values that drive and guide us in our therapeutic efforts at any particular time. Consequently, there is a need, a practical and ethical imperative, to examine our ideas and our values periodically and to strive to make them as explicit as we can. We owe it to ourselves and, more significantly, to our clients to be as clear as we can about the nature of therapy from our perspective.

The first portion of this chapter is devoted to stating the major assumptions and values that I hold regarding the treatment of persons in families. Following that statement are sections on the focus of the treatment (which includes a preliminary approach to establishing a decision tree for the clinician's guidance in determining the focus of therapy), form of the therapy, goals of therapy, and ethical issues in therapy.

ASSUMPTIONS AND VALUES

Certain assumptions and values that provide a framework and serve as guides for the integrative approach to family therapy offered in this book

75

have already been mentioned. These include the ideas of context and treating the individual in context. In this chapter I discuss assumptions and values regarding the client system, respectful treatment of clients, the relationship and alliance with clients, direct and indirect intervention, the responsibility for change, the principle of least pathology, the education and the motivation of clients, as well as gender and ethnicity considerations with clients.

The Client System

With whom does the therapist work? The preferred term here is "client" or "client system," whether one is working with one person, a marital or other subsystem of a family, or a total family. The term "patient," while respectable, implies passivity. A patient is one who receives care or treatment, someone to whom something is done. Although the term "client" historically has had similar connotations (e.g., formerly it meant one who was dependent on another and in a basic sense "leaned on them for protection"), today it embodies the meaning of "customer" and implies a more active participation in the therapy process by the client.

Systems intervention is aimed at effecting change so that the system is no longer functioning in a pathological or ineffective way that results in symptoms in one or more members of the system.

Adoption of a systems perspective does not mean that the total family must be present in order to perform family therapy. Family therapy does not depend on the number of persons present in the interview or therapy session. A therapist can intervene into the family process even if only one member of the family is present in the interview.

Even when more than one family member is present, it is possible to affect the family system and other members without directly working with them. Family therapy pioneer Murray Bowen (1978), for example, typically worked with one marital partner in front of the other or with one client in front of a family group. The witnessing client or clients can get something for him- or herself and the system can be altered through such intervention strategies.

In brief, one can affect the system by working with one member and, conversely, can affect the person by working with the system as a system.

Respectful Treatment of Clients

Within the therapy framework, clients are encouraged to exercise the greatest degree of self-determination of which they are capable, with the professional assistance of the therapist. My approach to therapy, in other words, respects the ability and right of the clients to participate as fully as possible in exercising their strengths and learning how to deal with their difficulties. Depending on the situation, this means enlisting of individuals, marital partners (as a couple), and/or the total family as collaborators in the therapy process. It also means that the therapist remains respectful of the client system's right to self-determination while attempting to maintain an appropriate balance between family/group rights and needs and those of individual members. Boszormenyi-Nagy (1966; Boszormenyi-Nagy & Krasner, 1986) has used the term "multidirected partiality" to refer to similar therapeutic attitudes and methods.

None of this should be construed as meaning that a therapist remains morally and ethically neutral. On the contrary, there are times in which remaining neutral means that the therapist is tacitly condoning inequitable treatment of one family member by another or others. Child abuse and spouse abuse are salient examples of situations in which a therapist is legally required to take a stand on the side of equitable behavior. The therapist who knows that one spouse is deliberately trying to convince the other that what is occurring is not happening (i.e., that he or she is imagining things) cannot morally remain neutral in view of such "gaslighting" (from the 1940s film of the same name) or "crazy-making" behavior (Zemon-Gass & Nichols, 1988).

The Relationship and Alliance with Clients

From experience, observation, and available research, it seems clear to me that the kind of relationship the therapist is able to form with clients is a crucial element in therapy. As Gurman and Kniskern (1981, p. 303) noted, the preponderance of evidence even from heavily technique-oriented approaches such as behavior therapy (e.g., Wilson & Evans, 1977) demonstrates the centrality of therapist–patient relationship factors in expediting positive therapy results. Establishment of a relationship of trust and the formation of a therapeutic alliance appear to be intimately related.

In the midst of the strong emphasis on the role of techniques in today's family therapy world (e.g., Nelson & Trepper, 1993), I am reminded of a statement about a famous football coach: "He'll take his'n [players] and beat you'rn, and he'll take you'rn and beat his'n." In therapy, it is not so much the availability of techniques, but rather the ability to relate empathically, sensitively, and sensibly to a client that matters most. As important as techniques may be, I am compelled to regard them as secondary to the therapist's ability to establish and maintain a trusting and effective relationship with clients. My therapy is inevitably "experiential" in the sense that the term is used by Napier, that is, the therapist's encounter process with clients is emphasized above technical intervention or rational understanding (Napier, 1976).

"The most basic intervention of all" is described by one family therapist as intervention based on his empathic understanding of the client, noting that he is no longer so interested in "what to do" but, instead, focuses on "how to be" with clients (McCollum, 1993).

Direct and Indirect Intervention with Clients

Closely related to the issues of the therapeutic relationship and respectful treatment is the question of whether the therapist intervenes directly or indirectly with the client system. Direct interventions include logical explanations, suggestions, tasks, and similar approaches. One version of a direct approach involves issuing directives to the clients that they are expected to follow in order to bring about change.

Some family therapists, including especially those labeled "systems purists" by Beels and Ferber (1969), have employed indirect approaches, emphasizing the use of paradox and, in earlier years, therapeutic double-binds. Watzlawick et al. (1967); Haley (1976); and Palazzoli, Boscolo, Cecchin, and Prata (1978) have been identified as being representative of therapists using such tactics. These efforts, which have been described as attempts to "outwit" families with a kind of "psychological judo," have been most highly developed in attempts to deal with severely dysfunctional and devious families (Skynner, 1981, p. 56).

The arguments advanced in support of using paradox with clients pertain primarily to power. With the development of what became strategic family therapy, the idea was advanced that the therapist was responsible for change. After assessing the family, the therapist devises a strategy to produce change and provides directives to the client system. If the therapist is in a position of power, he or she can tell the client(s) what to do in order to solve the problem. When a therapist is not in a position of power and, therefore, cannot expect the directive to be followed, paradoxical, indirect interventions are to be used in the strategic approach (Madanes, 1984).

Other underlying theoretical ideas, such as those embodied in a homeostatic model of family functioning, also affect the therapist's notions about the importance of needing to have power to move families. Breunlin et al. (1992), for example, point out that if a therapist believes a family resists change because it is currently maintaining a homeostatic position, it is logical for the therapist to believe in the necessity of using crisis induction in order to forcibly break the family out of the homeostatic phase. When the therapist adopts the idea that he or she is responsible for change and the corollary notion that he or she can bring about change, it seems that the pressure to "make it happen" can become a major dynamic in the actions taken.

Questions have been and continue to be raised about the necessity and wisdom of using paradox routinely. Even some therapists who favor this technique are careful to note that the use of paradox should be limited. There is no need to use indirect methods if people will respond to direct interventions, they indicate (Papp, 1980, 1981; Madanes, 1984). Williamson (1991) declares that "paradox is always the second choice [in psychotherapy]. It is always preferable to deal with clients in a straightforward way" (p. 81). Even when it is not possible or effective to deal with clients directly, Williamson prefers the use of playfulness in which both parties "are on the inside of the joke" to willful, intentional paradox, which he considers antithetical to intimacy (p. 81).

I certainly am in agreement with Williamson that willful, intentional paradox is antithetical to intimacy. Additionally, in my judgment if the other person(s) is not "in on the joke" and participating in the game with an adequate amount of "informed consent," the use of paradox and other contrived tactics borders on being unethical. In some instances, it may cross over the line.

Fortunately, there are other ways in which a therapist can deal with clients and their presumed resistance to change indirectly. Bowen (1978), for example, tried to focus on patterns and facts instead of feelings and to function as a kind of unbiased researcher, using stories, humor, and reversals to help clients perceive situations differently. As noted above, he also worked with one person in the system in the presence of one or more other members who were benefited indirectly. He worked especially with the person in the system he considered most likely to change (Anderson & Stewart, 1983).

The Responsibility for Change

How we relate to clients and what we believe about change and about the clients may considerably influence what we persuade them to believe and how they change; but we do not change others in therapy. Clients change themselves in therapy, which Prochaska and DiClemente (1992) call "intentional change." Intentional change is one of three mechanisms of change, developmental and environmental being the others. An informed and prudent approach to therapy would appear to be one in which the forces for change from developmental and environmental sources are recognized and, as possible, utilized within the intentional change process.

Andersen (1993) also makes the succinct point that a client cannot be changed but a client can change.

The therapist is a facilitator, rather than a director/manager who is totally responsible for change. Sullivan (1954), in stressing the role of the therapist as an expert in interpersonal relations, also emphasized that the patient (client) brings some expectation of gaining benefit from the interviews. Therapists are responsible for creating conditions (of relationship and of realistic hope) and for bringing appropriate knowledge and interventions to the client system and situation. This is done in order to help clients deal with their difficulties through therapy and through the use of their own resources as self-changers.

Change responsibility is closely tied with the client's growth. That is, clients or client systems get a major boost and increase their sense of achievement and control over their own life when they are primarily responsible for change. Whenever possible, clients should exit from therapy with an increased knowledge of how they function and how they can function better. Whenever their functioning has been hampered by unresolved trauma from the past (e.g., sexual abuse), by failure to resolve relationship problems with their family of origin, or by tangles in their present relationships, they should leave treatment, if possible, with those issues significantly ameliorated so as to remove the barriers to their future healthy functioning.

The Principle of Least Pathology

There are limitations to traditional psychoanalytic approaches, which often assume too readily that dysfunctional or maladaptive behavior stems from unconscious conflicts that require a reworking of personality structure and organization. The presumption that manifest problems indicate that individual clients harbor a mass of unresolved past issues in a seething cauldron of conflicting impulses that require intensive, long-term therapy is far from accurate in most cases. Although family therapists acknowledge that the problems that bring clients to treatment sometimes are based on significant amounts of underlying pathology, some of us doubt that presuming that this is the case at the outset is a productive way to proceed.

When we follow the principle of least pathology, we are guided by two questions: (1) At the outset, we ask ourselves whether that which is troublesome to a client necessarily arises from major pathology or whether a less complex and more parsimonious and commonplace explanation can be found for the behaviors, and (2) we also ask ourselves whether the problems necessarily require lengthy treatment or depth exploration and intervention. Whatever our conclusions about the origins of the problems, we try first to determine whether the problems can be dealt with in a simple and straightforward manner. If the more ingenuous and direct ways are not effective, then it may be appropriate to plan longer-term and more depth-oriented interventions.

Several experiences very early in my career taught me to question whether even some fairly dysfunctional behaviors call for an automatic assumption of major pathology and indicate that the client is in need of an extensive overhauling of his or her personality. Even after the passage of time, my embarrassment surrounding how I approached one case is lessened only by the fact that I learned from what occurred. At the conclusion of an initial exploratory session with a couple in which the major complaint was the wife's concern about her husband's drinking, I recommended a typical psychodynamic course of therapy to deal with the dynamics of the alcohol abuse. The couple did not enter therapy, but instead sought out their clergyman, who told the man to stop drinking. He did. Ten years later he was still abstaining. Not all situations are remedied that directly and easily, of course, but it should not take many such outcomes to suggest that direct, common-sense approaches may warrant careful consideration and application.

In fact, behavioral approaches sometimes work with both mildly disturbed and significantly disturbed/maladaptive situations.

The Education of Clients

People may not know what is needed. They may not know how to do what needs to be done. They may not know how to determine when it needs to be done. The therapist who helps them to become aware of what is needed and teaches them how to make the best possible determinations and decisions makes a significant contribution to their lives.

Sometimes, when people are aware of what needs to be done, they can do it. Frequently, however, they need to be taught how to acquire and use important skills. One task of a therapist is to help them learn new skills so that they can function as well as possible after therapy has terminated.

The therapist also has the task of determining what else—besides what has already been tried outside of therapy and in therapy—is needed in order to enable and empower individuals, couples, and families to do what needs to be done. This may include doing work with their families of origin (Framo, 1992; Williamson, 1991) and providing skill training in such important functional areas as communication. Not the least of the tasks of the therapist is the preliminary work of helping the client system to become free of acute and/or chronic anxiety so that the members can be as competent as they are capable of being in discharging their roles.

The Motivation of Clients

We do not motivate others. Some therapists talk about motivating people, but they may actually mean something other than motivation. Even Jay Haley (1976, p. 54), who talks about motivating people, points out that he is talking about persuading clients to take an action. We certainly can influence, encourage, and support many of our clients. Most importantly of all, we can strive to create conditions in which clients can develop the motivation to make the changes that are needed in order to function effectively and in a healthy fashion.

Beutler and Consoli (1992) espouse a helpful "philosophy that psychotherapy is a social-influence or persuasion process in which the therapist's operational theory forms the content of *what* is persuaded, and the therapist's technology functions as the *means* of influence" (p. 266). Furthermore, they point out that there needs to be adequate "fit" between client characteristics and therapy procedures. For example, persuasion should help the client to manage arousal levels and to focus efforts, the therapist should be a trustworthy and credible person whose perspective is considered knowledgeable and sufficiently different from the client's to induce motivation and to provide direction for change, and there needs to be an adequate receptivity on the part of the client to the therapist's direct persuasion efforts (p. 268).

Gender Considerations

Family therapy is still in the midst of altering its perceptions of gender considerations. Gender is used here to refer to issues pertaining to masculinity and femininity. Sex refers to whether one is male or female. Gender and sex are related in very complex interactions between social and biological factors (Unger & Crawford, 1993). Fairness requires that the therapist be alert to the possibility of gender inequities, recognizing their effects and working to change them wherever possible. Recognizing effects of sex and gender and providing descriptions of existing circumstances in this book do not imply condonation of inequities. The value and needs of children, women, and men are all valid and important.

Ethnicity Considerations

Family development is interpreted and dealt with in its cultural context. This means that ethnicity is a significant factor in evaluation and treatment. Ethnicity is used here in the general dictionary sense to refer to basic divisions of humankind as they are distinguished by customs, characteristics, common history, and language. When the reference is specifically to race, which is often lumped together with ethnicity, efforts will be made here to use the terms "race" or "racial."

Two standard sources of information and assistance for the family therapist regarding ethnicity are Papajohn and Spiegel's (1975) work on transactions in families and an edited volume by McGoldrick, Pearce, and Giordano (1982). Papajohn and Spiegel deal with generational conflicts and conflict resolution among Puerto Rican, Greek-American, and Italian-American families. A major focus is on the value orientations of these groups. McGoldrick and associates have collected chapters on Native American, Alaskan Native, black, African-American, West Indian, Mexican, Puerto Rican, Cuban, Asian, French Canadian, German, Greek, Iranian, Irish, Italian, Jewish, Polish, Portuguese, and Norwegian families, and provide a number of useful concepts for understanding and working with such families.

More recent material can be found in a special issue of the journal *Families in Society: The Journal of Contemporary Human Services*, which is devoted to the topic of multicultural practice ("Multicultural Practice," 1992). Especially useful are articles on clinical diagnosis among diverse populations (A. Solomon, 1992) and training racially sensitive family therapists (Hardy & Laszloffy, 1992). Solomon discusses four ways in which clinical diagnosis may be harmful to minority clients: through cultural expression of symptomatology (which is not understood by the clinician), the use of unreliable research instruments, clinician bias, and institutional racism. Hardy and Laszloffy analyze the culture of educational and training programs for marital and family therapy and make suggestions for reshaping programs in order to provide racially sensitive clinicians. The writers in the special issue strongly emphasize that clinicians must attend to both the general characteristics of members of minority groups and to specific idiosyncratic characteristics of the persons.

FOCUS OF THE TREATMENT

Where does the therapist focus his or her treatment efforts? Therapy in an integrative approach is flexible treatment. A variety of interview formats may be used and the focus may change during the course of the therapy. The therapist makes decisions to proceed on the basis of several factors. These include the initial assessment of the case, the ongoing assessment of the case, the changing needs of the case as different phases are reached, and the impinging external events that occur during the course of the therapy (Nichols, 1985a). Thus, I follow these principles throughout the course of treatment in making decisions and tailoring treatment to client needs.

System and Subsystems

Whether interviews are being conducted with the entire family, family subsystems, or with one person, the therapist keeps the system in mind at all times. What I am calling here system intervention or system-focused therapy involves treating the system directly and helping the system to explore issues and to nurture, support, and appropriately confront its members as members of the system. The therapist supports the system and intervenes in its functioning, rearranging its structure and redirecting its processes as required. Minuchin's (1974) structural approach, for example, rebuilds hierarchical arrangements and helps underorganized families (Aponte, 1976) become better organized so that they can function more effectively. Direct system intervention may take the form of working directly with the processes of interaction with the entire nuclear family. Some forms of family-of-origin work (Framo, 1992; Williamson, 1991) involve working directly with an adult and the assembled members of his or her family of origin.

Other forms of system intervention involve working with family subsystems such as the parent–child, the sibling, and the marital subsystems. Whatever the particular tasks undertaken in this approach, the therapist deals with the system or its subsystem as an entity rather than with persons as if they exist as isolated entities.

Persons Alone

This focus refers to treating persons more directly by providing exploration, nurturance, support, and appropriate confrontation in individual sessions, rather than intervening in a macroscopic fashion with an entire family system or with some of its subsystems. The client system in this focus consists primarily of one person. Initial treatment with the solo person may extend to therapeutic contact and work with his or her family of origin and, in instances in which the client is married, to work with his or her spouse.

Deciding on the Focus

How does the therapist determine the focus of the therapy? Assuming that a therapist is committed to a truly integrative approach rather than being wedded to a single model, there are a number of guidelines available. The following decision tree is not definitive because it is not possible at this time to be polished and precise within the boundaries of an integrative model. Instead, this preliminary approach is heuristic and subject to continuing refinements.

Availability of the Family System

Is the family system available for therapy participation? Does the identified client have a living family? Does he or she know its location? Is the family willing and able to be involved in therapy? Are there deficits in the situation or in the family itself that preclude the possibility of the person working with the family and receiving what he or she needs from it?

If the identified client is a minor who has no family system available for therapy, it may be necessary to construct a substitute or replacement family. This replacement family is needed not only in order to participate in therapy and provide current support and remedial assistance but also to furnish a family setting for completion of the minor's development and launching into the world.

Age and Status of an Identified Client

If there is an identified client, self-identified or nominated by the system, his or her age and status in the family are among the first criteria to be used in determining the focus of the initial therapeutic efforts. The age of the identified client typically is combined with the resulting influence of the system over him or her in establishing whether the initial focus is to be placed on the person directly or on the system primarily and on the person secondarily.

How directly and immediately is the system with its structures and processes affecting the person? If the identified client is still dependent on the family of origin, as in the case of a minor child, adolescent, or undifferentiated young adult, the initial emphasis of therapy is placed on treating the family unit. If an adult identified client's major problems are related to entanglements with or lack of differentiation from his or her family of origin, the focus is again on dealing with the family system.

If the identified client is no longer living in the family but is immediately affected—influenced and constrained—on an ongoing basis by the behaviors and current interaction of the family system, the decision typically is to start the therapy first with the individual client. Work with the family-of-origin system is undertaken secondarily and later.

Nature and Form of the Problem(s)

Increasingly, clients contact therapists with a request for therapy for the entire family. Even before making the initial telephone call, some potential clients have decided that their problems involve or affect the family as a whole and require professional assistance aimed at family functioning. When this is the case, it generally is a good idea to start with the entire family in the initial session. Sometimes a potential client will say things in the initial telephone contact that indicate to me that he or she is ascribing the problem to the family system in an attempt to blame others or to otherwise avoid focusing on him- or herself. Even so, the initial focus generally should be on the total family when the request for service is framed in total family terms.

A subsequent decision by the therapist to continue with family interview sessions and the focus on the entire family calls for attention to the developmental stages of the family. What are the current developmental stages and tasks with which the family is concerned? Has the family successfully completed stage-appropriate family life cycle tasks from the past? If not, the immediate focus must be on assisting the family to complete those family tasks as effectively and completely as possible. As well as being concerned with the extent to which problems and failures in family developmental tasks and stages contribute to the current dysfunction, the therapist needs to examine the extent to which family process and structure contribute to the positive support of the family members.

Some symptoms and disturbances require the involvement of the nuclear family—and sometimes members of the extended family—in order to ensure the likelihood of successful intervention. An example of such a case would be an emotional or mental disturbance that requires the use of medication and various adjunctive interventions. Schizophrenic reactions, for instance, can be treated through a psychoeducational approach (Anderson, Reiss, & Hogarty, 1986; McFarlane, 1983, 1991).

How successfully or adequately have varied parts of the family—such as a marital unit and/or individual persons—completed past stage-appropriate marital or individual life cycle tasks? If they have not done so adequately, or if they have done so and are deficient in current task fulfillment, the focus of therapy generally needs to be on them and their tasks before efforts are made to continue working with the family as a unit. That is, it frequently is necessary to deal with unresolved past stage issues of the adults in the family before focusing on the system's problems or on a child's symptoms that result from an extrusion of problems from the marital pair or from an induction of the child into enactment of adult issues. An example would be parents who have not completed the important work of differentiating from their families of origin. Still stuck in unresolved relationships with their own parents, they are not ready to be mature parents with their own children.

At other times, it is desirable to deal first with total family issues and to get things settled down before proceeding to work with individually focused problems or symptoms. The presenting complaint, for example, is the dating behavior of an adolescent female child. Working with the total family and effecting clear communication, functional negotiation patterns, and some reasonable mutually acceptable ground rules may diminish or eradicate complaints about the adolescent. Often, the focus then moves to the marriage or to problems of one of the parents, such as continuing pain over abuse or neglect in their upbringing.

The flexibility of an integrative approach, as noted previously, permits and often calls for the use of interviews with subsystems of the family. Brief illustrations follow of instances in which the focus may be placed on the parental, sibling, or marital subsystems of the family.

Parental Subsystem. When the therapist's assessment reveals that the marital partners are unable to function adequately as parents, the focus may need to be placed on the parents and their parental role in order to provide assistance for a child and for the family. The inability may stem from ignorance; interpersonal dynamics, such as avoidance of potential conflict, that cripple their ability to be parents (Colapinto, 1988); or from other sources.

Sibling Subsystem. There are a variety of issues that affect the decision to focus on the sibling subsystem (Bank & Kahn, 1982). Two examples follow in which the sibling subsystem could be used as the focus of therapy in family treatment. First, in an intact nuclear family it may be useful to arrange for a few sibling sessions in which the children are seen alone in order to provide support for and lessen the estrangement of a "rebel" child. Careful preparation of the parents and the children for such sessions is required. Attention also must be given to assisting the children to communicate their concerns to their parents in nonblaming and productive ways in subsequent total family sessions. When parents become aware that all the children, and not merely the identified client, share certain concerns, the way is open to consider those concerns as family matters and not idiosyncratic deviance on the part of the rebel, for instance.

Second, in situations in which the parents are separated or severely estranged so that the children feel isolated and confused, sessions with the children can be very useful in building support among the siblings and lessening the stress they experience. Particular attention needs to be given to helping the siblings to become aware of what their brothers and/or sisters are experiencing and to exploring ways that they can work out, where possible, reasonably satisfactory and separate relationships with their estranged parents. In the case of divorce, sibling sessions can assist children in coping with the pain and uncertainties of divorce adjustment (Nichols, 1986).

Marital Subsystem. There are several indications for focusing the therapy on the marital subsystem. Among the more salient are (1) when the initial complaint or request comes solely from the couple; (2) when the initial complaint comes from one of the spouses and it seems evident that the problems are linked to or are exacerbated by the marital relationship, or can be modified by changes in the relationship with the spouse, whether or not the problems appear to be stemming from the marriage; and (3) when the problems in a family relate primarily to the marital couple, particularly when the problems manifested by a child can be identified as stemming from issues extruded from the marriage.

FORM OF THE THERAPY

The integrative approach described here always features an emphasis on family systems. Specific factors affect the extent to which emphasis is placed on psychodynamic and behavioral or social learning theory aspects and approaches to therapy. Stated broadly, the indices for the three emphases or approaches include those below.

Family Systems Approach

The greater the degree to which the individual is affected by the system and reflects the system's functioning or malfunctioning, the greater the need to step in explicitly at the level of systems intervention and to emphasize systems processes and functions. The more important and influential the current ecological setting on the person(s) identified as the client, the more likely that one will work explicitly with the family system. Examples include working on structural problems by restructuring boundaries and hierarchies and dealing with total family issues such as coping with the demands of developmental stages, life cycle issues, and educational needs.

The greater the extent to which the problems manifested in the individual reflect "live" ties with the family of origin, the greater the need to deal specifically with family-of-origin issues. This is true whether or not the members of the family of origin are seen by the therapist. These

interventions involve dealing with intergenerational problems and relationships in any one of several ways (e.g., Boszormenyi-Nagy & Spark,
1973; Bowen, 1978; Framo, 1992; Nerin, 1986; Nichols, 1988; Paul &
Paul, 1975; Williamson, 1991).

Psychodynamic Approach

There are many points at which the clinician who understands psychodynamics can use that knowledge effectively in treating persons in families.
There also are several techniques such as dream exploration that may be
useful. Perhaps the most prominent of the indicators for employing a
psychodynamic approach, however, is the need to comprehend and work
with marital couples in the area of mate choice and expectations (Sager,
1976).

Object relations, especially in relation to marital choice and interaction (Dicks, 1967; Scharff & Scharff, 1991; Willi, 1982, 1984) but in other
areas of family life as well (Scharff & Scharff, 1987; J. S. Scharff, 1989;
Slipp, 1984, 1988), are exceedingly helpful to the clinician in both
assessment and treatment. The point of view here is that as important as
demographic and other general factors may be in determining the selection
of a mate, in the final analysis one must look to internal psychological
factors in order to comprehend both a person's choice (Nichols, 1978)
and much of the subsequent marital interaction.

Social Learning Theory Approach

Use of social learning theory principles can be helpful in a variety of
situations in which it is important to alter maladaptive and nonproductive
behaviors or to form new behaviors. Pointing out that "any response to
the behavior of another is a reward" that contributes to the continuation
of the undesired behaviors frequently makes sense to clients. This intervention, accompanied by coaching of clients to make no response if they
wish to extinguish the undesired behavior, has proven to be highly
productive in dealing with parent–child problem situations, for example.
Similarly, behavioral interventions with lone persons, marital couples, or
with the family system may be particularly useful in instances in which
skill training is needed.

In conclusion, which approach is emphasized and when depends on
the initial and continuing assessment of the problem(s) and the conclusion
("diagnosis") about what must be focused on in order to bring about
change. If it appears that providing information will help the person(s) to

change, for example, efforts may be made to provide such information and to teach the client(s) to change his or her actions. On the other hand, if it seems that the actions of an identified patient or client are resulting from the family structure and processes, the emphasis will be on altering the family system and processes. If the assessment indicates that there are lingering problems with differentiation from one's family of origin, intergenerational family therapy work is indicated. In cases in which there are physical medicine problems, use of medication and collaboration with appropriate medical specialists may be crucial.

GOALS OF THERAPY

Change and Relief from Pain

Change and relief from pain are the eventual foci of most, if not all, forms of therapy. At times the highlight may be on helping the client or client system to accept and adapt to a given situation. Nevertheless, people generally seek change and relief from their pain. The question is, what kind or kinds of change, in which system, or in which parts of the system. How extensive is the change that is sought or obtained? How lasting is the change that is obtained? What are the ways in which change can occur and/or be obtained?

Prochaska and DiClemente (1992), as noted earlier, indicate that there are five distinct but interrelated levels of psychological problems that can be addressed in psychotherapy: symptoms/situational problems, maladaptive cognitions, current interpersonal conflicts, family systems conflicts, and intrapersonal conflicts. These are interrelated in that (1) the symptoms frequently reflect interpersonal conflicts, and maladaptive cognitions often stem from family system rules or beliefs; and (2) change at one level of problem is likely to result in change at another level.

Five basic stages of change (precontemplation, contemplation, preparation, action, and maintenance) are described by Prochaska and DiClemente (1992, pp. 302–307). They also sketch the particular processes of change (consciousness raising, self-liberation, social liberation, counterconditioning, stimulus control, self-reevaluation, environmental reevaluation, contingency management, dramatic relief, and helping relationships) to be emphasized during particular stages of change. They illustrate where what they term the major systems of psychotherapy fit within an integrative framework. With family systems conflicts, for example, strategic therapy is used during the precontemplation stage, Bowen therapy during the contemplation and preparation stages, and structural therapy during the action and maintenance stages (p. 309).

First-Order and Second-Order Change

The concepts of "first-order change" and "second-order change" have become "coin of the realm" in family therapy. Any graduate student in the marital and family therapy field must learn to distinguish between them in order to prepare for academic or licensure examinations. Briefly, they were introduced to the field by Paul Watzlawick and associates (Watzlawick, Weakland, & Fisch, 1974), who drew on two abstract and general theories from the field of mathematical logic, the Theory of Groups and the Theory of Logical Types. The former theory is concerned with change that can occur within a system that remains the same. The theory of logical types provides a framework for regarding shifts between logical levels (e.g., member and class).

Watzlawick and associates pointed out that, following the basic distinction between the two theories, there are two types of change, one of which (first-order) occurs within a given system that itself remains unchanged and one (second-order) whose occurrence changes the system itself. First order change is quantitative, gradual, and continuous and does not exceed the rules of the second. Second-order change is qualitative and abrupt (Breunlin et al., 1992) and always involves a logical jump or discontinuity (Watzlawick et al., 1974).

The notions of discontinuous leaps and Ashby's (1954) "step-functions" have their limitations, as do some other concepts that family therapists have applied to human systems from other fields. Careful observation of the actions and behaviors of participants in family developments at various stages may lead to the conclusion that changes from one stage to another, often referred to as transitions, do not necessarily occur by leaps and in a stepwise manner. The changes that lead from one stage to another may be gradual. The attempt to describe them as leading from one class to another may not be applicable in the reality of human life, whatever the requirements in mathematical logic. Guttman (1991) is correct in the argument that the behavior of inanimate systems is not an appropriate model for use with human systems.

The Complexity of Change

Rather than regarding people somewhat mechanistically as elements in a system to be stimulated by the clever actions of therapists, the time has come to recognize that human beings and human systems are capable of thinking, feeling, and valuing and that they hold the keys to their own change. As Hoffman (1985) has noted, mental phenomena have become central again, returning from their banishment by early family therapists, who were themselves reacting against the excesses of psychoanalytic emphases. Apropos of the swing of the pendulum back to a focus on intrapsychic phenomena is the recognition that human beings do not have to change after the manner of mathematical logic or inanimate systems.

Papp (1983), who has been associated with the use of the directives and paradox brief therapy approach, argues that it is " impossible to assess all the elements that go into effecting change because of the complex, unpredictable qualities of human systems" (p. 215). She appropriately adds that in retrospect it is not possible to know with certainty what did work in therapy, what did not, or whether or not something worked. Papp also notes that on occasion nothing happens during therapy but expected changes occur later, although they may or may not be related to the therapy. All of this is reminiscent of Zuk's (1986) notion that therapeutic intervention is akin to dipping into a stream and that sometimes the act of dipping in diverts the stream. Nevertheless, I consider it important to try to understand what works.

Whose Definition of Change Prevails?

Just as there may be significant differences between the therapist's assessment of the complaint and problem and the client's assessment, so also there may be discrepancies between their conclusions and evaluations regarding what has occurred. Similarly, the client's feelings of satisfaction and/or dissatisfaction with outcomes of sessions and of the course of therapy as a whole also may be at variance with those of the therapist. Papp (1983) defines change in terms of the presenting problem. Has it been either eliminated or substantially modified? If it has not been altered, she defines the therapy as unsuccessful, even though other positive changes have taken place in the family (p. 215).

Does the client system feel the same way? Not necessarily. Client systems do not always define the results of therapy in terms of what has occurred in relation to the presenting complaint. Clients may say at the conclusion that "What we thought was the problem was not the most important thing troubling us. When we explored things, we decided that Johnny's problems with grades were not the problem; our marriage was. Johnny's grades have not changed very much, but things are much better in the family."

ETHICAL ISSUES IN FAMILY THERAPY

Family therapy has raised unique ethical issues since the time it first appeared. Traditionally, ethical issues and the clinician's responsibility were fairly clear for therapists who dealt only with individuals and who had no contact with the families. Treating members of a family, however, immediately brings forth potential conflicts that far exceed the concerns with confidentiality and privilege in traditional individual therapy. Family secrets provide an example of the increased ethical complexity in family therapy. Karpel (1980) describes three types of family secrets: individual (in which one member keeps secrets from other family members), internal (in which at least two members keep secrets from one or more other members), and shared (in which all members are aware of the information but agree to keep it from others outside the family). The needs of individuals and the needs of families can thus be in conflict.

Haley (1976) has declared that experienced therapists who have done therapy for many years know ethical behavior from unethical behavior. This may be an overstatement. There are certainly instances in which the ethical issues are clear. One, for example, is found in gaslighting situations, referred to earlier, in which one spouse is attempting to convince the other that "nothing [wrong] is going on. You're imagining things. You're crazy" when, in fact, the suspicious spouse's concerns are valid (Zemon-Gass & Nichols, 1988). Ethical imperatives compel a responsible therapist to take a stand in such circumstances in order to protect the gaslighted partner. Failure to do so provides at least tacit support for the abusive behavior and stamps the therapist as not being trustworthy. A therapist should not allow one family member to abuse another, emotionally or otherwise.

However, some common ethical dilemmas faced by the family therapist are not so straightforward. These include deciding whether to treat the entire family if a member does not wish to participate, interviewing one family member without the presence of other members, responding to requests for information from family members, manipulating a family for therapeutic reasons, securing informed consent from children, helping to preserve the family, sharing one's values with clients, and informing clients of the values implicit in the mode of therapy being used (Green & Hansen, 1989). The ethical course of action for the therapist is not always clearly marked out by statements and examples in ethical codes or mandated by legal statute.

Therapists continually face practical situations in which they must struggle to a decision without firm guidance as to what is legal, ethical, and appropriate. Sometimes they must reach the best decision that they can on their own. Counseling psychology (Kitchener, 1984) offers a situationally based model for making ethical decisions, a format whose use has been proposed for evaluating clinical decisions in marital and family therapy (Zygmond & Boorhem, 1989).

Kitchener's model distinguishes between two levels of ethical reasoning. The intuitive level consists of a set of ethical beliefs regarding what is right or wrong. The critical–evaluative portion has three different levels: ethical rules, ethical principles, and ethical theory. The levels in the critical–evaluative hierarchy become increasingly more general and abstract. A therapist who is unable to resolve an ethical issue at the lowest level will move up the ladder until, in some instances, the highest and most abstract level, ethical theory, is reached. Here, the theories of universalizability and the balancing principle prevail. The former implies that in order for an act to be ethical, it must be clearly generalizable to all similar cases. The balancing principle holds that when ethical principles are in disagreement, the ethical decision is one that produces the least amount of avoidable harm to all concerned (Zygmond & Boorhem, 1989). This approach attempts to implement the values of the physicians' ancient dictum, "First, do no harm."

Another, more comprehensive approach is suggested by Woody (1990). Her pragmatic model provides five decision bases that therapists can use in an effort to make a comprehensive analysis leading to a defensible decision. These are as follows:

- *Theories of ethics.* These provide a standard for making logical decisions on the basis of principles thought to be universal.
- *Professional codes of ethics.* These are general principles, norms, and rules that should become second nature for the professional. These seem to embody absolute principles and rules for professional conduct, but actually are subject to definition and interpretation.
- *Professional theoretical premises.* Therapies have different assumptions about and definitions of human nature, behavior, pathology, and health, which determine meanings for promoting client welfare.
- *Sociolegal context.* This includes sociocultural values and their evolution; public policy guidelines derived from statutes, regulatory boards, and case law; and the organizational context in which therapy occurs (e.g., prepaid therapy provided by health maintenance organizations; home-based therapy provided by social service agencies; and therapy offered by traditional family counseling agencies, private practitioners, and mental health centers).
- *Personal/professional identity of the therapist.* The therapist as a person makes intuitive and rational choices based on his or her beliefs and from ethical "character."

Concluding that clinical decision making "consists of an unpredictable mix of intuition and rationality," Woody offers the model in an effort to promote increased objectivity, generate sophisticated solutions, and contribute to prevention of some ethical problems.

Major ethical concerns in family therapy today appear to be related to multicultural issues and dual relationships (Peterson, 1992). Dual relationships pose a particularly cloudy picture and have brought forth controversy in the family therapy field over ethical codes. One specific question is whether the American Association for Marriage and Family Therapy attempts to make relationships "simple by legislation" in its ethical code rather than dealing with inevitable complexity (Ryder & Hepworth, 1990, p. 127). Such questions are not likely to be resolved in the near future. Complexity will continue.

5

FAMILY EVALUATION AND TREATMENT

All happy families resemble one another; every unhappy family is
unhappy in its own fashion.
—COUNT LEO TOLSTOY, *Anna Karenina*

Beginning work with clients from a family therapy perspective is both similar to and significantly different from dealing with a single person in an individual therapy approach. Typically, both family therapy and individual therapy approaches involve establishing a workable rapport, listening to the client, observing what transpires, determining the presenting problem or complaint, making some kind of assessment or diagnosis, determining the client's need and readiness for therapy, establishing goals, and formulating a treatment plan. Family therapy must go beyond those tasks, however, in that it involves not merely work with an individual but in addition the more complex tasks of multilevel evaluation and treatment planning.

THE INITIAL CONTACT WITH CLIENTS

Making some kind of effective connection with the client system is, of course, necessary in order to carry out the tasks of assessment, diagnosis, and therapy. The therapist must be able to establish not only a relationship with the client system that will permit him or her to gain information for an accurate assessment, but also an association that will enlist the client system in the pursuit of desired and necessary changes.

Family therapists have used a variety of terms to refer to the working relationship between the therapist and the family. Ackerman (1966) indicated that the therapist must establish a useful rapport; Minuchin (1974) described "joining" the family; Sluzki (1975) referred to the task of tracking and managing the "coalitionary process"; Napier (1976) called this the "engagement" phase; M. A. Solomon (1977) referred to "engaging families"; and Davatz (1981) wrote that the therapist's task is to "connect" with the family system (Pinsof & Catherall, 1986).

Joining

Probably the most widely used term in family therapy to describe the process of the therapist's beginning work with a family, marital couple, or family subsystem has been "joining." Minuchin (1974) describes joining as experiencing the reality of the family as the family member experiences it and becoming involved in the family's repeated interactions. Joining the family and becoming involved in its repeated interactions is somewhat different from the goals of those individual therapists who are concerned with remaining outside the individual client's actions in real life and assisting the client to join them in a "two-group" in pursuing change. Minuchin's intent is to form a partnership between two systems—the therapy system and the family system—with the goals of freeing the symptom bearer of symptoms, reducing conflict and stress in the family, and improving coping for the family (Minuchin & Fishman, 1981). He also refers to the accommodations, the changes and adaptations, that the therapist has to make in order to join the family.

Whether it is necessary or possible for most therapists to join a family in the sense in which Minuchin describes the process, (i.e., so that one feels "a family member's pain at being excluded or scapegoated, and his pleasure at being loved, depended on, or otherwise confirmed with the family" [Minuchin, 1974, p. 123]) is open to question. As frequently interpreted, this may represent an idealized version of what occurs and may be an overstatement of what is required in order to work effectively with a family. More modestly, the therapist needs to recognize that at best he or she may be "in the family" in terms of having an influential relationship with it but not "of the family" in terms of feeling so closely what the clients feel.

The family therapist may affect families in many of the same ways that live-in anthropologists impinge on the lives of families they study as participant observers. However, the family therapist and the anthropologist remain outsiders whose understanding is shaped by the personal and professional lenses they bring to the arena of interaction. These lenses include, of course, not only idiosyncratic aspects of the therapist but also significant issues of cultural diversity, which are only now beginning to be recognized as crucial factors in therapy.

Joining appears to be close to what Pinsof and Catherall (1986) mean when they refer to the therapist's relationship with the client system. They define this relationship with the client system broadly as encompassing all of the feelings, thoughts, and response predispositions that exist between the therapist and client systems.

The Therapeutic Alliance

As useful as the joining construct is, there is another term that is preferable for describing the working connections between the therapist and the family system. This is the "therapeutic alliance" construct, which has a long history and respected place in individual psychotherapy and which is readily adaptable to family therapy. Beginning in the early 1980s, Gurman (1982) and others began developing an explicit clinical theory about the place of therapeutic alliance in marital therapy (Pinsof & Catherall, 1986).

The concept of therapeutic alliance does not suggest that the therapist become part of the family, joining clients on their ground, from which position he or she can orchestrate change. Rather, formation of a therapeutic alliance implies that the family system comes into the therapist's world and the two systems interdependently construct the basis of trust and cooperation necessary for working together in an effort to achieve desired change. Specifically, the therapeutic alliance is "that aspect of the relationship between the therapist system [all of the people involved in administering treatment] and the patient system that pertains to their capacity to mutually invest in, and collaborate on, the therapy" (Pinsof & Catherall, 1986, p. 140).

Some writers have adapted the therapeutic alliance to family therapy by indicating that the therapist's task is to connect with the family system rather than simply with the individual patient, as in individual therapy. From the perspective of Bowen theory, the development of a therapeutic alliance with a single member of the family can be facilitated by placing that person within the context of his or her emotional system, increasing the individual's learning process, and rendering emotional concepts into interactional patterns (Davatz, 1981). If this is interpreted as connecting essentially with the family system as such, the idea seems too restrictive.

Instead, within the broader therapist–client relationship, it is necessary to form multiple workable therapeutic alliances—with the entire family system, with subsystems, and with individual members of the family.

Practically speaking, one needs to make personal contact with every family member and with the entire family system. This can be done in the first session if the entire family is present. In such sessions, as Napier notes (1976), the therapist tries to hear the view of every family member, including young children, by paying close attention. Children who are preverbal should be acknowledged in some fashion. Making contact with family members also can be done in stages. John Bell (1975) has described a pattern, for example, in which he meets first with the parents. He then meets with the entire family for what he terms "the child-centered phase" of family therapy. Making the session a safe place for the children to talk and encouraging them to express their concerns help the therapist to make a connection with them.

A typical way of opening in a phased approach such as Bell uses might be as follows. After introductions and brief getting-acquainted interchanges with the new members (children), the therapist may say something to the children along the following lines:

> "As you know, I met with your parents a few days ago. They are concerned with the fact that there is some unhappiness at your home. We have arranged for all of us to work together to try to make things better for everybody in the family. It's very important to know how you feel about things at your house: what you feel is wrong, what needs to be changed, what you like about the way things are. I have heard your parents. Now, I'm asking them to do something that is sometimes hard for adults to do—to be quiet and listen. We have a rule here that everybody speaks for themselves and nobody interrupts. So, they won't speak for you and you won't speak for them. They have agreed with me that it is important for all of you to try to hear and understand how the others feel."

The therapist then invites the children to speak and answers any questions they have. By the time they have been accorded a respectful and attentive audience, most children have, albeit grudgingly in some instances, started to enter into a working alliance with the therapist. Some children need help and permission from their parents before taking this step.

What, then, is the therapeutic alliance as the term is used in this book? Of course, it is a particular kind of partnership between the therapist and the client system (family, marital, and individual). But what kind of partnership? I find Bordin's (1979) operational definition in individual psychotherapy a useful way of thinking about what is needed between the family therapist and the client system. Bordin broke the alliance down into tasks, goals, and bonds. The bonds between therapist and client refer to the quality of the human relationship between them. From the side of the clients, it includes the feeling of being accepted and cared about by the therapist and the ability to permit the therapist to become an important figure in their psychological lives. The task aspect refers to the extent to which the approach and techniques of therapy fit with the clients' perceptions of their problems and complement their desire to change. Therapist and client share goals in the therapeutic alliance to the extent that they agree on what the goals are and concur that they will work toward accomplishing those goals.

It is difficult to overestimate the significance of the working partnership gained between therapist and client. A review of the psychotherapy research literature of the 1980s discloses that the therapeutic alliance is a key client–therapist factor in determining the outcome of therapy. Specifically, the quality of the client's participation in this tie with the therapist has the greatest effect of any variable considered on outcome. Therapists in the good-outcome category demonstrate high levels of helping, protecting, affirming, and understanding; and low levels of blaming and belittling behavior. The implication is that good-outcome therapists recognize early on the conflicts clients have with the therapist and explore those problems with clients (Marziali & Alexander, 1991). In brief, clients wish to be assured not only that the clinician is knowledgeable, competent, capable— an expert—but also that he or she is a person to whom they can relate with some degree of ease and intimacy (Parloff, 1986).

The therapeutic alliance is in a state of periodic alteration as treatment progresses. Rather than being set once and for all time, it has qualities of both stability and change, remaining constant so long as the trust prevails between therapist and client and altering as the various aspects and dynamics of the therapy process change.

The Client's Initial Anxiety and Uncertainty

Interwoven with the process of establishing an initial relationship is the task of bringing the client's initial anxiety and uncertainty under control. There is no reason why a family, couple, or individual coming to see a therapist should not be anxious. On the contrary, there are a variety of understandable reasons why taking one's problems and pain to the office of an outsider, who is generally a stranger, should create uncertainty, raise questions, and elicit specific fears.

Resistance in psychotherapy originally was conceived as an individual's reluctance to gain insight, and the concept was used with regard to the actions of a client in objecting to a particular interpretation by a psychoanalyst. Recently, resistance has become associated more with resisting change, whether behavioral or cognitive in nature (Wilkinson, 1993).

The family's "struggle over treatment" has been accurately described as "basically anxiety concerning change" (Napier, 1976, p. 3). The family wrestles with the question, "Do we dare expose our family to this stranger?" In their anxiety and lack of trust in the therapist/stranger, family members challenge the therapist, usually with indirect questions, about approach, procedure, or structure of the therapy. Napier suggests that the therapist work toward and look for a point somewhere in the first to third interview in which he or she senses a kind of subjective relief on the part of the family. That relief is a signal that the struggle is at an end and that the family has decided to be "in therapy" (p. 10).

Initial resistance from the family often stems most strongly from a reluctance to give up focusing on an identified individual as the problem source and to delineate the family as the unit of assessment and treatment (Anderson & Stewart, 1983; Napier, 1976). Furthermore, therapists may find themselves continually striving to keep the family focused on acknowledging that the problems that brought them in are family issues. Parents, for example, who originally wished to drop off their "problem child" at the therapist's door in order to get him or her "fixed" may continue to struggle with the notion that they need to be involved in change. Even those who were somewhat open to wider exploration early in the assessment process may revert, periodically and with heroic persistence, to trying to pin the problem on a single member of the family or on an external system such as the school.

Anderson and Stewart (1983) have made a number of suggestions for overcoming family resistance: (1) The therapist persuades families to accept therapy at the outset by demonstrating competence, understanding, and an ability to be helpful; (2) establishes a contract based on mutual and attainable goals; and (3) the client responds effectively to the therapist's competence. They describe a number of specific interventions that the therapist can make to respond to resistances during the ongoing course of therapy.

DIAGNOSIS AND ASSESSMENT

Family therapists traditionally were reluctant to use standard diagnostic terminology and, in some cases, even to do formal assessment. This was true for a variety of historical reasons. Rejection of the "medical model"; a focus on systems rather than individuals; and the action orientation of the early family therapists, especially those using a structural orientation, contributed to a general disregard for and neglect of the entire assessment process (Karpel & Strauss, 1983). Much of the structural orientation and focusing on systems to the neglect of the individual occurred in the California portion of the early family therapy movement in the 1950s and early 1960s. Links between Don D. Jackson's orientation and Harry Stack Sullivan's interpersonal view of personality were noted in Chapter 1. This attitude toward assessment is changing, particularly in view of the requirement for the diagnostic labeling and increased attention to treatment planning necessary to qualify for third party reimbursement.

Some distinctions need to be made at this point between diagnosis and assessment. Although they are related, they are not the same. Diagnosis is the more narrow and restricted of the two terms.

Diagnosis

"Diagnosis" comes from two Greek words: *dia*, which means between, and *gnosis*, which refers to knowledge or knowing. Literally, diagnosis has to do with "knowing between" or "distinguishing between" and implies that one classifies situations or conditions into types. Essentially, diagnosis is an individual concept and one related to an individual's disease or disorder.

Using individual diagnostic labels sometimes is necessary in today's family therapy environment. The widespread use of DSM-IV (American Psychiatric Association, 1994) and the *International Classification of Diseases* (ICD-9-CM; World Health Organization, 1979), both of which classify disorders solely in individual terms, requires that family therapists understand individual diagnosis in order to communicate with other professionals. Family therapists who work in medically oriented settings that use such classification systems have no choice about the use of individual diagnostic labels. They must be able to affix a standard diagnostic label on an identified patient or client. Clinicians of various persuasions and orientations who sign managed care contracts similarly have no choice but to use the DSM and ICD nomenclature.

Although historically associated with disease, physical medicine, and the treatment of individuals, the concept of diagnosis has been loosely adapted for use in other fields. In organizational study, for example, reference is sometimes made to organizational diagnosis. Similarly, the term "family diagnosis" is often used. This is an imprecise use of terminology and something of a misnomer. Reference to diagnosis in family therapy has been made by de Shazer (1982) in a broad sense as a special way of knowing that involves diagnosing, researching, and doing therapy.

Despite the fact that there have been some diligent efforts to classify families and their problems (L. Fisher, 1977; Kinney, Ravich, Ford, & Vos, 1987), no accepted nomenclature or nosology for classifying family disorders exists.

Although it may be hard to do so successfully, it seems sensible to try to restrict the use of the term "diagnosis" to the classification of individuals and their manifestations of problems and difficulties into psychological nosological categories. The term "assessment" may be used to refer to families.

Assessment

Assessment has to do with estimating or determining significance, importance, or value, rather than classification into categories of disease. Lacking as it does the specific rootage in the evaluation of the functioning of a lone individual that is associated with diagnosis, assessment is more applicable to systems. Hence, the concept of "clinical assessment" is used here primarily when the reference is to the family system and its subsystems, processes, and functioning.

Assessment includes what the persons affected believe should be done. This parallels individual psychotherapy in which the client's subjective reports determine in large measure when treatment will begin and end (Parloff, 1986). A formulation of the problem that also includes contextual circumstances "is a far more appropriate starting point for treatment" (Wynne, 1983, p. 252) than the symptom diagnosis approach provided by Axes I and II of the DSM.

Assessment is an ongoing process. One does not make an initial assessment of the problems, strengths, needs, and potentialities of a family and then forget about assessment from that time forward. Rather, assessment is something that is done continually, as the therapist works with the family. Assessment is undertaken for the purpose of understanding the problems of the family and of making suitable interventions both at the onset of one's contact with them and subsequently.

What Do We Assess?

The therapist who takes an integrative approach carries a heavy burden in the assessment—as well as in the treatment—process. He or she must comprehend a wide range of individual, marital, and family dynamics. Broadly speaking, individual (intrapsychic) and interpersonal (system) factors, along with the sociocultural context in which the systems function, typically comprise the most salient levels for assessment. These require attention to individual life cycles, to the marital life cycle, and to the family life cycle, and to interaction between the therapist and family.

The individual and interpersonal systems function in interaction and in patterns of mutual influence. "Ignoring or minimizing either level leads to an incomplete, and therefore potentially inaccurate, understanding of individual, couple, or family dysfunction" (Feldman, 1985, p. 358). The matters assessed include issues found in routine, relatively straightforward cases; they also include complicated collusive systems in which splitting and projective identification produce ongoing and additional collusion, rejection, and conflict, or excessive reactivity (Lansky, 1985).

Multilevel assessment can be described even more extensively as covering the individual level, the (family) system level, the system–therapist level, and, if necessary, the tissue/organ system level (biological/biochemical status) of the individual (Beavers & Hampson, 1990). Where indicated, the context in which the family functions (Feldman, 1985) also may be included.

With regard to assessing families, the clinician has some choice points in addition to those already mentioned. According to Reiss (1980), the therapist may choose to focus on developmental versus cross-sectional issues (longitudinal or current family functioning), family direction versus environmental direction (the impact of the broader network of relationships on internal patterns in the family or on the shaping forces inside the family), crisis versus character (immediate difficulties or the family's enduring patterns of defense and adaptation), pathology versus competence (disorder or the family's competence), and thematic versus behavioral (the underlying experience and motives or the surface phenomena).

Assessment as interpreted here involves emphasizing and giving attention to pathology and competence, to problems and strengths, and difficulties and coping competencies. Choices can be made on other points in light of the particulars of the problem brought in by the client system.

How Do We Assess?

In the broadest terms, two approaches to assessment prevail: a standardized approach and a tailored approach. The standardized approach involves taking the path of systematically assessing all families or couples in the same manner (e.g., following structured interview guides, using formal assessment devices, and covering the same points with all families). Tailoring the assessment to each family means that one covers those issues that appear to be most significant on the basis of what has been initially presented. The course taken by the clinician depends on a variety of factors, including the following:

• *The orientation, abilities, and purposes of the clinician.* Some clinicians prefer to move directly into interaction with the client, making interventions from the first few minutes of the initial interview. Their assessment proceeds concurrently with the interventions into the processes of the client system. If they are concerned with securing change immediately, they may have some degree of impatience with obtaining information from areas that are not directly affected and that do not appear to be essential to effecting change.

Many experienced clinicians who are comfortable with their ability to reach valid judgments on the basis of a quick reading and synthesis of salient information from a few prominent keys will not consider it necessary to map the entire family landscape before proceeding with treatment. Clinicians who are more interested in measurement, adherence to a treatment manual method, and such factors as demonstration of treatment efficacy and outcome research will be more concerned with treating each client system in a standardized way and "mapping the territory" rather thoroughly at the outset.

• *The setting in which the evaluation occurs.* Assessment conducted in research or training centers in which there is attention to teaching students about family assessment in a standard, comprehensive fashion, and in clinics in which there is a concern with adhering to a treatment manual approach will more likely be more extensive and standardized than assessment done in independent practice locations.

• *The presenting problem(s) of the client system, including the nature and severity of the problems.* If the family is in a crisis when it contacts the clinician, practical concerns may dictate the assessment and intervention stance that one takes. The need to get the situation under control may call for intervention first—on the basis of generally accepted crisis intervention strategies—with a more complete assessment conducted later. If the family indicates that there is no crisis but that it is coming in because of chronic conditions, assessment may get attention first. It is sometimes possible in such situations to forego crisis intervention because one may be able rely to some degree on lower anxiety on the part of the family due to familiarity with the condition that prevails as opposed to the situation when a condition is strange and novel.

The practical approach that I advocate as a working clinician dealing with families, couples, and individuals from the community on an outpatient basis involves tailoring the assessment process to the clientele and to their presenting complaints or problems. It is also an approach in which assessment and therapy occur concurrently. There is no separate assessment procedure in which tests are given, except in exceedingly rare circumstances in which their use clearly has clinical relevance, such as the need to ascertain the current intellectual functioning of one of the clients.

If a choice has to be made between client needs and research interests in a session, the needs of the client get the nod without hesitation. Our commitment to furthering knowledge is not what we are being paid for by clients. They have the right to expect that we be committed first and foremost to helping them deal with their problems and to accomplishing the goals we mutually establish for their benefit.

(Different priorities may prevail in training settings in which the clinician is a supervisor. With the clients informed that their therapist is a trainee, the supervisor has the primary task of helping the supervisee learn how to help the clients deal with their problems and accomplish the goals the supervisee has mutually established with them for their benefit. Although I as a supervisor am ethically committed to protecting the clients, I also have the responsibility of maintaining the integrity of the learning–teaching process in which my primary task is to supervise a learning therapist, not to treat the clients through the supervisee.)

METHODS OF ASSESSMENT

Data gathering in family assessment involves three broad approaches: interviewing, observing, and using formal assessment instruments. In some instances, one also gathers reports from outside sources such as schools and physicians.

Interviews

The interview remains the most widely used method of clinical assessment. This is probably the case because it gives the clinician opportunity to observe client behavior as well as to learn about family members' subjective views and beliefs (Wilkinson, 1993). Unlike methods in which families are assigned tasks or clients complete questionnaires, interviews provide both the clinician and the client system the opportunity to interact directly and to get "a flavor of each other" so as to begin forming a therapeutic alliance from the outset.

Individual and Conjoint Sessions

Interviews with individuals are used routinely by some clinicians as part of the assessment process and not at all, or very seldom, by others. The chief advantage of individual interviews, according to Feldman (1985), is that they are useful for obtaining information that may not be readily available in conjoint sessions. They may allow for detailed searching of an individual's significant feelings, thoughts, and behaviors that he or she would not disclose or discuss in a conjoint interview. These may include an affair, homosexual behavior, plans to divorce the spouse, family violence, and other issues. Awareness of such feelings, thoughts, and behaviors permits their use by the clinician in developing a comprehensive treatment plan.

The major drawbacks to using individual interviews are, first, that they do not permit the clinician to observe family or couple interactions in relation to issues described by the individual. This limits the clinician's ability to assess such interactions and to obtain consensual validation of the issues from other family members. Second, they may create practical and ethical dilemmas. For example, a client may disclose in an individual session information that is not known to other family members, but which the clinician believes must be shared with them in order for therapy to proceed effectively. This second factor makes it essential for the clinician to enunciate clear and explicit guidelines regarding confidentiality early in therapy (Feldman, 1985).

Genograms/Family Maps

A genogram or "family map" (Minuchin, 1974) is used routinely by some clinicians. Skillful employment of the genogram can provide important suggestions and hypotheses for further study of a family system. McGoldrick and Gerson (1985) provide an extensive and helpful treatment of genograms and their use in family assessment.

It is possible to get much of the data required to construct a partial genogram by having clients complete a background information form of the type that I have used for nearly 30 years (see Figure 5.1). Clients are requested to arrive 10–15 minutes prior to the scheduled first appointment so that they can complete the form before the session. They are advised that completion of the form will save time in the session. The data provided on the form and the ways the form is completed typically provide guidance regarding questions that need to be asked and leads that should be followed by the clinician (see Nichols, 1988).

Kinds of Questioning

Tailored assessment in family therapy follows the same path as in other forms of therapy in terms of the kinds of questions and other requests for

**BACKGROUND INFORMATION
FORM**

Date _____

Name _____ Home Telephone _____

Home Address _____
(CITY AND ZIP CODE)

Business Address _____ Business Telephone _____

Height _____ Weight _____ Date and Place of Birth _____

Education _____

Occupation _____ Annual Income _____

Religious Affiliation _____ Childhood Religious Affiliation _____

Military Service (Date and Branch) _____

Name of Person Who Referred You _____

Previous Counseling or Psychotherapy (Dates and Names of Therapists)

_____

_____

_____

MEDICAL

Name of Physician _____ Last Medical Examination _____

What Medical Problems or Illness Do You Have? _____

_____

What Medication Are You Taking? _____

MARITAL

Mate's Age _____ Education _____ Religion _____

Mate's Occupation _____ Date Married _____

Children _____ Name _____ Sex _____ Age _____

_____ Sex _____ Age _____

_____ Sex _____ Age _____

_____ Sex _____ Age _____

_____ Sex _____ Age _____

-over-

FIGURE 5.1. Background information form.

Have There Been Previous Marriages? If So, Was Marriage Ended by Death or Divorce?_____

Were There Children by Previous Marriages? _____ Number_____ Sex_____ Age_____

PARENTS AND SIBLINGS

Brothers and Sisters (Include Any Deceased)

Age	Sex	Education	Marital Status	Occupation
____	____	_____	_____	_____
____	____	_____	_____	_____
____	____	_____	_____	_____
____	____	_____	_____	_____
____	____	_____	_____	_____
____	____	_____	_____	_____
____	____	_____	_____	_____

Father   Birthplace_____   Education_____

Occupation_____   Religion _____

Present Age_____   If Deceased, When_____

Mother   Birthplace_____   Education_____

Occupation _____   Religion _____

Present Age _____   If Deceased, When_____

Was Either Parent Married More Than Once? Please Give Details_____

_____

_____

_____

information used by the clinician. One asks general or "projective" questions, such as "What brings you in?" "What are you looking for from therapy?" The client is free, and indeed encouraged, to answer in whatever terms desired. From that starting point, one can begin to focus more specifically on pertinent areas.

"Focused" questions are an intermediate form of asking for information. They lie between the general, projective questions and highly specific requests for information. For example, the therapist may use the following, or similar, requests for background information. "Tell me about your family." "Tell me about yourself." "What is your communication like?" "How has your marriage changed over the years?"

Specific questions are similar to questions posed in many of the standardized approaches to family assessment and individual diagnosis. Specific information is requested. Some questions can be answered in "yes" or "no" terms or quantified (e.g., "Six years." "Grade 10." "Age 15.").

The clinician who is seeking to fit the assessment to the client system in a tailored fashion seeks treatment relevant information as quickly as possible. In this kind of parsimonious approach, one typically moves back and forth between general questions, focused questions, and specific questions. Once an area has emerged as pertinent, either through the verbal and other contributions of the clients or by obvious omission, the clinician is in a posture to pursue information through focused or specific questions. Similarly, once an area has become a matter of interest, one can ask general questions, fishing for the meaning it has to the client.

Observation

All clinicians, except perhaps the most inexperienced beginners, typically glean a considerable amount of information from informally observing their clients when they come in for interviews. Inferences can be made from observations of how the clients respond to this new and generally alien situation. How do they arrange themselves in seating, in the reception room and in the clinician's office? What kinds of facial expressions are seen? What kinds of gestures occur? How do they address, or ignore, each other? What kind of atmosphere exists among them? General tension? Hostility? Hopelessness? Apathy? Confidence tinged with anxiety? Who takes the initiative in talking? Who appears to be in charge? Do they strike the observer as a fairly cooperative unit or essentially as unrelated or barely connected individuals? In some instances the ambiance is so ponderous that it feels as if "it couldn't be cut with a sharp machete." At other times, there may be obvious anxiety but an overall mood that contains hope and some degree of openness to the occasion.

Although videotaping a session permits the clinician to observe the family's interactions and behaviors subsequently, either with or without the family being present at the viewing, the use of this technique is not recommended during the initial assessment phase. Although the family's permission to record the opening session(s) frequently can be secured, the price that it extracts in trust does not appear to match the gain from using the procedure. All forms of recording can be assumed to introduce a distracting and artificial element into the clinical session. This element probably can be better tolerated later in the course of therapy, after trust has been established between the family and the therapist.

Structured situations can be established for the observation of families. Two examples that can be used as part of either the original assessment or the ongoing assessment are observation of the family in a problem-solving process (Feldman, 1985) and family enactment (Minuchin & Fishman, 1981). Both approaches essentially involve structuring a situation in which the members deal with issues (e.g., problems the family has previously identified) in the presence of the therapist, who is then able to observe their transactions and to discern functional and dysfunctional patterns as the members attempt to work out mutually acceptable solutions.

A family, for example, may be instructed to decide how to deal with the question of setting hours for an adolescent member and proceed with the task. The therapist can intervene as necessary and can also make additional observations regarding how the family functions and how its members deal with the problems. The interventions may include not only instructions to make changes, to do something different, but also may involve positive, encouraging comments. The therapist may state, for instance, "You made a start before you came in, when all of you got together over the weekend and made a list of things that you want to see changed in the family. You came in with some successful experience in cooperation."

Formal Assessment Devices: Rating Scales

There are many formal assessment devices available that can be used for various purposes with families and couples, (see, e.g., Touliatos, Perlmutter, & Straus, 1990; L'Abate & Bagarozzi, 1993). Family rating scales can be helpful in furnishing a general understanding of current family functioning by assessing various dimensions of family life such as problem solving, communication, and so forth. These dimensional approaches also have the advantage "that in principle *all* families can be assessed on these dimensions" (Wynne, 1988, p. 102). Unfortunately, as Wynne (1988) notes with regret, they do not assess the presenting problem(s) for which the family seeks help.

Two of these rating scales that are clinically based and have demonstrated clinical usefulness are the Family Assessment Device (FAD), which was developed by a team at McMaster University, and the Beavers Family Systems Model, developed by W. Robert Beavers (Beavers & Hampson, 1990). The FAD is completed by families. A companion scale, the McMaster Clinical Rating Scale, designed to be completed by a trained rater after an interview with a family, is in the research stage and reportedly has been found to correlate significantly with the FAD (I. W. Miller et al., 1994). Although both the FAD and the Beavers model have shortcomings and have been criticized as being unlikely to provide anything other than crude distinctions (Wilkinson, 1993), some therapists and researchers consider them the most complete approaches to family assessment available (I. W. Miller et al., 1994; Beavers & Hampson, 1990).

Family Assessment Device

The FAD is designed to be a screening instrument only. It is used to collect information on the various dimensions of the family system as a whole— problem solving, communication, roles, affective responsiveness, affective involvement, behavior control, and general functioning. A paper and pencil questionnaire for use with family members over age 12, the FAD is based on the idea that the family's functioning depends more on the transactional and systemic properties of the family system than on intrapsychic characteristics of individual family members (Westley & Epstein, 1969). The underlying McMaster Model of Family Functioning is said to describe family structural and organizational properties and patterns of family transactions that distinguish between healthy and unhealthy families (Epstein, Baldwin, & Bishop, 1983).

The FAD's chief use for most clinicians, therefore, may be to provide a description of various aspects of family functioning from the perspective of family members. Rather than gleaning information about the presenting problem(s), the clinician can develop, from those descriptions, guidelines regarding therapeutic focus and interventions in general family functioning. If the FAD results show, for example, that there are similar magnitude problems with both communication and family roles, it becomes a matter of clinical judgment, of course, whether to intervene first in one of those areas or to tackle them simultaneously.

Beavers Family Systems Model

Attempts to relate individual diagnostic categories and disorders to families and family process have not been particularly successful or significant, although some rudiments exist for continuing and refining such work. One recent attempt, noted earlier, is that of Slipp (1988), who has provided an object relations-based typology in which specific family transactional patterns are related to specific forms of psychopathology in a family member. The Beavers model provides some additional assistance in the effort to link family patterns with individual pathology or problematic behaviors and symptomatology. Certain family types in the Beavers family assessment schema frequently produce offspring with particular kinds of symptomatology.

Beavers (Beavers & Hampson, 1990, p. 47) places families along a health/competence dimension (horizontal). The scale includes Severely Dysfunctional, Borderline, Midrange, Adequate, and Optimal. Adequate and Optimal are both deemed Healthy families. Families also are described in terms of a stylistic dimension (vertical), ranging from Centripetal families (which have virtually impenetrable outer boundaries and little room for individuality) to Centrifugal families (which have weak outer boundaries and little internal cohesiveness). Between those two styles are Mixed families (which combine a mixture of centripetal and centrifugal forces). From this schema Beavers describes nine groupings that are clinically useful, six of which frequently produce offspring with clinical problems. As adapted, those that often produce such offspring are as depicted in Table 5.1. Beavers notes that optimal, adequate, and midrange centrifugal families are seldom seen in therapy.

Beavers's (Beavers & Hampson, 1990) provision of clear descriptions of the pertinent family types can enable an experienced clinician to make a quick assessment and placement of a family into the appropriate category even without using formal rating scales.

TABLE 5.1. Selected Family Types and Problems (Beavers Family Systems Model)

Family type	Problems often found in offspring
Midrange Centrifugal	Behavior disorders
Midrange Centripetal	Neurotic
Borderline Centrifugal	Borderline
Borderline Centripetal	Severely obsessive
Severely Dysfunctional Centrifugal	Sociopathic
Severely Dysfunctional Centripetal	Schizophrenic

Combining Elements in Assessment

Whatever is gained from observation of the family is mixed with what one gains from questions and discussion of topics to form the basis for evaluation. Combining information from several different perspectives increases the likelihood of gaining a more complete picture of the client system. Beavers emphasizes, for instance, that assessment often includes the integration of materials from family "insiders" and observing "outsiders" (Beavers & Hampson, 1990, p. 7).

It is important to assess with both family and individual approaches. This is the case even when the clinician uses standardized tests to assess family functioning. For example, using the FAD, Sawyer and colleagues (Sawyer, Baghurst, Cross, & Kalucy, 1988) found adolescents in both clinical and nonclinical families rating their families as significantly less healthy than their parents rated them. Those results emphasize the need to consider separately reports on family functioning obtained from different members of the same family.

Others would argue that it is necessary to return to assessing individual and dyadic characteristics, instead of total family functioning (L'Abate & Bagarozzi, 1993). This perspective certainly has validity and is quite consistent with an integrative approach.

How Does Individual Diagnosis Relate to the Family?

The diagnostic and statistical manuals regard symptoms as stemming from inside individuals, whereas family therapy views them as coming from processes arising within family systems and other systems. Both approaches have their limitations, as noted above. Fortunately, as Denton (1990) observes, the rigidly held assumption that individual symptoms always serve family functions is beginning to be questioned by some family therapists (e.g., Goldner, 1985; James & McIntyre, 1983; and others), who indicate that family systems should be viewed within broader social contexts. Greater care needs to be given to comprehending how familial and nonfamilial systems are related. It is also true that attention needs to be given to biological, temperament, and personal factors. Treatment does not have to be, nor should it be, restricted to a single level of functioning, as Wynne (1988) has emphasized.

It is important to look for and to understand ways in which symptoms and complaints fit with both family and marital, as well as individual, development and how they fit with interaction of developmental cycles. For example, one looks at the current family life of the child for comprehension of how it helps to create and maintain problems in the child. Beavers's model (see Table 5.1) provides some guidance in this pursuit.

Similarly, how does the adult's current family life help to maintain problems and symptoms? How does the family of origin create and help to maintain problems in adults?

Parenthetically, dropping the widely used term "identified patient" (IP) has been proposed by Wynne (1988). Wynne's idea is that "identified patient" is an ambiguous and outdated carryover from the earlier concept of family scapegoat. Sometimes it is taken as indicating that therapists are insensitive and demeaning in their attitudes toward clients. He would use "patient" when a family member has been formally diagnosed by a professional, "index patient" for record-keeping purposes, or "problem person" when a family member is perceived by other family members as having a presenting problem. The "problem person" may or may not have been formally diagnosed by a professional as a patient. Presumably, the careful approach advocated by Wynne would help to avoid casual and premature labeling of individuals, and convey more respectful and sensitive attitudes toward families, thus keeping the way open for more appropriate assessment.

THE PRESENTING PROBLEM(S)

How a family initially views the problems that they bring in can be classified in several different ways. Wynne (1988) notes that some families present with relational problems or with a problem person. The individual deemed the problem person by the family can be carrying a psychiatric or medical diagnosis or manifesting undiagnosed distress or problematic behavior (Wynne, 1988, p. 105)

The clinician starts with the presenting complaint—for example, a child at school—and examines this in terms of developments in the life cycles and family system. What tasks are the child and other family members facing in their life cycles? What is impinging on the person's life? For example, is the child's life affected by marital separation, death of a family member or friend, or other occurrences or processes?

The term "complaint" is used here deliberately in order to reflect the fact that what is presented at the outset as the family's problem(s) frequently is not what turns out to be the problem(s) that becomes the focus of therapy.

Conjoint Family or Marital Interview

One typically asks each family member, in turn, what they see as the problem(s). In the process, the clinician secures information about each family member's observations, thoughts, and feelings about the presenting complaint (Falloon, 1988).

Once the presenting complaint(s) has been stated and agreed to by the family members, the way is clear to understand the origin of the complaint(s).

Problem History

The next step is to trace the course of the family's or couple's history, determining what things were like before the development of the problem(s) and how things have been changed by the presence of the problem(s).

Events Associated with Problem Development

What has been the progress of the problem process? What events have been associated with the development of the complaints? These may include transitions in the life cycles of the family, such as births, deaths, moves, and illnesses.

Problem-Solving Abilities of Client

Attempts at solution are an early focus of attention by the clinician. "How have you tried to deal with the problems?" "What have you tried?" "What were the outcomes?" Possible answers to some of these questions can be anticipated in part from information provided by clients on the background information form (Figure 5.1). For example, has there been any previous therapy? Is medication being used? What other attempts have been made at solution?

Feldman has aptly observed that the clinician can use the presenting complaint as a starting point for analyzing how the family functions as a unit (Feldman, 1985). Wynne also underscores the value to the clinician of an assessment of the family or marital system's "ability to cope as a relational system" (Wynne, 1988, p. 93).

Feldman (1985) refers to problem stimuli and problem reinforcers. Problem stimuli are interpersonal (behavioral) and intrapsychic (cognitive, emotional) events that lead to appearances or exacerbations of symptoms or dysfunctional family interactions. Problem reinforcers are interpersonal or intrapsychic consequences of symptoms or dysfunctional family interactions that have the effect of maintaining or increasing the probability that such symptoms will recur. In true systemic fashion, he sees problem stimuli and problem reinforcers as combining to establish and maintain a problem-maintaining loop.

Positive Elements

If information is not provided by the clients on strengths, one asks such questions as the following: "Have things always been like this, or was there a time in which things went pretty well and you felt good about the relationship?" "What was it like in the early stages?" or "What was it like then, when things were going well?"

This approach provides data for delineating any positive elements of the family, couple, or individuals that currently are evident, and any positive elements that have disappeared or have been overwhelmed by the problem(s). Feldman (1985) notes that in addition to providing useful information, exploring positive aspects of the family or couple's history "contributes to the creation of a positive, change-promoting therapeutic climate" (p. 361). If information on current positive functioning is not volunteered or otherwise derived from the exploration, the therapist specifically asks about current coping and satisfactions. "How are things going now? Tell me about what is going right."

FEEDBACK TO CLIENTS

Feedback to the clients is an important element for both the clients and the therapist, in my opinion. It helps the clients to understand how the therapist is perceiving their difficulties and to correct what they perceive as omissions or errors in those perceptions. It also helps the therapist to judge how the clients comprehend what he or she communicates to them and to form an estimate of their ability to enter into therapy cooperatively.

A golden rule of successful assessment and therapy is "a continuous negotiation with the client/s about the aims and ongoing process of therapy" (Wilkinson, 1993, p. 228). Wilkinson (1993) uses the term "customerhood" to refer to motivation for change on the part of the client. He also emphasizes the importance of focusing on using the family members' views in selecting and discarding options from among those available in therapy.

Behavior therapists consider the family members a vital resource in their problem-centered treatment approaches (Falloon, 1988). Although the choice of a response to problems will be affected by many factors, the assumption is that the client will choose the perceived "best" option under the circumstances (Falloon, 1988, p. 102)

Feedback, therefore, is a two-way process. The clinician asks the family members for their reactions to the interview(s) and explores with them how well he or she has understood what they presented during the session(s). Additionally, the clinician shares with the clients his or her impressions of their problems and strengths.

Feedback on particular issues may begin fairly early in the session. This depends on what is being conveyed by the clients and on the therapist's impressions regarding how important it is to secure clarification at that point.

Finally, near the end of the session, the clinician shares with the family his or her recommendations regarding treatment. All of this is part of the entry into the goal-setting phase of the clinical process.

GOALS OF THERAPY

The family sets the treatment goals in agreement with the therapist. During the process of assessment and feedback, the clinician should have received an answer from the client to the question, "What would you like to see changed?" The therapist is primarily responsible for planning therapy, based on his or her expertise and knowledge, and obtaining the family's agreement and participation.

Goals, like assessment and other parts of the therapy process, are not static. Both distal (distant or terminal) and proximal (near or proximate) treatment goals are distinguished by Gurman and associates (1986). The treatment goals may undergo three types of change:

• *Evolving goals.* These occur when the therapist reframes presenting problems, typically early in the therapist–client contact. (I have made a distinction between the client's presenting complaint and the presenting problem to cover instances in which the early assessment interaction disclosed such a discrepancy between what was initially verbalized as a reason for contacting the therapist and what emerged once the client–therapist contact was underway [Nichols, 1988].)

• *Emerging goals.* These do not represent reframing of the original goals but the addition of new goals that the participants consider worthy of therapeutic attention. That is, as therapy progresses, it may become evident that something that was not included in the original goals deserves attention.

• *Reordered goals.* This designation alludes to the "reordering or reprioritizing of multiple initial goals." Adult clients may decide, for example, that it is desirable to work on differentiation from family-of-origin enmeshment before attempting further alteration in the marital relationship.

TREATMENT PLANNING

Clinical assessment is, by definition, the process by which clinicians gain the understanding necessary for making informed decisions (Korchin, 1976). Adapting Feldman's (1985) description of the treatment planning process in integrative family therapy provides the following pattern: Taking the observations and information gleaned in interviews, the therapist develops a diagnostic formulation for the individual, where pertinent, and an assessment of the marital partners and/or the family and their problems. This picture also includes the factors stimulating and maintaining the problems and the strengths of the individuals and couple and/or family. All of these parts of the picture form guidelines for treatment planning.

Assessment may or may not lead to family therapy, or to therapy of any kind, for that matter. One of the purposes of clinical assessment is to determine what kind of help, if any, is needed. Wynne and associates (1986) have made the point that in many instances families need only assessment and are not seeking therapy. Thus, some families have a "family consultation" and use what they learn about their situation from the assessment procedure with the clinician to solve their own problems without further outside assistance.

If therapy is indicated, what kind and with whom? Is another kind of intervention required and, if so, what kind and with whom? Careful assessment may lead to the conclusion, for example, that an adolescent who has been marked by his parents as "a problem" or as having problems needs academic tutoring and other forms of practical help and not therapeutic assistance.

Treatment planning can benefit from attention to Olson's (1988) schema on family therapy studies. He defines the systems level as including five variables: the individual, the marital relationship, the parent–child relationship, the family system, and the community. I have adapted the symptoms/presenting problems of the various levels:

Individual: DSM symptoms
Marriage: marital problems
Parent–child: parent–child problems
Family: nuclear family and extended family problems
Community: social and community factors

Specific treatment goals would be developed for each level. The goals would be problem solution and change in the presenting problems/symptoms of the individual and appropriate change in each of the other levels.

The techniques selected in an integrative approach to therapy depend primarily on the nature of the problem(s) being addressed. Some of the general guidelines are discussed below.

If the assessment contact indicates that there is a discrete problem, it is more likely to respond to a direct and straightforward intervention such as a behavioral approach (Wilkinson, 1993). The principle that has evolved for me in connection with the assumption of least pathology is the assumption that therapy begins with the most straightforward and simple approach. If the suggestion that a client stop drinking works, it works. And it has worked with some clients across the years, as it did with the client I mentioned earlier who accepted the suggestion of his clergyman. When the more overt, straightforward approach does not work, the clinician moves to the next level of intervention with the system.

When the problems deal primarily with communication, the therapeutic interventions selected first are behavioral and educational in nature. Underlying behavioral family therapy approaches to improving communication are the assumptions that every member of the family is attempting at all times to do his or her best to maximize pleasant and minimize unpleasant events, and that improved communication skills typically must be accompanied by specific training in constructive problem-solving skills and conflict resolution skills (Falloon, 1988).

According to Falloon (1988), there are neither contraindications to behavioral family therapy nor case descriptions indicating that competently applied behavioral family therapy produces major negative effects. Some of the areas for which specific behavioral approaches have been developed for specific problem areas include marital enrichment, parent training, behavioral marital therapy and sexual therapy, and divorce mediation (Falloon, 1988).

When the problems relate basically to attachment between persons (e.g., selection of a mate, the nature of the attachment, and patterns of personality needs), the first therapeutic choice is likely to be psychodynamic in nature. Depending on the form and extent of individual symptomatology, a mix of marital subsystem and individual therapy may be indicated. Determining when a combination of marital and individual therapy is appropriate is much more a clinical art than a science.

If the presenting problem is a complex one with indications that family system patterns maintain it, there is a greater need to comprehend the family system and interaction and to intervene at that level. When the issues pertain essentially to the maintenance of symptoms and problematic behavior in the present, the initial focus is likely to be on dealing with and altering the family system. Alteration of family patterns involves family-of-origin work when there are indications from the assessment that transgenerational issues are maintaining symptoms and problems.

Therapy in an integrative approach inevitably involves juggling interventions. This means that at times we focus on selected areas for active intervention while holding others in abeyance or putting them temporarily on hold. The major guidelines, which must be incorporated into the treatment plan, are (1) focus first on the "hot spots," that is, things that have to be handled on a crisis basis; and then (2) focus on systemic factors, that is, family system interventions that will affect both the family functioning and the symptoms of individuals.

Not only the nature of the presenting problem and the problems subsequently uncovered during the course of therapy but also the stage of development of the family, marriage, and individual may significantly affect the treatment planning and interventions. The use of a general developmental framework in terms of a family life cycle helps to determine how we will focus on issues of sequence and causation (Wilkinson, 1993). For example, if we are dealing with a young married couple early in their relationship, the issues typically found in that stage of life and development are the need to establish oneself in a vocation, the need to more adequately differentiate oneself from family of origin, the need to establish adequate boundaries around the marital relationship vis-à-vis all outsiders, and the need to establish workable patterns of intimacy, trust, and dependency between the partners. These provide starting points for our assessment of the strengths and problems of the clients and indicate where intervention may be needed.

6

THERAPY WITH FAMILIES
IN FORMATION

*Marriage is that relation between man and woman in which the
independence is equal, the dependence mutual, and the obligation
reciprocal.*

—LOUIS KAUFMAN ANSPACHER

*Marriage: a community consisting of a master, a mistress, and two
slaves, making in all two.*

—AMBROSE BIERCE

Developmentally and systemically oriented family therapy with young
adults, whether single or married, addresses issues relative to their families
of origin. Differentiation and separation problems are likely to be encountered from two perspectives. One is from the outlook of the young adults
as they struggle. The other is from the viewpoint of the parents as their
difficulties are manifested in dealing with the contraction of the nuclear
family through the departure of offspring. The focus of therapeutic
intervention in this chapter begins with young adults, as individuals and
marital partners, and expands to include other systems.

Marital therapy is discussed in depth in this chapter. Individuals
become part of a couple or dyadic relationship through mate selection.
The addition of children brings about the formation of a family. Hence,
both mate selection and the early problems of marriage including

preparation for adding a child are included. For the sake of convenience, some generic features of marital therapy—in later stages of the life cycle as well as in the early stage—are also considered. The issues obviously change as time passes and the partners enter subsequent phases of their marriage.

Family therapy that pays attention to systemic and developmental perspectives focuses on parallel and interrelated patterns. The family therapist tries to view and interpret pictures on parallel and overlapping screens simultaneously. With young adults who marry, the pictures that the therapist needs to understand may involve the following:

1. The developmental and practical living tasks/problems of the young adult vis-à-vis the mate, his or her own parents, siblings (if any), the mate's family, and the outside world.
2. The developmental and practical living tasks/problems of the partners as a couple in relation to each other inside the relationship and to others outside of the marital unit.
3. The developmental and practical living tasks/problems of the parental generation, that is, each mate's family of origin, vis-à-vis their spouses, their children, the outside world, and their own mortality.

Among the broad questions the therapist seeks to answer are the following:

- What are the major tasks of the couple at this stage, and how well is the dyadic unit accomplishing its tasks? What kinds of function and dysfunction are the couple exhibiting?
- Where is each person in his or her development and individual life cycle? What strengths and symptomatology are individuals exhibiting?
- What are the overlaps between the individual's life cycle stage and tasks and those of other parts of the larger family systems?
- How have the young adults been affected in their development by their family? How are they currently being affected?
- What do the couple or the individuals need in order to proceed effectively with their development?
- What resources do the individuals, the couple, and the extended family have for aiding the couple?
- To what extent does the therapist have to provide direction, education, nurturance, and support (including dealing with past events and their impact)? What is the educational and reeducational role of the therapist?

THE FAMILY LIFE CYCLE, STAGE 1–FORMATION:
MATING AND MARRIAGE

Although young persons in North America are marrying on the average at a later time in their lives than did several preceding generations, the majority still wed in early adulthood. Hence, the family life cycle schema used here begins with family formation (mating and marriage) as the first stage.

The mating and marriage stage of family formation actually is concerned with three life cycles: the marital life cycle (which at this time is synonymous with the part of the family life cycle that typically will become a new family unit); the individual life cycle—young adulthood (for the two persons who separate from their families of origin and enter into the mating and marriage process); and the family life cycle for each of the families of origin of the mating partners. (See Stage 4 of the family life cycle for the postparental tasks of the parents of the young couple [see also Chapter 9].)

The tasks of the individual life cycle (see Table 6.1) provide guidelines for assessing the functioning of the young adult and potential indicators of problematic areas, whether the person is single or married. Failure to achieve adequate functioning in any one of the five areas listed in Table 6.1 can be the source of individual and/or marital problems. Similarly, assisting the person to deal with the incompletely or inadequately mastered tasks sets the client on the path toward establishing of adequate functioning. The tasks overlap functionally and are discharged simultane-

**TABLE 6.1. Family Life Cycle, Stage 1–Formation:
Mating and Marriage**

The individual life cycle—Young adulthood

The young adult's major task is to learn to be a relatively independent adult vocationally, educationally, and socially.

Tasks

1. Differentiating sufficiently from family of origin to become a relatively autonomous single person.
2. Making appropriate progress toward establishment of self as vocationally and economically independent adult.
3. Establishing appropriate and satisfactory sexual outlets and identity.
4. Establishing appropriate and adequate social and personal relationships.
5. Beginning to demonstrate ability to function interdependently and in a socially responsible manner while manifesting a firm sense of personal and social identity.

ously, as should be evident in the discussion of mate selection and marriage that follow.

Mate Selection

Mate selection in North America is officially a matter of open choice and personal preference. Young people ostensibly are free to "marry for love." Although there is considerable room to select a mate on the basis of personal attraction, the idea of free choice in mate selection is about as valid as the notion of free will in human behavior generally. We are surrounded and deeply influenced by a number of social and demographic factors, as well as being influenced by our own psychological and emotional factors.

Social and Demographic Factors

These factors generally shape and influence the choice of a mate in demonstrable ways. As reflected in the popular adage that "like marries like," sociological researchers have long demonstrated that individuals typically select a mate from a similar racial, religious, educational, and sociocultural background (Hollingshead, 1950). Although there has been some diminishing of barriers between potential partners from different sociocultural groups in recent decades, the pattern of similarity still holds true for the most part. Propinquity, opportunity, and the emotional factor of being comfortable with the familiar are a few explanations for the tendency to marry a person from a similar social and cultural background.

Psychological and Emotional Factors

These factors apply in mate selection in a variety of complicated ways, for which there are no simple and clearly delineated theories. Some of the more widely accepted ideas stem from Sigmund Freud, Henry V. Dicks, Murray Bowen, and Clifford Sager.

The idea that individuals select a mate on the basis of need complementarity has been a significant part of psychological theory from at least the early part of this century. Freud theorized that the selection of a love object (person) often occurs because people strive to gain a perfection perceived in the lover that they have not been able to attain on their own. He indicated that narcissistic persons select anaclitic (dependent) persons and conversely. Similarly, the classical psychoanalytic view that mates are selected on the basis of a combination of conscious and unconscious needs and perceptions has been widely expounded. The discrepancy between the conscious and attainable and the unconscious and unattainable in one's expectations has been regarded as a major, if not the main, factor in subsequent marital discord (Kubie, 1956).

The theory of complementary needs was given a significant boost in exposure by sociologist Robert Winch (1958). Viewing the selection process as varying in the degree of conscious and unconscious awareness present, he suggested that the complementarity operated in a reciprocal fashion. That is, a dependent person would likely be attracted to a nurturant individual because of the dependent needs that the nurturant partner could gratify. Reciprocally, the nurturant partner would receive gratification in the process of taking care of the dependent partner.

Winch posited with four types of complementary couples and relationships: the Mother–Son marriage in which the husband is childishly dependent and the wife, nurturant and dominant; the Ibsenian couple in which the husband is dominant and nurturant in a "motherly" fashion and the wife, childishly dependent; the Master–Servant Girl pattern in which the husband, holding a traditional view of the status of women, is overtly dominant and covertly dependent and the wife, subservient and strong; and the Thurberian marriage in which the husband is inhibited in the expression of emotion and the wife, highly expressive. Those complementary patterns can be witnessed clinically in some couples.

Dicks (1967) described a process of selection in which partners enter into an unconscious, interlocking collusive process in order to make certain that unresolved issues from earlier in life are never resolved but that the marital relationship is never ended (an unsatisfying but enduring "cat and dog" marriage). Napier (1971, 1978) postulated that individuals tend to marry someone who seems to represent an opportunity for them to master their fears. This is very close to Kubie's (1956) statement about marrying to wipe out old pains or to settle old scores, for example, marrying the alcoholic friend of one's alcoholic brothers at whose hands suffering had been experienced, thereby attempting to achieve mastery of an old problem.

Bowen (1966) theorized that persons tend to marry someone who is functioning at approximately the same level of personality differentiation but whose defensive patterning is organized in an opposite fashion. The defensive patterning difference is basically consistent with what some others have observed in terms of "marital complementarity."

Beavers and Voeller (1983) also noted that it is difficult for a person to move in his or her individual development much beyond the level of competence of his or her family of origin. Further development can occur if the individual is fortunate enough to encounter a particularly helpful environment, a family with greater possibilities, or a therapeutic relationship that is helpful.

The idea of a marital "contract" based on one's expectations has been used as the basis for an approach to marital therapy by Sager (1976). He points out that each partner enters marriage with three levels of expectations for the relationship, spouse, and self. Some expectations are conscious and verbalized. Others are conscious but not verbalized (being withheld from the spouse because of embarrassment or a fear that they will not be fulfilled even if they are communicated). Still others are held outside of awareness. Some of those that exist outside of awareness may not come into effective operation until the marriage moves into a particular stage of the life cycle. One's expectations constitute a kind of unspoken but powerful contract in which each spouse expects the mate to fulfill a reciprocal part of the assumed bargain.

The thesis that the need pattern of each person in the selection process is complementary rather than similar remains an intriguing idea but one that is far from being demonstrated definitively as a central rule in mate selection. Some authorities have suggested that the individual tends to marry someone with similar, rather than complementary, needs (e.g., Murstein, 1961). Framo (1980) has attempted to reconcile conflicting opinions here by pointing out that both the need complementarity and the need similarity theses may be accurate and true, depending on the depth and length of inference one is making about mate selection.

A Transitional Process

Viewed developmentally and dynamically, mate selection serves important differentiating purposes for the young adult. Functionally and symbolically, it becomes an attempt to replace the attachment patterns from one's family of origin and developmental years with fulfillment in an adult relationship, and to integrate the residues of the past with present experiences and relationships. For the young adult, it represents a dramatic psychosocial transition from parental identifications and family dependency to the establishment of a new level of attachment and expected intimacy as an adult. For example, John may expect that his new spouse, Mary, will help him separate from his family of origin or will replace a nurturing parent. The process of selecting a mate, although colored by cultural romanticism and social/family expectations, nevertheless serves to link each individual's personal development and historical need patterns with those of a selected mate in a new dyadic process.

The way individuals make this transitional process to marriage provides the clinician with critical data with regard to marriage and family formation and subsequent function and dysfunction. Characteristics of this process are identifiable and clinically predictable and have been described more fully elsewhere (Nichols, 1988; Nichols & Everett, 1986).

Marriage

Marital relationships are different from other kinds of relationships. Individuals are different when witnessed in relation to and in interaction with their spouse than when they are seen alone. A seemingly sensible, reasonable, and mature man or woman who is otherwise a social or vocational success may become irrational, unreasonable, and immature in attitudes and behaviors when involved in interaction with his or her spouse. There are explanations that answer the question of why the nature of intimate relationships is different from other human relationships (Dicks, 1967; Fairbairn, 1952, 1954; Framo, 1970).

Both object relations theory and multigenerational family theory provide explanations for the fact that in marital interaction the feelings that operate between the spouses are not confined to the present situation. From the multigenerational perspective, for example, mate selection can be explained in terms of individuals seeking to regain a lost parent through marrying a person who seems to embody some crucial attributes of the lost parental object. By replacing the missing parent, one strives to rebalance obligations and loyalties in the family ledger (Boszormenyi-Nagy & Spark, 1973).

From an object relations standpoint, one projects onto the individual with whom one is intimate certain important images from earlier relationships with parents. This is particularly evident in conflict areas, where one may project part of the earlier conflict onto the mate and act out the other side of it. Psychologically, one acts both defensively and in pursuit of satisfaction when seeking a mate. Even if a therapist has difficulty understanding all of the object relations patterns that may be present with a couple, he or she should be able to note how individuals seek out what is familiar when they pursue close interpersonal relationships.

How the partners leave their families and what they bring with them form an important part of the mate-selection and marriage process. When mating evolves into marriage, there is a coming together of more than simply two individuals. Marriage involves the joining of two families and two ways of life. Each partner brings from their family of origin not only issues in relating that were not resolved but also ways of believing, thinking, valuing, and acting. In other words, the relationship issues and tasks involved in mate selection are not merely those of dealing with parents, but also those of dealing with an entire family unit.

Clearly, successful resolution of the relationship issues with one's family of origin is essential to the formation of a marital relationship that has adequate opportunity for growth and resolution of its own tasks and problems. Optimally, the joint marital and individual task here appears to be that of securing and maintaining an appropriate distance from the family of origin that involves some contact and closeness but not so much that it interferes with individual and marital development.

Marital Problems

There is no available taxonomy of marital problems. Most of the early research in that area (e.g., Goodrich, 1968) has not been pursued in a systematic fashion by family researchers. The few efforts made in recent years to classify marital difficulties have been the work of clinicians.

Framo (1980) described four sources of marital discord: discrepancy between conscious and unconscious demands, relationship between the intrapsychic and the transactional, secret agendas of marital partners, and family problems repeating themselves from one generation to the next. He also made a preliminary classification of marital problems. Martin (1976) delineated four pathological marriage patterns—the "love sick" wife and the "cold sick" husband (hysterical wife and obsessional husband), the "in-search-of-a-mother" marriage (hysterical husband and obsessional wife), the "double-parasite" marriage (hysterical–hysterical or dependent–dependent), and the paranoid marriage (including the folie a deux, paranoid, and conjugal paranoid patterns). All of these patterns involve significant amounts of interlocking pathology.

Two psychoanalytically oriented marital constructs have been offered by Giovacchini (1958). The first is a "character object" relationship in which the partners have made a tenuous reciprocal relationship. They share an elemental intrapsychic bond and defensive traits or symptoms. In those senses, there is a homogamous marriage. The second is a "symptom object" relationship in which the partners do not have a deep form of attachment and are characterologically heterogamous. Different forms of treatment have been recommended by Moss and Lee (1976) for the two types—individual therapy for the homogamous and conjoint or group psychotherapy for the heterogamous.

From the work of the family therapists at Palo Alto came some early attempts at classifying marital relationships. Haley (1963) described a complementary marital relationship as one that occurs when the spouses exchange different kinds of behavior. For example, one partner gives and the other receives. He also depicted a symmetrical relationship as occurring when the partners exchange the same behaviors, as when both partners receive. He saw a marriage as being limited in its functioning capabilities to the extent that the marital partners were unable to form either a complementary or a symmetrical relationship.

Don Jackson (Lederer & Jackson, 1968) also attempted to construct a classification based on exchanges of behavior between marital partners that resulted in a "more or less workable" relationship. "Workable" was used to define a marriage that was maintained without great personal loss or damage to the mental or physical health of either spouse. To the two basic modes of relationship described by Haley, Jackson added a third, the parallel mode of relationship. Marriages were then described by Jackson as Stable–Satisfactory, Unstable–Satisfactory, Unstable–Unsatisfactory, and Stable–Unsatisfactory. Each of these had two subtypes, the Stable Satisfactory having the Heavenly Twins and the Collaborative Geniuses; the Unstable–Satisfactory having the Spare-Time Battlers and the Pawnbrokers; the Unstable–Unsatisfactory having the Weary Wranglers and the Psychosomatic Avoiders; and the Stable–Unsatisfactory having the Gruesome Twosome and the Paranoid Predators.

Rather than attempting to construct a taxonomy of marital problems, I have identified a number of concepts from the marital life cycle that are useful in making a broad assessment of how a marital relationship is functioning (Nichols, 1988; Nichols & Everett, 1986). The tasks of the marital life cycle, along with individual diagnosis, provide guidelines for assessing and intervening when marital discord is presented to the clinician. The five concepts of commitment, caring, communication, conflict and compromise, and contract have proven to be useful over the years in working with couples. They can be used both by clinicians and by couples, partly because they refer to important areas of marital interaction and partly because they conceptualize those areas in everyday language that is easily understood.

1. Commitment refers to the degree of attachment and degree of intent to stay involved with the spouse and/or the marriage.
2. Caring has to do with the kind and amount of cherishing, love, and similar feelings that one has toward the spouse.
3. Communication refers to the kind, quality, and range of communication that exists between the marital partners.
4. Conflict/compromise relates to how the partners are able to deal with differences, including their ability to compromise over genuine differences in order to make the relationship remain functional.
5. Contract pertains to the explicit and implicit agreements each partner holds regarding the spouse and the relationship between them.

The particular forms and tasks of couples in the early marriage stage are described in Table 6.2.

TABLE 6.2. The Marital Life Cycle, Stage 1–The Beginning: Mating and Marriage

Separating from families of origin and establishing a couple identity, including developing a mutually satisfactory affectional–sexual relationship.

Core tasks

Commitment
Developing an initial commitment.

Caring
Discerning whether there is sufficient and appropriate caring to warrant marriage.

Communication
Beginning to establish workable processes and patterns of communication and constructing a shared universe of discourse.

Conflict/compromise
Beginning to learn how to resolve conflicts and effect compromise.

Contract
Working to explore and clarify expectations and establish a good interactional contract.

THERAPY IN THE FAMILY FORMATION STAGE

Treatment, of course, must be done in context. It is not limited to the individual, but includes that part of his or her systems that it is deemed most necessary or desirable to include in order to bring about change most effectively. Marital therapy typically is the treatment of choice for an integrative family therapist who is working with couples in the early stages of a marital relationship. Marital therapy is intended to treat both the marital partners and the marriage (i.e., the transactional system in which the partners are involved). Individual pathology may be a result of marital/family dysfunction and may clear up following amelioration of difficulties in those systems.

Why Not Individual Therapy?

Some therapists have given extensive lists of indications and contraindications for the use of marital therapy. For example, it has been suggested that the partners should be treated together when the presenting symptoms relate almost entirely to the marriage and when both mates are committed to the marriage (Grunebaum & Christ, 1976). Otherwise, the partners presumably would be given individual psychotherapy or, in some cases, group therapy.

However, individual treatment may have negative effects on the person's marriage—it may dislodge the marital collusion and shift the complementarity between spouses. The same risk prevails when one spouse is in group therapy in which the other spouse is not involved. The therapist also should be cautious to advise clients that change, including growth, experienced in therapy by an individual may exacerbate present marital dysfunction and place the marriage in further jeopardy. A systemic orientation anticipates reciprocal changes throughout the system.

The therapist needs to help the client to understand the impact of both the system on the spouse and the spouse's role and function in the system. This often involves exploring with him or her a paradigm of change, which goes as follows: If you change your behaviors, then others in the system react to accommodate the new behavior, and you must respond to them in order to effect a change in the system. Change is aborted and the system remains the same if, when you start to change and others react in ways that say, "Don't change," you drop your new behaviors and resume the old behavior patterns.

Where the presenting problems of one spouse are major and overriding, attention may need to be given to those difficulties before work is begun explicitly on the marital relationship. Assessment may also disclose that one of the partners is sufficiently symptomatic to require the major focus both at the beginning and throughout the course of therapy. In some extreme cases, such as those in which one partner has a manic-depressive disorder, marital therapy may be used in conjunction with other forms of therapy (Greene, Lee, & Lustig, 1975).

Marital therapy was the treatment of choice, for example, in one of my cases in which the presenting problem was a paranoid psychotic episode experienced by one spouse. The person was treated in the context of home and family rather than being hospitalized. The mate served to reinforce reality and to provide support for several weeks until the acute phase of the episode had passed. Subsequently, the focus shifted primarily to the marital interaction with some attention being devoted to the lingering paranoid ideation.

In other presenting individual disorders such as borderline symptomatology, it may be desirable to focus on the nuclear family system rather than on the marriage because of the intensity and splitting present in the marital relationship (Everett et al., 1989).

In cases in which individual therapy is used and the decision is made not to involve the spouse, the therapist should attempt to have the other spouse attend at least one session in order to establish a preliminary acquaintance and rudimentary relationship of trust with him or her.

Marital Therapy

Marital therapy may be the treatment of choice for a variety of diagnosed conditions with individuals such as reactive depression, anxiety reaction, and certain personality disorders. There are marital cases, of course, in which there is no presenting individual pathology. In those cases, marital problems result primarily from ignorance, lack of maturity, or situational factors culminating in a marked degree of friction and discord in response to the stress. Therapy in such an instance would consist not of individual psychotherapy but of interventions aimed at restoration of balance in the system (Christ, 1976). Difficulties in the marital system in such cases may be viewed as stemming from an interactional imbalance or from a diminishing of emotional satisfactions for the partners.

When there are marital problems present, some clinicians suggest (Sager, 1966) that the only genuine contraindication to the use of marital therapy is the inability of the therapist to prevent destructive behavior on the part of one member of the marital pair toward the other in the therapy sessions. We can certainly add to this the inability to prevent the spillover of discord into violence at home. However, working with the spouses in such situations not only may help to contain the symptomatology but also may provide a better view of etiological factors than other modes of treatment.

The approach advocated here is very much in line with the broad stance taken by Willi (1984). That is, in deciding to use marital therapy, one takes into consideration the couple and their relationship, along with their marital situation and problems; the limitations and potential of the modality of treatment; and the therapist's own preferences, attitudes toward marital difficulties, and competence to perform marital therapy. In addition to these criteria, it is crucial, of course, to determine the reciprocal relationship between the marital partners and their respective families of origin vis-à-vis the presenting problem.

MARITAL THERAPY IN THE FAMILY FORMATION STAGE

Marital therapy at the mating and marriage/family formation stage, as emphasized above, focuses basically on the primary marital tasks of the couple and the core tasks of this stage of the marital cycle (see Table 6.2). Secondarily, as indicated by the deficits in functioning brought to the marriage by the individual partners, marital therapy focuses on individual developmental tasks (from the individual life cycle) as these affect individual and marital functioning.

The preference in treating marital complaints is to have both spouses participate in the therapy. As noted above, it is risky to assume that changes that one partner may make in therapy can correct marital dysfunctions and successfully rebalance the dysfunctional relationship. In addition, it is likely that the absent spouse will sabotage therapeutic change, which may be seen as threatening the dynamic balance of the marital relationship. However, it often is the case that only one individual is available or motivated for therapy. This may not only reflect the marital dissonance but may also imply that separation and divorce are pending.

Some therapists emphasize the transference aspects of the client–therapist relationship even when conjoint marital interviewing is being used (e.g., Willi, 1984). Most couples presenting themselves for marital therapy can be worked with effectively without extensive exploration of transference reactions of the clients to the therapist. As Sager (1976) has pointed out, such phenomena can be handled more directly by focusing on the marital relationship rather than on the couples' relationship with the therapist. Avoiding the deliberate fostering of regression in the clients is a significant factor in maintaining a therapeutic relationship that remains appropriately focused on the marital relationship and the clients. Family therapy emphasizes dealing with the life situations of persons as directly as possible, rather than imposing a therapist as a screen on which conflicts can be projected and then analyzed.

The therapist's major task, especially during the early stage of therapy, is to help the clients "settle down" so that the therapeutic process can be helpful to them. This includes giving careful attention to the feelings and behaviors of clients, the therapist's own feelings and behaviors, and the ways in which the context of the treatment facilitates or hampers progress toward therapeutic goals. At all times during the assessment/treatment, it is important to monitor not only the content of the sessions but also the process factors. That is, it is necessary to keep in view how the clients are responding and how therapy is proceeding so that the therapist can make the necessary alterations in order to deal effectively and sensitively with the clients.

Marital therapy methods have been characterized as fitting into two basic categories: growth-oriented techniques that focus on the conflict, including individual problems and difficulties; and problem-oriented, systems, and communications techniques (Willi, 1984). Treatment can include elements of both approaches or follow basically one or the other of them, according to what is found in the assessment work with the couple.

Conjoint marital therapy probably is the most widely used interviewing format in marital therapy today, although it often is combined with occasional individual sessions at both the initial assessment and ongoing treatment stages.

Couples group therapy in which three to five couples are seen together is chosen by some therapists. Framo (1992), for example, who relies heavily on such an approach, tells couples that, by participating in couples group therapy, they can reach any therapeutic goals that could be reached otherwise. He combines the group work with family-of-origin sessions in which an individual is seen with his or her parents and siblings but without the spouse being present.

Treatment of the marital unit may be entered into through one of several doors. That is, marital therapy may be asked for directly or may come about as a result of an original request for another kind of therapeutic assistance. One or both of the marital partners may seek assistance for marriage and family relationship difficulties, asking for marriage counseling or simply for help. Marital therapy also may become the treatment of choice after one of the partners either has been in individual treatment or has asked for individual psychotherapy.

Assessment

The focus of the assessment of the individuals and the marital unit and their relationship to multigenerational family processes will vary according to the needs of the individuals and of the system, as well as the particular phase of assessment/treatment with which one is involved. Assessment typically differs according to the point of entry through which the partners initially pass on their way to meeting with the clinician. When they begin by asking for help with the marriage, the assessment begins at a different point and with a different focus than when their initial contact is made in relation to individual concerns, for example. When the initial contact is made for marital help, at least one of the partners has delineated certain marital difficulties that he or she considers troublesome. Those problems may or may not be the major sources of difficulties affecting the partners, but at least the focus of the therapeutic endeavor has been placed on the marriage. As a colleague has aptly put it, "When one marital partner says that there is a marital problem, there is a marital problem."

Although to call the marriage a "third personality," as some leading marital therapists have done, is to go too far; a marital system is present that forms the core subsystem of the nuclear family typically founded by the spouses. Rather than making a facile assumption that marital problems are a reflection only of systems dysfunction or of individual pathology, it seems more accurate to assume that marital problems typically are an amalgam of several processes. We need to understand the marital subsystem and the partners as well as how transgenerational family functioning affects what is going on with them and in the marriage. It is not always easy to determine the couple's commitment to the marriage or their motivation for change early in therapy; likewise it may be difficult to ascertain at the very beginning how transgenerational issues affect the couple.

Effective assessment must deal with both the marital unit and the individual/personal subsystems. As Framo (1980) has pointed out, the relationship between the intrapsychic world and the interpersonal world provides the greatest understanding and the most promising therapeutic leverage. By this he means "how internalized family conflicts from past family relationships are being lived through the spouse and children in the present" (p. 58).

The therapist, in other words, needs to spend some time exploring the background of each of the partners. Such exploration is concerned not only with the past, with the childhood and developmental experiences of the man or woman who is being interviewed, but also with the current, active relationships with family members, and, still farther, with the carried-over issues from the past that are affecting present relationships with his or her family of origin.

Out of such exploration may come an awareness that the therapist is primarily concerned not with how an individual related to his or her mother or father but with the "models of relationships" that existed in his or her family of origin. Those models of relationships include interactions between his or her parents and, perhaps, between the grandparents or in other marriages to which the person was exposed during childhood.

The concept of models of relationships can be used descriptively with clients. Once the concept has been presented to them in simple terms, they can grasp how they may have picked up ideas of what is desirable and normative during the course of growing up. Similarly, many people can comprehend the possibility that they may have made some definite, conscious decisions to avoid certain patterns that they witnessed in their parents' marriage while retaining an unconscious adherence to other parts of the patterns. For example, a therapist asks a client: "Do you ever find yourself growling at your wife [or scolding your husband] in the same tone of voice, with the same inflections perhaps, that you disliked in your father [or mother]?" The client may nod in agreement and then begin talking about other manifestations of the same phenomenon.

Focusing on such developments as a normal part of living, as something that happens with most people rather than as something strange or pathological, enables many people to open themselves up to the possibility that such behavior occurs with them. It thus prepares them for learning about themselves and how they function in marital and family relationships. It also helps to elucidate how transgenerational relationships affect their functioning. In other words, when the focus is placed on the models of relationships that existed in a client's family of origin, the spotlight is taken off the individual, and the stigma of being viewed as pathological is removed. Instead, the clients are helped to look at the relationships in which they formerly lived and at those in which they currently live. Through this single set of concepts, clients are helped to become learners about things that have been of interest to them since childhood. Meanwhile, the therapist helps them to keep the present marital and family relationships in mind, rather than getting bogged down or lost in exploring the past or the intrapsychic functioning of one partner as if their partner were living in a vacuum.

The Initial Interview

The actual procedures followed in the first interview will vary from one situation to another, depending on the therapist's assessment of the needs. When a telephone request is made for marital help, some brief information is obtained in order to determine the suitability of the request for marital treatment. "Can you tell me a bit about your situation?" is a common question for prospective clients. Other questions may also be asked, including whether either of the spouses is currently receiving psychotherapy and whether the mate is willing to come in for marital help. Information also is provided to the prospective clients regarding office location, fees, length of appointment (which may be limited to the usual 45- to 50-minute time slot or scheduled for a longer initial meeting if the time is available); if requested, information may also be given concerning therapist qualifications.

When the clients come to the first interview, the opening gambit typically is a simple one. After getting them seated and perhaps after a pleasantry or two, the therapist may say something along the line of "I know what you sketched out for me on the telephone, but let's start off as if I know nothing at all about you. What brings you in?" (If only one of the partners has talked on the telephone, the therapist may repeat what was written down during that conversation and ask for confirmation from the partner who called regarding the accuracy of what is being said in the session, e.g., "Is that about it?")

The therapist pays close attention to both what they answer and how they respond. Do they agree? Are they there for the same reasons, at least insofar as they verbalize their reasons for being present? What are those reasons? To change their spouse, dump their spouse on a therapist and leave the marriage, find out what their difficulties are, get marital therapy, get divorce therapy, or something else? A variety of responses typically come from the partners in terms of both content and mode of responding.

How the partners answer generally helps the therapist to begin forming a view of how they relate and interact.

A considerable amount of useful information can be obtained from most couples in a short time by posing a few simple questions. If they have not already provided some descriptions of how things have developed and changed in talking about their problems, the therapist may focus on those questions in the initial interview. "Tell me about yourselves. I wonder if things have always been this way. How did you meet? What attracted you to the other person? How did your dating go? How did you decide to get married? How did things go when you were first married?"

If they do not do so automatically, each partner is asked to respond from his or her own point of view. The therapist looks for the areas of agreement; for the areas of difference in perception, motivation, and understanding; and for any assessment clues that may be available with regard to the nature of personal and marital strengths and difficulties. Some individuals have never thought consciously about what attracted them to their future spouse and find this an intriguing question. It often makes for a smooth transition into talking about expectations.

Responses to the cluster of questions posed above vary widely, as one would expect. Some couples disclose that there were significant problems from the beginning of their relationship, for example, "We fought like cats and dogs from the start." Others demonstrate amazement that particular feelings were felt by the other spouse, "I didn't know that you felt like that. I always thought that you. . . . " Still others indicate that the relationship started off well, only to encounter difficulties later. Sometimes this change can be traced to certain events, most of which pertain to disappointments because the mate failed to live up to certain expectations and broke the (conscious or unconscious) contract (Sager, 1976).

From even a brief discussion with the partners, one may be able to gain two important pieces of information for the assessment. First, some understanding of the degree of chronicity of the problems can be obtained. That is, the therapist can gain a picture of how long the partners perceive that they have had difficulty, also whether the problems are chronic or of an acute, crisis nature. Second, a range of material may be forthcoming on how the partners have attempted to deal with their problems, on the degree of difference or similarity in their feelings about the relationship, including their optimism or pessimism about its history and future; one may also gain some rudimentary grasp of the motivations of the partners. Both sets of information have important prognostic implications.

The intent in the first session is to get the best picture possible of what the partners have brought in and what the therapist and couple may be able to accomplish together. Was it a crisis or a chronic set of problems that brought them to the appointment? Whose idea was it to come to therapy? What do they desire from the therapist? How do they interact? How committed are they to each other and to working constructively on their problems? How willing and able are they to change? What is the prognosis for them and for the marriage? The last question may not be answered as quickly or easily as some of the others. The therapist may not be able to answer it even tentatively at the end of the initial session. Particularly in instances in which ambivalence is high and commitment unclear, a prognostic statement may be formulated only after therapy has been attempted for some weeks. A more pressing question, perhaps, at the outset is that of what needs to be done with and for them before they leave the first interview.

Some therapists, such as Greene (1970), have emphasized the significance of the first few minutes of contact with clients in beginning to establish hope in them and to launch a working alliance between clients and therapist. Harry Stack Sullivan (1954) stressed the importance of having a client leave each interview with a sense of having derived some benefit from the experience. Both points of view are valid, although initial errors in dealing with a couple may not prove fatal. One can get off to a slow start on occasion and recoup before the end of the interview, particularly if the errors or omissions are clearly recognized by the therapist and the errors corrected.

The emotional/motivational picture may be quite complex. Traditional psychodynamic psychotherapy has emphasized the resistances that the client manifests to treatment. Some marital and family therapists recently have stressed that dealing with resistance is not effective when an adversarial approach—one in which the client is viewed as being deliberately or pathologically obtuse—is assumed between therapist and clients (Wile, 1981). Others have pointed to concerns about change and changing as a source of anxiety for clients and thus a basis for resistive behavior on their part (e.g., Napier, 1976, as noted in Chapter 5).

Therapists need to maintain a balance among assessment, alliance formation, and intervention that is appropriate for the particular couple and situation. Certainly, in the first interview, the therapist should do enough assessment to know what he or she is dealing with in order to respond intelligently. If there is time for an extended assessment period during the first appointment, the clinician initially may see the spouses conjointly, then split them for short individual sessions, and then bring them back together before closing the first session. Some clinicians prefer to see each spouse individually for a full session the week following the initial conjoint session. Others do not see the spouses separately at all.

There are cases in which a couple requires immediate intervention. The problems are too acute and too pressing for them to accommodate themselves to an extended assessment process. That is, there may not be time for the clinician to hold several interviews and make leisurely decisions before attempting to intervene.

Whether the therapist decides to split up the first session and see the partners separately for a period of time as well as together depends on more than time considerations. It also depends on the clinician's impression that the partners may be able to open up and reveal their concerns more freely and openly in the absence of the spouse, there being issues that they cannot discuss in the presence of their mate. The following case exemplifies the utility of separate sessions.

Mrs. Farmer, a 27-year-old teacher, who had been married for a little more than a year, sat silently in the opening minutes of the first appointment. Her husband did almost all of the talking. Her body postures and nonverbal language bore mute testimony to the fact that she was constrained and inhibited by her mate, rather than simply being a passive individual. Sensing that she would be different when seen alone, as individuals frequently are, the therapist interrupted the session after 10–15 minutes and indicated that he wished to see them separately. When Mrs. Farmer was seen alone the therapist started by asking, "Is there anything that we haven't talked about that you would. . . . " Interrupting, she spewed out in staccato bursts her fears of her husband's violent and erratic behaviors, the details of one public outburst that had resulted in his arrest, the salient factors in his recently disclosed bisexuality, her feeling that she had been misled, and the certainty of her intention to seek an annulment of the marriage. When Mr. Farmer was seen alone, he also opened up with his concerns about whether to come out of the closet publicly. When the conjoint meeting was resumed, it was possible to move directly and quickly into an examination of the salient issues.

There are pros and cons regarding seeing individuals separately during the initial assessment phase or at any other time during treatment, as opposed to using only conjoint interviews. For example, while it is true that a considerable amount of learning about each other can take place when history is gathered from each partner in the presence of the other, it also is true that important pieces of history may be omitted from conjoint sessions, particularly if such information relates to sexual histories, extramarital relationships, and other matters that may be embarrassing, guilt producing, or conflictual to the marital relationship.

On one hand, not seeing the partners separately does entail some risk of missing important information. Early individual sessions also can effectively establish rapport for the therapist with each spouse, thus bypassing the spousal collusion and give each partner the opportunity to be him- or herself with the therapist, as was the case with the Farmers. A thoughtful statement on the individual interview as a treatment technique in conjoint therapy has been provided by Berman (1982).

On the other hand, some clinicians conclude that the gains from individual sessions are not worth the possibilities of creating loyalty and confidentiality conflicts on the part of the therapist and of raising suspicion on the part of the absent spouse (Framo, 1980). Individual interviewing certainly can cause some suspicion on the part of individuals who are extremely frightened and anxious and who manifest tendencies to be untrusting in the situation.

Settling In

Although therapy probably begins when the partners start to consider getting help, treatment itself starts with the first contact with the clients, usually during a telephone call. From at least that point onward, what transpires is part of a process leading either toward entry into an ongoing therapy process or toward an abortive movement out of contact with the process. This phase is referred to here as the "settling in" phase of treatment.

Zuk (1969) has suggested that a major goal of treatment has been accomplished when the therapist has gained the commitment of the family to be treated on the therapist's terms. He refers to the settling of the terms of the commitment to be treated as a major determinant of outcome in family therapy.

Some common issues begin to emerge in conjoint marital therapy during the settling in phase. These issues vary to some extent from case to case, of course, but a considerable amount of similarity is to be found in the early responses of couples in conjoint therapy. One of the first things couples generally do in conjoint marital therapy is to seek to find the boundaries of permissible behavior. Some family therapists describe this process in terms of establishing the power relationship. This concept can be widened a bit and referred to as "finding the parameters." Getting into treatment often permits the mates to release anger and hostility that previously were held back entirely or were partially restrained, seldom released fully. Having a third party present may encourage the mates to engage in an emotional sparring match in the fashion of two boxers who feel each other out and then begin to throw punches, secure in the knowledge that a referee is present. Each may be seeking to get the referee to be a protector, advocate, or ally, but there generally is a more complex set of issues involved.

The therapist may be viewed at times as benign and at other times as unfeeling, depending on the particular salience that he or she has for the clients involved. Just as the therapist's presence may enable some couples to feel that they can release anger, so it also may make it possible for some other marital partners to probe the possibilities of getting closer to each other emotionally and behaviorally. The anger that emerges may be a mixture of pent-up feelings and defense against anxiety and fear. Similarly, in the early sessions spouses often will move toward establishing a coalition with the therapist. Such efforts at establishing a coalition may range from simply behaving in a way that is intended to make the therapist like them to more overt manipulations aimed at getting the therapist to side with them against their mate.

Whatever form it takes, the clients' anxiety arises and protective mechanisms emerge against experiencing uncertainty and possible pain. What has often been described as resistance in therapy can be interpreted in many instances as apprehension against proceeding into the unknown. The prospect of changing, even if the alteration is being accomplished in the company and presence of a benignly viewed therapist, can be unsettling for many persons.

Management of the exposure of feelings, as the marital partners seek to find acceptable parameters in, as well as out of, the sessions, is one of the early tasks of the therapist. As the partners begin their sparring or other behavioral and psychological probing, the therapist should attempt to adhere to a tight line between supporting appropriate exposure and encouraging adequate restraint. The couple should not be allowed to expose their feelings to the extent that they become unduly anxious and frightened over either the release of their own positive or negative feelings or possible rejection or retaliation by their mate. At the same time, the therapist needs to facilitate the clients' emergence from behind the bulwark of their defenses so that they can engage their spouse in sharing, communication, and problem solving.

The task of supporting appropriate exposure and risking behavior while simultaneously encouraging restraint is an art, rather than a precise science. How well the therapist handles those matters does not depend on observing others and picking up an abstract collection of strategies and techniques to use in any situation that comes along. Rather, it depends to a significant degree on his or her ability to comprehend the nature of the marital subsystem and the personalities of the marital partners with whom he or she is working. Much of the understanding and skill required for such work will be acquired in the beginning therapist's supervised clinical experience, although many years of experience are required in order to hone one's functioning to a high degree. Whatever the extent of one's experience, only an ongoing assessment of the meaning of the actions of the partners enables the therapist to deal intelligently with the behaviors.

We need a normative model for workable relationships against which the varied early behaviors of clients are assessed. It is important to recognize that clients are normally anxious in therapy. Early in treatment, the couple may be moving too rapidly or too slowly. They may be "windmilling their punches" wildly on the one hand and "shadowboxing" and sparring cautiously on the other. Or, they may be shifting from one modality of interaction to another. During the initial appointments, the reluctant client may be able to hide behind his or her more overt defenses, throwing up a smokescreen of words and behaviors that obscure the issues. Similarly, those sessions may give the client opportunity to vent his or her more pressing concerns. Venting may alleviate some anxiety and bring the client back to a state of relative quiescence. Once the initial anxiety has been lowered, there may be little or no desire to continue with therapy. That is, with some persons, once the immediate tension has been eased, there is not enough residual pain or overt conflict to push them toward continuing with therapy. Recognizing their behavior for what it typically is—manifestation of anxiety—makes it possible to intervene appropriately.

My clinical impression is that it is a major mistake on the part of the therapist to remain inactive or to be primarily reflective during the early sessions. To acknowledge explicitly that entering therapy, especially for the first time, can be difficult appears to be essential to launching and continuing with effective treatment. One may say to clients, "These are difficult matters that you are dealing with; it is not easy to talk about them, especially with somebody that you had never seen until a short time ago. Let's all try to be sensitive to what's happening and try to deal with things in measurable doses."

There is a noticeable change in many cases by the 6th to the 10th session. With the passage of time and the development of trust from continued contact with the therapist, a kind of crisis occurs for some clients. At the least, most clients reach a point of decision about continuing in therapy. The simplest explanation is that the partners begin to care about the therapeutic relationship and what it brings them. Perceiving at some level of awareness that trusting the therapist can help them to risk more exposure of themselves in therapy, they are faced with a choice between really committing themselves to a process of change or stopping treatment.

This stage is one of those times at which I consider it appropriate to explore with clients their goals. "We have accomplished some things [specifying what they are]. We could go ahead and work on the areas that we have discussed where there seems to be more work that could be done. Or, we could stop for now and you could decide later whether you wish to set some new goals and objectives and work on them." The first purpose here is to affirm as honestly and clearly as possible what has been accomplished. A corollary is to pave the way for continued therapeutic work if desired by the client(s) in the future.

Some couples stop before the 10th to 15th session, particularly in those cases in which immediate problem-solving approaches and crisis intervention are the treatment of choice. Those who continue beyond this point move into longer-term treatment that may last for a year or two, although the average time involved in marital cases is usually less than a year.

Exploring Dimensions of the Marital Relationship

Where there is difficulty in determining what is transpiring with a couple, it may be helpful to move away from their self-directed and often global explanations of their problems. Instead, the clinician concentrates more explicitly on the various dimensions of the marriage. What follows is a description of one useful way of proceeding, using a framework adapted from Berman and Lief's (1975) work.

Boundaries of the Marital System

Exploring the boundaries involves helping the couple to focus on their relationship and on who is to be included within the boundaries of the relationship. This approach has three interrelated factors.

Inclusion. Who is included in the boundaries of the relationship and, hence, who needs to be included in their work on the marriage? This approach is aimed at helping the couple to focus on dealing with the marriage and marital interaction. It becomes clear that for the immediate purposes of exploration and work in therapy, the focus is not on the job, the in-laws, or other things, but on the marriage and how the partners deal with one another. Detriangulation from involvement with one of these other relationships may be a necessary step in order to move forward. (As it becomes appropriate to do so, the focus is widened in the therapeutic sessions.)

Extrusion. This involves exploration and discussion of what is being extruded from the marriage. Discussing who and what are to be included in the marriage relationship brings about in a normal progression the question of which problems are extruded from the relationship and, when there are children, assigned to the children. This is often how the therapist begins to learn about parentification of children, for example, as well as about other ways in which a couple is dealing inappropriately with marital issues.

Intrusion. Similarly, discussion of inclusion tends to bring about a consideration of intrusion. What persons, events, or other things are intruding into the marriage and in what ways? Are friends, in-laws, or overinvolvement in work driving a wedge between the partners? Is the husband still "going out with the boys" as he did prior to marriage and using his weekends for hunting and fishing or other activities that do not include the wife, leaving her with the feeling that his friends and leisure time pursuits come before her in his interest and commitment?

Asking the couple to take a normative position in the discussion, that is, asking them to take a stand and to spell out who/what is to be included in the marriage, rapidly brings into the open their expectations and the issues that currently are causing disagreement or agreement, conflict or coopera- tion. Also, asking such questions as what needs to be put out, fended off, or brought back into the relationship gives some rough indication as to issues that may be problematic in therapy. How the partners deal with such questions also provides some indication of the power dimension of the marriage. Does one of them set the agenda for discussion, determine the course the discussion takes, and determine the conclusions while the other defers to the course taken, or are they more flexible, perhaps negotiating the agendas, course of discussion, and conclusions?

Power Dimension

What is the nature of the power relationship between the husband and wife? How has it changed over time? Have there been recent alterations in the dominance–submission patterns, for example? Changes in the individual life cycles and in the family life cycle frequently result in problems in the marriage; for example, increased striving for autonomy by the wife may bring about negative reactions on the part of the husband, as witnessed so frequently with the recent rise in women's consciousness.

Intimacy/Closeness

Difficulties in tolerating and responding to the needs and wishes of others for closeness or lack of closeness frequently form the major issues under- lying a considerable amount of marital discord. Not infrequently, appre- hension regarding getting close to the mate leads to games of "uproar." They argue over minor things. Neither is willing to discuss issues ration- ally. So long as they emphasize the differences between them and continue to express their disagreements, "safe" distance can be maintained. John's inability to be sensitive and caring is not challenged, for example. Mary is protected against her fears of being disappointed if she relies on John emotionally. Until such dynamics are identified and appropriate interventions made, the partners are likely to keep shifting from one set of disruptive, sometimes argumentative actions to another. Hence, it is important to identify the intimacy/closeness issues early in the assessment process.

The beginning therapist may not recognize the issue of intimacy/closeness because it often is camouflaged by a broad array of external symptoms and complaints. For example, a man who gets into arguments with his children and "hassles" them when he comes in from work may be (1) displacing anger and frustration that spill over from work; (2) consciously or unconsciously setting up a psychological fence around himself as he approaches home that shuts out not only his children but also his wife; (3) acting in accordance with a model of relationship behavior internalized when he was growing up (e.g., his father acted that way, or he thought that his father should have come home and "taken charge"); (4) acting in accordance with a cultural pattern in which "macho" male behavior is enhanced and held up as an ideal type of behavior; and (5) influenced by combinations of the foregoing.

In this example, the immediate task for the therapist is to focus on the most likely path to follow in order to obtain clarification and then to move the spotlight so that it shines on the question, "What are the basic issues for the marriage and the family in the problematic behavior?"

Tactically, one may start by offering or seeking understanding of the man's job and by establishing a beachhead of sympathetic rapproachment with both the husband and the wife. Similarly, if that is the case, the therapist can further establish with the man that he does not wish to continue a relationship with his children in which there is estrangement; angry, hostile behavior; or hurt feelings prevailing between himself and them. The therapist does this with the awareness that there may be other issues involved, for example, a need on the part of the wife to maintain a fence or a cloud of confusion between herself and her husband through the hostile and confused interaction with the children. That can be kept in mind by the therapist but not necessarily noted explicitly or mentioned to the clients. As conditions for change are created on the part of the husband, the therapist can begin to help the wife diminish her reluctance to change. This generally will involve doing some work with the family-of-origin issues that are carrying over into the marriage and contributing to the present problems. Frequently, exploring with the wife in a hypothetical way what it would require from her if her husband changed his behavior opens the way for understanding and acknowledgment that getting close is not easy for the couple, and that they do have some problems as a couple in getting close.

Although the therapist could assess the state of the ego of each of the partners in an extended assessment approach, such tactics generally are not as productive as moving in to help them experience closeness to the degree that they are able to handle intimacy. The clinician does need to be able to assess the nature of the partners' anxiety about closeness, including the rigidity or permeability of their personal boundaries. For example, if there is strong anxiety about being swallowed up in relationships or fears about one's own solidity and separateness (as in schizophrenic or border-line personalities) the boundaries constructed by the person will be rigid, in an attempt to keep out what is perceived as external danger. The firmer the sense of self and the more internally secure about selfhood a person is, the more freely he or she may be to relate to others in an intimate manner and to allow the existence of permeability in relationship boundaries.

Kris's (1934) concept of regression in the service of the ego may help the clinician to work with the intimacy problems of couples. It also may assist the marital partners themselves to become more comfortable with the idea of risking. Such regression is temporary and is allowed for purposes of pleasure and growth. The idea that one can temporarily regress, as in play or in sex, and then move back to a position of rational behavior and control is one that many individuals can comprehend. With some clients, there may be unconscious fears that prevent such regression.

In addition to Berman and Lief's constructs, the five "C's" of the marital life cycle also provide important assistance in the marital assessment process.

Commitment

Marriage is the sole voluntary relationship in the family, and therefore the most fragile. The partners can, of course, decide to leave the relationship and divorce, a possibility that probably is considered by the majority of individuals at some time in their marriage. As an heuristic device, it is useful to think in terms of persons being either preambivalent, ambivalent, or postambivalent in their commitment to the marriage. The first of these, the preambivalent stage, is found with individuals who have not seriously struggled with the question of getting out of the marriage. Their earlier positive feelings about the marriage have not been sufficiently disturbed to cause them to give serious consideration to ending the relationship. Hence, they assume that it will continue. With some persons, this stance takes the form of denial. They are, in other words, positively committed and have not significantly questioned the relationship, even though there may have been serious adjustment problems.

Ambivalent individuals look toward the mate and the marriage with a mixture of positive and negative feelings, often genuine love–hate mixtures, and move back and forth between the two extremes. Large numbers of our clients fit into this category. Some make the decision to leave the marriage as a means of breaking out of the tension that grips them.

The postambivalent stage is found among those who have seriously questioned whether they wish to remain in the marriage and have resolved their feelings one way or the other. Those who are postambivalent–positive have decided on staying. Those who are postambivalent–negative have decided to leave the marriage, a fact that they may or may not have communicated to their spouse. In some instances, if they have attempted to convey their decision, the mate may not have been willing or able to receive the message.

Some typical patterns with regard to commitment include the following:

- *Mr. and Mrs. Donald.* She was committed to the marriage, had not seriously considered leaving the relationship (preambivalent). She was unaware that her husband was ambivalent and was moving toward making a definitive decision regarding his continuation in the marriage (postambivalent).
- *Mr. and Mrs. Sloane.* Months of hard work in marital therapy could not get them off dead center (both ambivalent). Mrs. Sloane finally filed for a divorce, saying that she needed to get on with her life. While working as a paralegal, she began going to law school at night. Eventually she earned a law degree and began a new career.
- *Mr. and Mrs. Harold.* He had essentially made a decision against continuing the marriage but had not completely reached that stage (postambivalent–negative). She was somewhere between being naively committed to the marriage (preambivalent) and undecided about it (ambivalent), and was being pulled away from her unquestioning commitment by his ambivalence and his budding wishes to get out of the marriage.
- *Mr. and Mrs. Charles.* She had definitely decided to get out of the marriage (postambivalent–negative). He was undecided (ambivalent) and attempting to be unquestioningly committed (preambivalent). Individual divorce counseling or therapy was recommended for each of them, along with attention to completing the emotional detachment on his part.
- *Mr. and Mrs. Daniels.* Both were unquestioningly loyal to the relationship (preambivalent) and planned to stay in the marriage, but wished to make some changes. This was the basis for conjoint work with an essentially normal couple who manifested no obvious symptomatology other than garden variety adjustment problems.

What kind and level of commitment to the other do the partners have? What commitment to being married? Do they intend to remain in the marriage? Is there enough commitment to give the therapist something to work with, to provide a basis for marital therapy? How does the clinician find out where the partners are with regard to their commitment to being married and with regard to their willingness to work on their marriage and to change personally? The following suggestions are offered:

1. Explore with them their feelings and assess their motivation as well as possible from both what they say and what they do. This involves assessing the object relations capacities of each partner, for example, the emotional bases on which they need the other person and the level of maturity in their object choice, including their ability to give emotionally to their mate.

2. Ask them in a separate individual session where they stand, feed back to them the therapist's impressions of where they seem to be at the present in their commitment and where they seem to be heading, and subsequently secure their reactions to those impressions.

3. Ask them together about their commitments. There are contraindications to this approach, such as the obvious inability of one partner to accept an ambivalent or postambivalent statement by the other, and the therapist's need to gain some time for the strengthening of the dependent partner or for more complete and extensive examination of the stance of the partner who is considering leaving the relationship.

4. Share one's impressions with the partners together and get their reactions to the impressions and analysis of them and their situation. This can include as much straightforward explanation of an assessment on the matter of commitment as the marital partners seem able to absorb. (The issue of secrets will be discussed subsequently.)

5. Observe what the partners do after the therapist has given observations/recommendations regarding their needs and therapy. (Needs may include practical steps that may be indicated and/or recommended to them regarding seeking legal advice and other practical matters.)

6. Push on the emotional boundaries of their relationship by raising in a casual and yet sensitive manner issues that would challenge or threaten the protective collusion; for example, "Have you seriously considered or talked about separation?" Observe how they respond to such questions and pushing.

Sometimes, a firm determination of their commitment to marriage or to marital and personal change cannot be made until after marital therapy has begun and the partners have attempted to change.

Caring

This is another significant component of the assessment, caring is the ability to lay aside one's concern with oneself and to be concerned with the welfare of the partner. How much does each partner care about the other? This question can be asked in either conjoint or individual sessions. It generally is a better question to ask than whether they love their spouse. "Care" or "caring" is used here rather than "love" because care is an emotionally laden term, but it does not carry the prevalent ideology about love: "I don't love him or her any longer and, hence, there's no reason to stay married." In marriages of relatively short duration, this kind of thinking emerges at the time in which the initial idealization of the mate has given way in the face of the onslaught of reality testing in close, everyday living.

Are the partners capable of dealing with each other on a mutual, reciprocal basis? What degree of mutuality exists between them? Do they value their mate primarily as someone who can gratify their wishes and serve their needs? Or do they value the spouse for him- or herself alone, apart from their own needs or desires? Do they see the partner as a "service station?" In object relations terms, are they functioning primarily at some point in the need-gratification stage in which "the need is primary and the other person exists only to serve it?" (Blanck & Blanck, 1968, p. 70). At the need-gratification level, one partner can be exchanged for another fairly easily if the partner does not gratify or fulfill one's needs. Or are they at the level of object constancy or object love, so that they see the partner as a loved object whether or not he or she is fulfilling a particular need or desire at a given time?

Both levels of object relations represent part of the ego functioning and development of the individual persons. There are various degrees to be found in both the need-gratification and the object constancy/object love levels. One partner may be at a more mature level than the other, that is, may be more able to share and to consider the mate's wishes and needs as well as his or her own. The difference in maturity between the partners may be a significant factor in the prognosis for the individual and for the marriage.

The major point here is that caring is related to the level of object relations development attained by the individuals in the marriage, and that the degree and kind of caring existing in the partners has major implications for the future of the therapy and the marriage. Such caring can be observed in nearly all of the partners' interactions and attitudes involving the other, from their division of roles to their sexual relationship. By definition, this kind of caring is not the same as the self-sacrificing found in codependency relationships in which one partner "parents" the other in ways that reinforce the other's immaturity and dependency.

Therapists cannot create caring, although they can help one or both of the partners to clear away some of the barriers to caring for their mate. Such barriers include poor communication, difficulties in dealing with differences, faulty "contracts," apprehensions regarding risking oneself in a relationship, and various unresolved traumata.

Communication

During the early phase of treatment, therapists generally move beyond dealing as explicitly with the commitment and caring components of the marital relationship as they did during the assessment/engagement phase. This occurs after an assessment of commitment and caring have been determined to be strong enough to provide a realistic level of optimism and a positive prognosis for the couple. Although those components continue to be of concern in therapy, two more components—communication and conflict/compromise—now move to center stage. During the middle phase of treatment, and especially during the time that we are seeking to repair, restore, or establish adequate communication between the partners, we can use virtually everything that we have ever learned about communication. We can clarify, offer feedback, make observations, interpret not only the message that one partner is beaming to the other but also the intentions of each partner as we can understand them. Serving as a mediator or go-between who persuades each as legitimately as possible of the benign intentions of the other, we try to remove barriers and permit the flow of communication to be as clear as possible.

Combining the study of marital communication and decision making by married couples, Thomas (1977) has devised step-by-step procedures for the assessment and modification of problems in both the communication and decision-making areas. There are self-help materials available, such as the 20 rules devised by Wahlroos (1974) and the popular work of Miller and associates (S. Miller, Wackman, Nunnally, & Saline, 1982). Miller and associates provide a practical couples communication program that has been taught to thousands of couples over the past 25 years. The "four fears" that they help persons to face—the fear of speaking out, the fear of fighting, the fear of intimacy, and the fear of commitment—are quite compatible with ideas expressed in this book. In broad terms, they deal with the following:

- *The style and substance of communication.* This includes attention to several kinds of style (e.g., small talk, control talk, and search talk), becoming aware of one's "inner you" and acting on that awareness, engaging in straight talk, and matching style to situation.

- *The skills "to say what you really mean."* This includes sending straight talk messages, listening attentively, attending to style, building esteem (I count me/I count you), discovering the roots of conflict, and reaching creative solution through talking out problems.
- *Connecting.* This focuses on connecting in bed, connecting with kids, and connecting with work.

As husband and wife begin to communicate more effectively, it may become evident that communication is no panacea. The partners may start to communicate clearly and find that, as they understand the other, they disagree profoundly. Also, clearing up communication may reveal the presence of deeper levels of wishes and needs that are discrepant with the partners' ability to respond. Our efforts to help the mates improve their communication may get us into the area of conflict/compromise.

Conflict/Compromise

As better communication uncovers differences, the issue becomes that of how the partners deal with those revealed differences. The differences may include not only their variant values and discordant ideologies but also their discrepant relationship wishes and needs. George may really wish to be primarily and essentially dependent on Mary, while she wishes him to be more independent.

The therapist's first task here is to observe and understand how the clients respond to conflict and differences as they emerge. Does the appearance of conflict frighten the couple? Often it does. Hence, the immediate need may be to help them become more comfortable with the fact that differences exist in all marital relationships. How therapists deal with such matters depends in large measure on their assessment of the situation. How have the clients responded to differences and conflict throughout their life cycles? How have they dealt with conflict with persons intimately related to them? Can the partners be helped to face the issues directly? Must they be helped first to establish patterns of trust in less conflicted areas?

There are several important facets to dealing with conflicts and obtaining the compromises necessary to secure accommodation or resolution. The first is usually the removal of major amounts of fear and anxiety in connection with the presence of differences. Another involves deciding how the particular problems that they are facing can be resolved, or if they can be resolved. Frequently, it is helpful to explore the problems patiently and in detail, delineating differences as well as agreements between the partners and examining how one or both of them may change in order to obtain a workable degree of agreement and possible harmony. Sometimes, marital contracts or agreements can be used productively in dealing with differences. However, beginning therapists need to recognize that such contracting should not be undertaken while differences are still obscured. Premature introduction of marital contracts may not only lead to failure because of sabotage by one or both of the spouses but also it may inhibit crucial system and relationship growth.

During this stage, treatment often seems to take three steps forward and one backward. A therapist may need to work doggedly and determinedly to help marital partners deal one by one with the issues that are raised. Often it is not only a question of reworking and resolving old problems and hurts, but also of helping the couple reach a level of functioning that opens the possibilities for new ways of relating. As new ground is broken, new anxieties and new fears may arise.

Once the therapist and clients are solidly working on such issues as communication and conflict/compromise, therapy has moved into the middle phase. This presumes that the therapist has been able to secure a sound working alliance with the clients. During the middle phase, things typically go more smoothly in that the clients know what to expect, have moved past some of their earlier and more noxious anxiety, and are more likely to come to appointments ready to work productively than they were at the beginning. Nevertheless, in some cases the therapist may still be dealing with a client situation that moves back and forth between eruptions of anger and misunderstanding on the one hand and greater understanding and competence and the consolidation of therapeutic gains on the other.

Sometimes, it may appear that a stage of productive working has been reached when, in fact, it has not. For example, Mr. and Mrs. Jerry went through a series of hysterical scenes both in the therapist's office and in their life outside during the early period of attempted conjoint marital therapy. The therapist finally was able to get them past the point of exploding in anger about unresolved conflicts from the past. By that time, the wife was ready to work on reestablishing their relationship and so, ostensibly, was the husband. Presumably, each of them was committed to working on the marriage and committed to the treatment process. However, every time something was worked out, some concession made by the wife or some overture of affection or conciliation made by her, the husband would become evasive so that they got no closer together than they had been previously. It soon emerged that he had not terminated his extramarital affair, as he had sworn he would, and that he was doing a number of other things that were counterproductive to the development of a workable marriage. In brief, he was trying to hold on to a life pattern that was very disturbing to his wife and to maintain the marriage at the same time. A part of himself certainly did not wish to make the marriage work on her terms of fidelity, and wished her to know that he was having an affair. Evidently, he had been going along in an effort to see if he could work things out so that his wife would tolerate his extramarital liaisons while he tried to buy time to get some of his considerable financial assets concealed in case there was a divorce. When his wife finally saw what he was really like in contrast to the idealized version of him that she had maintained over the years, she moved ahead with divorce action, extricating herself from a relationship that had long been a mixed blessing for her. This case provides an example of a marital situation that required therapy efforts and the passage of time before it was possible to ascertain the truth about the marriage. Until that point, no firm prognosis was possible.

In this case the therapist and the couple got through the anxiety and parameter-establishing phases, but they were not able to work on longer-term and more serious issues after the couple had settled down in treatment. It was not possible to get a solid working alliance with the husband because his personality organization and character structure would not permit it.

Contracts and Complementarity

Both in commitment and in caring, one of the major factors in the creation of discord is the amount of discrepancy between the positions or expectations of the partners. A number of clinicians (e.g., Kubie, 1956; Martin, 1976; Sager, 1976) have emphasized the problems arising from differences between the conscious, attainable expectations and the unconscious, unattainable expectations of marital partners. Sager (1976) in particular has affirmed the importance of expectations, as noted above, indicating that people who are marrying feel that they have the equivalent of a contract with the spouse that he or she will meet their expectations. Martin (1976) similarly has said that marital disharmony results when one of the mates fails to honor the contract because of either inability or lack of willingness to do so.

Marriages sometimes hold together with minimal discord and minimal caring because the expectations regarding what each of the partners is to do personally for the other are low. This can be found in marital relationships in which there is permissive extramarital involvement and marital stability at the same time. The amount of "fit" between the expectations of the partners in several areas such as affection, power distribution, and leadership is a major factor in the degree of satisfaction and, often, of stability in the relationship. Discord following marriage frequently comes from differential growth rates. This has been called "the most common toxic process in marital disharmony" (Martin, 1976, p. 63).

It is exceedingly important for the therapist to learn something about the complementarity of the spouses, that is, how they are matched, how well they fit together, and where changes have taken place over time in their marriage. If they are mismated, were they mismated at the beginning, or did it occur later? If they consider themselves mismated currently, to what extent does each feel that this is the case? The therapist's own assessment of how well the partners were matched and where the difficulties lie may differ from that of the clients, but that becomes a matter for future consideration in therapy. Clients act on the basis of their own, not the therapist's, perceptions, feelings, and reactions to events and processes in their relationship.

The major question, of course, for the therapist and the couple is not necessarily how the process of developmental mismating has come to pass—"schismogenesis," as Bateson (1972) termed such processes—but whether or not a workable balance can be reestablished between the marital partners. The issue of whether a new balance or a new complementarity can be established often is one of the major problems with which the therapist must grapple during marital therapy.

Midwiving the Relationship

"Midwiving the relationship" is a descriptive term covering a variety of sensitive and often subtle techniques, interventions, and other actions and stances taken by the therapist in order to help the marital partners attempt the following:

1. Discern what they are seeking from the partner.
2. Resolve their ambivalence about whether they wish to be in the relationship.
3. Reduce their destructive interactions.
4. Improve their communication.
5. Elucidate their differences and effect viable compromises and accommodations.
6. Either establish a workable marital relationship or consider getting get out of the relationship in as nondestructive a way as possible.

"Midwiving the relationship" is a more inclusive term than one referring only to techniques or strategies. It refers also to attitudes and a general atmosphere of warmth and support maintained by the therapist.

One does serve as a go-between, as Zuk (1976) has indicated one can do in family therapy, while remaining in control of the sessions. Being a manager and staying in control are essential to any form of therapy, but particularly in any kind of systems therapy. Beyond this, however, we use the term "midwiving" to indicate that the therapist who performs the task of maintaining a growth-producing, reconciling, and problem-solving atmosphere skillfully must deal intelligently and sensitively with the needs and personalities of both partners as well as with the marital subsystem.

Once the therapist has determined that the couple has the ability and wish to continue the marriage, midwiving a relationship includes urging the spouses to take certain steps toward enhancing and deepening the relationship. This may include such direct interventions as asking one of the partners in a conjoint session how he or she feels about the other and then patiently and supportively leading that person to communicate his or her feelings to the spouse. For example, a client will sometimes finally tell the therapist that he or she loves the spouse. The therapist may respond, "Then, why don't you tell her (or him) right now how you feel?" Such apparently simple techniques, used with appropriate timing, enable the spouse to reveal him- or herself and to risk being rejected or accepted by the partner in a relatively safe environment. Obviously, it is important for the therapist to be able to know when to be warm and accepting, when to be tender, and when to be bold.

Mr. and Mrs. George, for example, were slowly reestablishing a relationship after an exceedingly bitter estrangement. The husband indicated in one session that he had come in with the intention of asking his wife to accompany him to a significant political event the following week. But, he said, he was not extending the invitation because of something that she had done in that therapy hour. Having time to do so, the therapist decided to extend the hour and to see if it would be possible to get them to go to the gathering together. It would be significant in many ways, including the fact that it would be a symbolic statement to many of their friends and acquaintances that they were reconciling after a publicly messy separation of several years duration. First, the therapist helped the husband to "get out of the corner" and to extend his invitation, while pointing out to Mrs. George what a gift and piece of volunteering behavior the invitation would be on the husband's part. Then it was necessary to discuss with both of them the meaning of their public appearance together. It was particularly impor-tant to point out to Mrs. George that she could survive some possible embarrassment and apprehensive feelings at the prospect of facing friends and acquaintances at the gathering. By this time in the session, the husband was helping the therapist to convince the wife that those present probably were not all that concerned with spending the evening gossiping about the Georges' reconciliation. Therapy then was focused on dealing with some of her fears about public gatherings, which dated from her adolescence. The therapist finally said, "I'm going to do something that you know is very unusual for me to do, and that's to urge you to go. If it turns out badly, Mrs. George, you can come in next week and call me whatever you like, and I'll take it as my due." A little later, Mrs. George turned to her husband and said, "I'd be honored to go with you." The session ended there, and the couple embraced and left in a close, tender mood. They ended up going not to one but three political gatherings in the next week. Subsequently, Mrs. George engaged in some very important giving and volunteering behavior, offering to help her husband with a major business problem, an action that made him feel deeply touched and appreciative.

A "Pollyanna" tactic may be another aspect of midwiving a relationship. It also can be called "accentuating the positive" or "reframing." In this context, it means that the therapist helps the couple to recognize the positive thing or things they have done, rather than to permit them to seize on and magnify their failures to do things perfectly. This is part of the therapist's efforts to try to help clients avoid self-defeating actions as much as possible and to recognize realistically what they have done that is successful. Instead of letting them consider their efforts a total failure because they did not succeed in doing perfectly whatever they attempted, the therapist points out to them as realistically as possible what they have succeeded in doing, and labels that endeavor a successful effort. Sometimes, this refers primarily to the fact that they have tried to do something, that they have been willing and able to take an appropriate risk.

As indicated, midwiving also involves facilitating growth by providing a benign atmosphere and minimal interference. The therapist, on some occasions, primarily provides an understanding presence that enables and facilitates, instead of uncovering pathology or undoing old hurts. Mr. and Mrs. Daniel, for example, decided to keep coming in for assistance after they had worked through most of their worst marital tangles. They would come in every 3–4 months and talk as they seldom talked at home. They felt that the pattern of regularly scheduled appointments was necessary at that time in order to ensure that they continued to work at maintaining their improved communication and at obtaining greater flexibility and depth in their marriage. By the time that this way of dealing with things becomes the characteristic pattern of the sessions, the clients usually have reached the point at which they can consider termination. The therapist has almost succeeded in reaching the treatment goal of putting him- or herself out of a job.

Terminating the Therapy

A case involving a combination of therapeutic modes illustrates the closing phases of treatment. Mr. Chrysler was seen individually once a week at the beginning and subsequently every other week, and the partners were initially seen conjointly once a month and later were seen every other week. This case passed through most of the difficulties of the first phase of treatment mentioned earlier in the chapter and then settled into a middle phase that had its problems, its ups and downs. Several of the conjoint sessions were very tense hours, filled with recitations of arguments and confrontations in the everyday life of the couple, situations that were worked on and reworked in the treatment hours.

Mr. Chrysler was seen alone at first for several reasons. He had never communicated easily and had developed a number of patterns of relating and reacting that were causing him difficulty in interpersonal relationships. At the beginning, the therapist made the assessment that changes in Mr. Chrysler were the key to changes in the marriage. The man had the courage to accept the recommendations that were made about a combination of marital and individual therapy and committed himself rather wholeheartedly to treatment. It is unusual to have someone approach their problems with the problem-solving attitude of Mr. Chrysler. Both the client and the therapist worked very hard in the individual sessions and all three participants put a considerable amount of effort into the conjoint sessions as well. In the husband's individual hours, examination was made of how he dealt with other persons and with various situations not only in his marriage but also in his work life. A large part of the time was spent in dealing with family-of-origin issues, most of which he would not have been able to deal with at that time in the presence of his wife.

By the final phase of the combined therapy, the clients had resolved several of the issues alluded to above and had succeeded in coping with difficult situations. They now had a reservoir of success experiences that gave them confidence in their ability to face and deal with problems together. They were basically individuals of solid integrity and, hence, as their hostilities and anxieties receded, it became increasingly easy for them to trust what they had accomplished together. Both were at the object love/object constancy level of development, although he had regressed from it in some ways prior to entering treatment.

The decision to terminate with the Chryslers was reached in an ideal way. The therapist and the clients independently concluded that the time to stop was near. Mr. Chrysler mentioned it first in his individual hour, noting that he did not feel that he had much more to work on. The therapist agreed that he was doing well and added that the marital interaction also seemed to be going well and that it seemed time to consider termination. As things worked out, the couple went on vacation and had a period of approximately 3 weeks away from therapy before they came in for the next conjoint appointment. At the termination time, the wife confided to the therapist in her husband's presence, "I've never seen as much change in a person as I've seen in Jim. He's a much happier person." The session involved some conjoint exploration of what had brought the couple in originally and where they were in their relationship at the present time.

Change had occurred that both partners could see and assess for themselves. The therapist and clients looked at the changes and the fact that the clients felt that the changes would be durable and lasting, as well as at some of the things that had contributed to the alterations. It was noted by the therapist that there had been a tapering-off process in that the clients had been entirely on their own for 3 weeks and had had opportunity to test their new relationship. The brief period of "swimming for themselves" had worked well. Given other considerations, it was enough of a trial period for the therapist and clients to conclude that they were ready to terminate without additional sessions.

Several concepts discussed earlier—commitment, caring, communication, conflict/compromise, and contract, along with volunteering—provide a guide for both the therapist and the clients in assessing preparedness for ending therapy. (Volunteering refers to behaviors taken by a spouse on behalf of the other partner freely and without expectation of immediate benefit, simply because one wishes to do something that is helpful or pleasing to the partner.) These are used, of course, along with other criteria such as the amelioration or resolution of interactive problems and symptomatology. A brief depiction follows of the use of these concepts in the case example.

With the Chryslers, *commitment* to the marriage and to therapy was strong, and it increased during the course of treatment, especially after things moved out of the first phase. Mrs. Chrysler in particular had been ready to leave the marriage at the beginning if things did not improve, but her preference had been to stay in the relationship. *Caring* for each other was strong and solid. It was necessary to work through the hurts and to get past the defensiveness of each partner, but the quality of feelings was relatively benign underneath the exteriors that originally were alternately cold and stormy. One of the early things that was pointed out to the partners was that they were far from indifferent toward each other and that the relationship was troubled but still very much alive. Removing the barriers to the caring proceeded very well during therapy.

Communication was a major focus in the case. It was necessary to do a lot of interpretation and educational work with the husband in his individual sessions in order to help him function better in his work (a less threatening arena for him) and in his marriage. His increased ability to open up in his communication in his marriage—something that he tested out on the job and found worked well there—was the key to lifting Mrs. Chrysler's depression. His new communication skills paved the way to discuss their differences in ways that led to accommodation and to more dialogue that, in turn, led to deeper understanding and appreciation of each other's feelings. With regard to *conflict/compromise*, most of the backlog of problems that they brought into therapy were worked out and a functional pattern for dealing with differences and conflicts in general was established. During the course of therapy, additional conflicts arose and were adequately resolved. The Chryslers felt, as noted, confident enough about their ability to deal effectively with problems in the future. The couple's *contract* became clear and was agreed to by both partners.

Volunteering, a major sign of a mature relationship, began to be a significant part of their relationship. In reality, they had resumed some of the volunteering behavior that had been present in their marriage before things had knotted up and become unsatisfactory. Volunteering, a kind of behavior that goes beyond the quid pro quo or "I'll do this if you'll do that" kind of interaction, means that the spouses act for at least a good part of the time in relatively nondefensive ways. The Chryslers did that; they were able to stick out their necks and risk being misunderstood, rejected, or unrewarded and to continue volunteering until it once again became a part of their life pattern together.

Confidentiality and Secrets

What is the therapist to do with material that one partner reveals that presumably is unknown to the other partner? Some therapists avoid such dilemmas by dealing with the partners only in conjoint sessions or by stating at the outset that there are no secrets, that whatever is communicated by either spouse belongs in the therapeutic arena to be shared with all three parties, husband, wife, and therapist.

Another approach involves handling each case on its own merits and making decisions in terms of the best judgment of the therapist. An ongoing extramarital affair might be treated differently, for example, from a one-night stand of several years ago. Among the pertinent questions are the following: As best the therapist can determine, what is to be gained by exposure of the secret, by the sharing of it with the other partner? Does the second partner *really* already know or strongly suspect the secret? Does the second partner manifest a desire to know or not to know the secret? Does hearing the secret compromise the therapist and pull him or her into an ongoing conspiracy with the partner who has revealed the secret? Such questions are not easily answered or handled.

A third approach that is successful for some therapists is to offer a conditional confidentiality to each spouse. This means saying to them that the therapist will not report issues or information gained in individual sessions (or via the telephone) to the second spouse in conjoint sessions. However, if an issue emerges that would directly inhibit or jeopardize the therapy process, the therapist and the reporting spouse must deal with it together and achieve some resolution. In the case of an extramarital affair, for example, the resolution may include agreement by the involved spouse to suspend the affair while the marital therapy proceeds. If the secret is a family-of-origin matter that is not known by the second spouse, resolution may involve an agreement to report the secret in a conjoint meeting so that it can be addressed by both partners with the therapist.

Keeping individual sessions confidential in this way can be precarious but often the early data that are obtained under such a framework can outweigh the therapist's concern by providing for a much more rapid elucidation of issues than would otherwise be possible. An example would be a postambivalent–negative spouse who is involved in a serious extramarital relationship but cannot move to end the marriage. Processing such data in the second hour of therapy can save the therapist from struggling for weeks with the couple in treatment and not being certain why there are difficulties with commitment and therapeutic movement.

The therapist is not in a position to keep confidential all information given by clients individually. Increasingly, therapists are being held accountable and liable if they do not warn a potential victim of threats made by their clients. Similarly, legal and ethical constraints require that therapists report to appropriate authorities knowledge of such illegal activities as homicide and, in some cases, child or spouse abuse.

The Sexual Relationship

Sexual relating, including sexual satisfaction and sexual problems, may or may not be a significant part of a particular marital therapy case. Although some exploring of the sexual relationship is part of the initial assessment, it generally is not necessary to take formal sexual histories or to focus specifically on the sexual area unless it is problematic. Generally, the sexual relationship is a fairly valid barometer of the quality of relatedness and satisfaction for many married persons. Nevertheless, couples who manifest a considerable amount of difficulty and discord in their relationship do not automatically encounter sexual problems. In fact, some experience dissatisfaction and discord in other parts of their relationship and still indicate that they are quite satisfied with their sexual life. At the same time, sexual problems seldom appear to be a major source of difficulty without reflecting problems in other parts of the couples' life and relationship.

Although there are many good sources available on human sexuality and human sexual behavior, Helen Singer Kaplan's three volumes, *The New Sex Therapy: Active Treatment of Sexual Dysfunction* (1974), *The New Sex Therapy, Volume II: Disorders of Sexual Desire and Other New Concepts and Techniques in Sex Therapy* (1979), and *Sexual Aversions, Sexual Phobias, and Panic Disorder* (1987), generally are acknowledged to be the best resources for the clinician who seeks well-researched information.

Sex therapy traditionally has been regarded as a specialized area and not as part of marital therapy as such. Most marital and family therapists probably deal with sexual problems in marital therapy but primarily in terms of how they fit into the marital relationship and the general marital subsystem. A major step toward bringing together marital therapy and a Masters-and-Johnson-oriented sex therapy approach has been made by David Schnarch. A massive amount of substantive material and treatment description are included in Schnarch's (1991) *Constructing the Sexual Crucible: An Integration of Sexual and Marital Therapy*. The reader is referred to that volume as well as to the Kaplan sources.

7

THERAPY WITH
EXPANDING FAMILIES

The dreams of childhood—its fairy fables; its graceful, beautiful,
humane, impossible adornments of the world beyond: so good
to be believed in once, so good to be outgrown.
—CHARLES DICKENS, *Hard Times*

This period begins with the birth of the first child and lasts until the last
child leaves home. For families not altered by divorce or death, the
period of family life from expansion to launching typically begins when
the partners are in their middle to late 20s or early 30s and lasts until
their middle adulthood. Beginning with the first child, the nuclear family
expands so long as children are coming and then has a period of
consolidation before the launching of the children into the outside world
begins. As the children begin to depart, the nuclear family begins the
process of contraction that continues until death eventually takes the
partners and marks the end of that unit in the family chain. The
children's development and that of other members of both the nuclear
and the extended family—the families of origin of their parents—are
tied together in what can be described as a "cogwheeling of generations."

From a family transactional point of view, change in parts of the
family system, such as alteration in the parent–child subsystem or the

marital subsystem, can result in shifts that affect the entire family system. Functioning in one part affects other parts, functioning in the whole affects the parts, and functioning in one part may affect the whole system. For the stage of the family life cycle addressed in this chapter, the following questions (adapted from Rosman, 1986) are important:

- How does the developing child affect the family system?
- How does the family context (its organization and functioning) affect the child's development and functioning?
- How does the development of individual members affect the family system and, therefore, the development of all the family members?

The expansion stage of the family life cycle (see Table 7.1) involves a significant increase in the complexity of life in the home. Five types of life cycles are involved: the family life cycle, the marital life cycle, the adult individual life cycle (for each of the adults), the child individual life cycle (for the new infant/child), and the family life cycle of the families of origin of each of the marital partners in this family (the older generation's life cycle). Each time an additional child becomes part of the new family, another life cycle adds to the mix and the family's complexity.

Table 7.1. The Family Life Cycle, Stage 2–Expansion: Parental Beginnings and Subsequent Years

Family developmental tasks of the expansion stage

1. Incorporating new family members appropriately: Making room for an addition(s) and adjusting to the realities of being part of a new nuclear family and not simply a couple (see parental tasks in the marital life cycle, Stage 2).
2. Providing for the physical and economic needs of family members.
3. Establishing and maintaining socially acceptable ways of interacting, communicating, expressing sexuality, and providing for the primary emotional and developmental needs of family members: Balancing the differing developmental needs of family members.
4. Providing for the socialization of the members into their family roles: Learning to fulfill parental roles as a couple (see parental tasks in the marital life cycle, Stage 2), providing for inclusion of grandparenting roles, and guiding child/children's learning of family rules, roles, and expectations. Appropriately facilitating and supporting family members' socialization by external agencies: Encouraging and supporting child/children's development of learning abilities and educational competence.
5. Affiliating satisfactorily with the extended family and the kinship and friendship networks.

ENTERING PARENTHOOD

Generativity

Although marriage today is occurring later than formerly and parenthood is being postponed in many cases, having a child typically becomes part of most marital partners' life experience during their 20s or early 30s. Therefore, at the same time that young adults are concerned with intimacy, power, and other issues in the marriage (see Table 7.2) and their individual life, they are also, in Erikson's framework, dealing with the individual struggle of generativity. Primarily, generativity has to do with one's concern for establishing the next generation (Erikson, 1950). This is the side of parenthood that has to do with caring for the offspring rather than merely being identified as a parent. Parenthood has, along with its pain and toil, the potential to help men and women tap into growth-producing

TABLE 7.2. The Marital Life Cycle

Settling into the marriage, rerelating to own parents, and taking a new place in extended family networks as a couple. (Floating task of reworking authority/power relationship with own parents.)

Core tasks

Commitment
Deepening internal loyalties.
Dealing with external attractions and threats.
Dealing with internal threats, including possible discovery of original
   or subsequent mismating.

Caring
Reworking caring definitions and meanings.

Communication
Enlargement of range and depth of communication.

Conflict/compromise
Dealing with "floating" marital task of rebalancing the power relationship
   in marriage due to shifting of roles.

Contract
Reworking the coexecutive relationship.

Parental tasks

(As related to or influencing marital life cycle)

Childrearing
Making room for an addition and adjusting to the realities of being part
   of a new nuclear family and not simply a couple.
Learning to fulfill parental roles as a couple.

experiences and activities that are not likely to be found elsewhere in their lives.

Generativity is not the property of one sex or the other. Rather, it is an experience that can be enjoyed by both parents and may be crucial to the maintenance of marital satisfaction. In current North American society, however, there is an underinvolvement of many fathers in the experiences and processes of childrearing, leading to divergent developmental paths for fathers and mothers that can leave them in different developmental positions (Hawkins, Christensen, Sargent, & Hill, 1993). To the extent that men are underinvolved in the socialization and caring activities with their children, they not only are shortchanged on this dimension of growth in their own personalities, but this underinvolvement also tends to affect their marriage negatively. The trend that started in the 1960s for men to be more involved emotionally and practically as parents is changing the picture to some extent. Clinicians cannot predict how men will be involved in parenting nearly so easily as they could three decades or so ago. Reactions against placing career and commitment to one's employer first and opting for "quality of life" on the part of many men help to make the picture more complex than it was during the era of the Great Depression, World War II, and the early postwar period.

Adjustment Issues

The birth of the first child transforms the relationship of the couple from dyadic to triadic in nature, from a twosome to a threesome. It was once characterized as a crisis (LeMasters, 1957), but more recent family scholars have referred to the birth of the first child less spectacularly as constituting a time of transition in the life of the couple (Rossi, 1966; Hobbs & Cole, 1976).

Childbearing, which ushers in a period of childrearing covering approximately one-half of the family life cycle (McGoldrick, 1980), does bring new adjustment problems for the couple. Advice long given to young couples to have a baby in order to help them cement their marriage or otherwise cope with adjustment problems flies in the face of research which shows that the addition of a child brings more, not fewer, coping issues and stress. The childbearing and childrearing years are the times in which couples have reported low levels of marital satisfaction, for example.

Research in the 1960s and 1970s found marital satisfaction highest in the early stages of marriage, before the addition of children (Campbell, 1975); dipping with the advent of children; and rising again after the children departed (Rollins & Feldman, 1970). More recent research has emphasized the influence of multiple factors (Belsky & Rovine, 1990) in the changes in marital relationships during the transition to parenthood. These include the partners' family-of-origin experiences (Lane, Wilcoxson, & Cecil, 1988), prior marital adjustment, and perceived parenting stress (Wallace & Gotlieb, 1990), not simply the addition of a child.

From clinical experience, Bradt (1988) concludes that no stage brings more change or challenge to both the nuclear and the extended family than the addition of a new child. He emphasizes that marriage with children generates a "collision of paradigms" between the attitudes and beliefs of men and women, as well as those of older generations and the work world. This collision includes clashes regarding the belief in sexual equality, the egalitarian marriage, cultural norms and attitudes, social policies on working families with dependent children, and the balance of home life and work life (p. 237).

Clinicians need to give careful and sensitive attention to the differential meanings of the transition for women and men. Similarly, differences in marital satisfaction between women and men warrant more consideration than they generally receive (Kazak, Jarmas, & Snitzer, 1988). More than two decades ago, Bernard (1972) pointed out differences in marriage between men and women, graphically noting that there are two marriages, his and hers, and concluding that "hers makes her sick."

Readiness for Parenthood

Some research has bolstered the common clinical impression that the important question is not whether the child comes early or late, but the quality of the readiness of the husband and wife for the experience of parenthood (Daniels & Weingarten, 1982). Adequate separation from one's family of origin, possession of a clear sense of identity, and establishment of a strong relationship of intimacy with one's mate are important ingredients in readiness for parenthood.

The partners need to establish and maintain clear and firm generational boundaries in order to rear children adequately and to produce healthy relationships and appropriate autonomy in their offspring. The maintenance of boundaries is not an easily accomplished matter. For the couple in their late 20s and early 30s, there may be temporary disruptions in the marital boundaries while the partners seek to make up their minds about each other, vie for power and dominance, or, perhaps, become restless and suffer a commitment crisis (Berman & Lief, 1975).

Decision making about having a child may follow any of several paths, from not making a conscious decision to deciding not to have

168   EVALUATION AND TREATMENT

children at all. Some partners simply "let nature take its course." Others
defer childbearing for a variety of reasons. The major difficulties between
the partners are likely to come when they have different expectations or
wishes. For example, one wishes to have a child later or not at all and the
other desires to have a child as soon as possible. Similarly, problems arise
when there is poor communication or no communication between the
spouses about their wishes, and the issue is not clarified.

At any given time in the United States, an estimated 15% of married
couples in the childbearing years have fertility problems, the great majority
of which have a physical basis (Daniels & Weingarten, 1982). Among
those who are childless, a small number, which is difficult to ascertain
precisely, are voluntarily childless. Professional literature has given an
increasing amount of attention to those married persons who do not wish
to have children (e.g., Veevers, 1973, 1974, 1975), as have popular writers
(Peck, 1971; Silverman & Silverman, 1971). Pressure to have children has
lessened, but certainly has not disappeared. A recent study comparing
voluntarily childfree adults with parents, for example, found the childfree
men and women feeling significantly more negatively stereotyped by their
relatives than the parents. The childfree women particularly were negatively affected in comparison to the parental women (Somers, 1993).

Clinicians need to pay more attention to the feelings of both partners
about having or not having children. Feelings of stigma, particularly those
of blame for not having children or having too many and reactions of
resentment about being stigmatized, can play significant roles in marital
and individual adjustment.

Reactions to the birth of a child may need to be explored with a couple
prior to the birth of the child. Sometimes, later difficulties in marital or
personal adjustment that contribute to family problems may be traced
back to dislocations in the family system that occurred at the time of the
birth of a child. Such dislocations as the need for the spouses to give time
and attention to the new infant/child at some cost to their marital
relationship or personal time may go largely unexamined at the time, but
surface later as sources of unresolved problems.

Many reactions can be felt by either the mother or the father with
regard to the birth of a child. Particularly if the child is unwanted or is
obviously physically damaged, there may be denial, embarrassment, guilt,
failure feelings, or grief. In subsequent years, reactions of overprotection,
scapegoating, or even emotional and physical abuse may be forthcoming
toward a damaged or disabled child (Tymchuk, 1979). Even among
parents of presumably desired and healthy babies, reactions of anxiety in
mild to moderate forms are not uncommon.

Both parents tend to view the birth of subsequent children differently
from the arrival of the first. Common observation shows that a couple

may not be ready for a second child, or may be upset by the arrival of a child after having thought that their family was complete. Just as the addition of the first baby may put a strain on a marital relationship, so may the advent of a second, third, or subsequent youngster. An insecure husband, for example, may be able to cope reasonably well with the addition of the first child. However, he may be unable to share any more of his parentified wife with a second child and may begin to exhibit symptomatic behavior that may or may not fracture the marriage. A number of factors typically enter into how the newborn's addition to the marital or family unit affects the husband and wife.

Obviously important to the family are reactions of the child or children already present to the arrival of a sibling. Much of the parenting material in the popular pediatric materials and mass circulation magazines is devoted to helping young parents find ways of making the experience an acceptable and nontraumatic one for the children already in the family. Preparation of the child and such actions as bringing the child a gift from the new sibling are common parts of this picture. As Toman (1993) has pointed out from his extensive research into family constellations, attitudes toward the arrival of a sibling may vary according to the number of years between the siblings, the sex of the newcomer, the number of children already present, and the position of the child already present. These attitudes and affects emerge and change over the years. Sibling relationships are just beginning to be studied seriously on a significant scale with respect to the lifelong impact that such connections have among brothers and sisters (Bank & Kahn, 1982).

According to Toman, the age difference between the children tends to produce some definite patterns of reaction. If the baby arrives only 1 or 2 years after the older child, the older typically sees the sibling as a rival for the affection, care, and attention of the parents. If the second child comes 3 or 4 years after the first, the older seems to be less threatened in his power and control over the parents. If the older child is 4 or 5 by the time the baby makes its advent, the older youngster generally has learned how to respond to the different sexes, and the reactions depend in large measure on the gender of the baby. In brief, the older child tends to be considerably more secure by this time in its life (Toman, 1993).

Family balance is affected by the gender of the new arrival; a family of two males and two females generally functions more smoothly than one in which there are three members of one sex and one of the other. In the latter case, the older child, aware that his or her role as the youngest is over, is likely to seek the affection and attention of the parents more strongly. If the age difference between the children is 6 years or more, they belong, in my terms, to different generations. The older child is hardly affected by the younger. As a general rule, a small age difference tends to pull siblings more strongly together (Toman, 1993) and may create more rivalry.

Toman's research is an excellent resource not only for understanding the meaning of new arrivals but also for comprehending many other feelings, attitudes, and behaviors that stem from the particular ways in which families are structured on the basis of age and sex differences and similarities among the children. This research may be helpful not only for the clinician or student but also for the client. For a client, the knowledge that his sister has certain "mothering behaviors," for example, because of her ordinal position sometimes provides a beginning point for effecting attitudinal and behavioral change. "Migawd! That's us!" has been the reaction of more than one client to the reading of a few paragraphs of Toman's descriptions, and this reaction has been followed by less defensive and more protective behaviors.

Clinical Issues

The marital pair in the nuclear family link together three generations: themselves, their children, and their own parents. Much of the change required to alter the lives of children—to free them from being either parentified or scapegoated—comes about through effecting changes in the marital subsystem and relationships between the parents. Similarly, much of the work of facilitating positive change in the lives of the marital partners frequently comes from helping them to resolve issues of differentiation from their own parents and families of origin. Therefore, clinical work with the marital subsystem often is central to systemic transgenerational family therapy.

During the parenting stage, the young adults tend to be engaged in reworking the relationship with their own parents. A new stage of the family life cycle, referred to as the "termination of the intergenerational hierarchical boundary," has been proposed by Williamson (1991). During approximately the fourth decade of life—the 30s—the adult seeks to terminate the hierarchical boundary between self and the older parents. Power is redistributed and the younger generational member seeks to give up a need to be parented and also attempts to relate to his or her parents as a peer. This process involves accepting the older generational members as they are while giving them up emotionally and psychologically as parents. Williamson has spelled out a number of specific guidelines for working with those clients who can be helped to achieve a successful negotiation of this proposed stage and can thus be freed up to become more effective partners and parents.

Williamson's construct is similar to the first task set forth in the individual life cycle—adulthood (Table 7.3; see also Nichols, 1980; Nichols & Pace-Nichols, 1993). Rather than being located specifically in the 30s, as with Williamson's schema, the task of reworking the authority/power relationship with one's parents is viewed in the individual life cycle as a floating task. That is, it probably is handled by most persons in their 30s, but it may be accomplished by some individuals in their late 20s, by others in their 40s, and by some seemingly not at all.

During their 30s, while the husband/father may be settling down vocationally (Levinson, Darrow, Klein, Levinson, & McKee, 1974), the wife/mother may be undergoing a crisis of her own as an individual. She frequently goes to work or returns to work outside the home shortly after the birth of a child or when the youngest child enters kindergarten or begins to stay at school all day in the first grade. Not infrequently, by the time she hits the mid-30s, today's middle-class wife/mother in particular may be asking the now familiar questions, "Is this all there is?" and "Who am I?" As a result of the changes that she requires as a person in order to find a secure personal identity, a firm sense of self, and a sense of meaning and satisfaction, a marital crisis often occurs. At the very least, if the wife/mother does not abort her struggles and striving, a new marital task surfaces for the couple. Briefly put, it becomes necessary for the couple to restructure their marriage so that there is room for both the husband and the wife to have their own identities (Zemon-Gass & Nichols, 1981), rather than to be identified primarily in terms of the husband and his occupation.

TABLE 7.3. The Individual Life Cycle–Adulthood

The adult's major task is that of learning to be an adult who is interdependent vocationally and socially.

Tasks

1. Reworking one's authority relationship with parents so as to be an "orphan" in the sense of being able to take one's place in world as an adult who is responsible for one's self and being able to relate to one's parents and family-of-origin members as an adult and no longer as a "child" of the parents.
2. Deciding about one's commitment to vocation and work, deepening vocational (and personal) commitments, and pursuing long-range goals.
3. Maintaining appropriate and satisfactory sexual outlets and identity.
4. Maintaining appropriate and adequate social and personal relationships.
5. Demonstrating the continuing ability to function interdependently and in a socially responsible manner, while manifesting a firm sense of personal and social identity.

Unfortunately, both the wife/mother's struggles and those of the husband/father (see Chapter 8) often occur at approximately the same time that one or more of their children has undergone or is undergoing puberty's changes and the later vicissitudes of the teenage years.

At all stages through the childrearing years, it is important for the clinician to be alert to the relationship between the expectations of the parents regarding their children and the actual behaviors of the children (see Table 7.4). Typical social expectations of parents for children beginning with the school years and subsequently may include good performance in school during the elementary period; during the years 12–18, continuing advancement in school, some interest in the opposite sex, and an increasing evidence of responsibility and self-sufficiency; and at approximately 18, increased separation from the parents, greater self-sufficiency, departure from home, and perhaps marriage (Tymchuk, 1979). There are, of course, social-class, ethnic, and individual family variations on those themes.

How the boundaries of the marriage are maintained with regard to the children and in relation to other systems in their environment seems to be strongly related to how the partners deal with the issues of intimacy and power. The power task of spouses in their 30s pertains to establishing "definite patterns of decision making and dominance." In "good mar-

Table 7.4. The Child's Individual Life Cycle

The child's major task is to secure an appropriate base of experience as a totally dependent being and building on that base to make satisfactory incremental progress toward the relative independence appropriate to subsequent developmental stages.

Tasks

1. Learning to give and accept affection and learning to participate in family in cooperative and increasingly responsible ways and to demonstrate an expanding ability to meet family requirements and expectations.
2. Developing cognitive abilities, that is, speech and an ability to communicate with a growing range and number of others, and the basic skills required in the educational system.
3. Developing physical skills appropriate to one's age and forming conceptions of gender identity and sex role for present and future living.
4. Learning to interact with peers as a social being, to expand cooperative abilities, and to meet social expectations appropriately.
5. Developing a sense of morality, internalizing impulse control, and developing autonomous living guides suitable to social living.

riages" there is a notable increase in intimacy during those years and in "bad marriages" a gradual distancing between the spouses (Berman & Lief, 1975). Conflict in the marriage is likely to come from different approaches to productivity in terms of how the couple deals with their children, work, and friends, as well as their marriage during those years (Berman & Lief, 1975).

At the end of that decade and into the 40s, there is a simultaneous need to evaluate where things are and a tendency to question and to consider leaving marriage, changing job, and making other changes in living. It truly is a time of transition for the marriage. If the wife/mother has a career of her own, a midlife transition question probably will occur regarding vocation. Women's participation in the labor market is moving from a "double-peak" to a "single-peak" pattern. That is, women are becoming less likely to work outside the home prior to childbearing, drop out of the labor market during childbearing years, and return later. As noted by Roos (1985) and others (Baber & Allen, 1992), there is a transition toward a single-peak pattern like the men's (i.e., increased labor force participation into the 40s and then a trailing off).

At the least, these trends toward more traditionally male labor force participation, especially by better educated and better paid women, challenge men's dominance in the home and marriage.

FAMILY THERAPY FOR CHILDREN

When is family therapy contraindicated for a child? Bernice Rosman's response of "never" (Rosman, 1986) seems valid. The following guidelines regarding goals and interview forms for child and preadolescent clients are adapted in part from her work.

Child Clients

Treatment goals vary with age and stage of development of a young person; the younger a child, the greater the emphasis placed on working with the parental subsystem.

Preadolescents

With preadolescent clients and their families, the primary goal is likely to be strengthening the parental coalition and increasing parental effectiveness. Such treatment starts with conjoint family sessions—although in some instances the parents may be seen prior to the initial family session.

Typically, the focus shifts to sessions with only the parental subsystem present. Therapy may in some instances also involve sessions with the sibling subsystem. (Therapy with adolescents will be addressed in Chapter 8.)

Symptoms and Family Processes

Two closely related family processes are likely to be found behind much of the symptomatology that appears in children (and in adolescents). These are parentification and scapegoating. Both generally are related to triangulation within the family. Many family systems tend to have children who play such roles, sometimes interchangeably.

Parentification

Children who are parentified frequently manifest such symptomatology as adolescent depression, problems with self-differentiation, school phobia, separation problems, or emotional cutoff from other family members. Parentification is a process in which typically a child is pulled into a caretaking role for one or both parents as well as for the siblings (American Association for Marriage and Family Therapy, 1992). It often comes about when threatening stress occurs and the marital subsystem facing potential breakup or overwhelming stress triangulates the child into the group in order to restore balance or to maintain the continuity of the marital unit. Contributing factors include diffuse internal boundaries in the system, a poorly defined spousal subsystem, and overly strong ties on the part of the parents to their families of origin, with a resultant inability to perform the executive parental function for the system. The child who assumes the parentified role, particularly if he or she is forced into the role at a early age, is pulled out of the normal developmental experiences, becomes a pseudoadult, and may give up childhood play and peer attachments. Sibling rivalry often appears as an associated symptom. The parentified child may be unusually vulnerable to physical abuse or incest (Boszormenyi-Nagy & Spark, 1973).

Given the fact that the child gains a certain amount of status and emotional reinforcement as a result of playing the parentified child role, it is not surprising that not only may the parents be reluctant to give up this pattern but the child also may resist returning to an age-appropriate position in the sibling subsystem. When the role is given up by one child, it may be assumed by another child in succession.

As adults, persons who were parentified as children often manifest an inability to relinquish control in adult relationships. Consequently, parentification may occur between adults when one spouse "parents" the other. Similar roles may be assumed in intergenerational patterns such as those between mother, child, and grandparent, as well as in nuclear families.

Scapegoating

The symptomatology resulting from scapegoating typically is manifested through depression, school misbehavior, inappropriate sexual activities, or a variety of delinquent actions.

Like parentification, scapegoating involves a systemic dynamic in which one member is triangulated into a subsystem in order to alleviate stress and rebalance the total family system. Unlike parentification, where the parentified child functions within the troubled spousal subsystem, the scapegoating process involves an attempt to dissipate or remove the stress by pushing it away and placing it outside of the subsystem. While scapegoating may occur throughout the intergenerational network, it most often is seen in a parent–child triangle. In such situations the scapegoated child takes on or absorbs the stress from the marital dyad and carries it away from that family subsystem.

The classic statement on scapegoating was made by Vogel and Bell (1960). They identified "an emotionally disturbed child as an embodiment of certain types of conflicts between parents [and recognized that members of the family] are able to achieve unity through scapegoating a particular member . . . " (p. 412). Ackerman (1964) defined a similar three-person process that embodied roles of "persecutor," "victim," and "rescuer." The victim performs the scapegoat role, thus seemingly binding the family together. As that role takes on greater proportions, however, it begins to impair family functioning significantly.

A scapegoated child typically is brought to clinical services as the identified client, the source of the presenting problem. The parents often are willing to relate repeatedly stories of the child's misdeeds, carefully keeping the focus away from themselves and representing their own relationship as calm, reasonable, and stable. Typically they will resist all efforts to have them take a close look at their own relationship. The role of the scapegoat in the family is accepted and reinforced by the siblings who see their brother or sister as "bad" or "crazy."

Similarly, many therapists and treatment programs do not comprehend at the outset the systemic etiology of the presenting problem and proceed to accept the parents' designation of the scapegoated child as the source of the family problems. They then treat the child and his or her behaviors in either individual or group therapy.

The system's power to resist change should never be underestimated. Despite the parents' complaints about the child who is identified as the major problem and their pleading to the therapist to correct the behaviors, there typically is great resistance to change, particularly when the remainder of the family is not involved in therapy. In fact, it is to be expected that as the child's behavior improves, the parents will attempt to sabotage the therapy, either overtly (by changing therapists, dropping out of therapy, and so on) or covertly (by aiding the child to commit additional inappropriate behavior).

Removal of the scapegoated child from the family is not a panacea. In addition to the trauma to the removed child, such actions may set off a reactive sequence of negative events within the family system. First, it may result in instability and some degree of chaos in the family system. Second, the marriage may begin to manifest stress and conflict may erupt. Some marriages may be so vulnerable once the extruded stress and conflict have returned that the partners move quickly to divorce. Third, there generally is a move to restore balance to the family system by parentification or scapegoating of another individual.

WORKING WITH THE MARITAL PAIR

Two different sets of tasks form the basis of intervention and therapeutic work in sessions with the adults: parental tasks and marital tasks.

Parental Tasks and Education

The major parental task once a child has arrived consists of learning to fulfill parental roles as a couple. Many parents today need guidance not only about what the child needs but also about how to do what needs to be done. A considerable amount of the therapist's effort may be expended in parent education. This can take the form of modeling, bibliotherapy in which readings are assigned and discussed, and didactic work. Clients also can be referred to groups for parent education when appropriate groups are available. The preferred pattern is to work on skill training where it is needed and to deal with underlying dynamics that interfere with the learning when it becomes obvious that the clients are not able to carry out the assigned tasks and roles.

The notion that "where there is a parent–child problem, there is a three-generational problem" guides a considerable amount of the therapeutic/educational work with parents. Explaining to parents that much of their stress regarding childrearing is related to their own childhood experiences is only the first step in helping them to comprehend their tensions in dealing with their children. Most seem to grasp fairly readily the idea that their childrearing practices are affected by a concern with "who is looking over your shoulder, literally or figuratively." They recognize that they are affected by the actual contemporary involvement of their own parents in their childrearing or by their strongly held although not always entirely conscious, ideas about what is "right" or "wrong" gleaned from their upbringing.

For those who are caught in a loyalty conflict, a web of feeling that they must do as well as their parents or do what their parents did, the immediate therapeutic task often is respectfully to disqualify the parent as an omniscient and omnipotent authority. By comparison, the client feels inadequate and unsuccessful. These feelings frequently lead to reactions of frustration that result in harsh treatment of the children in the client's attempt to overcompensate for the perceived failure.

A woman was struggling alone to rear her children in a large metropolitan area and doing what appeared to be a reasonably competent job, but she continued to berate herself for being "a bad parent." Her therapist raised the obvious question of why she considered herself a bad parent. "Because I can't control my kids," she replied. "I tell them to do something and they ask why. They want to argue about it. They say their friends don't have to do it." She paused, and then resumed, "If I had done that. . . . My father said, 'jump' and we just said, 'how high?' We didn't dare question."

The therapist responded, "With all due respect to your father, he could not be 'Father' in that way today. When you were growing up way out in the country, your father didn't have to contend with drugs, television of the kind you have today, gangs, and the influence of peer groups that hold values quite different from his own. You didn't have a lot of choices. Your father had a comparatively simple task compared to yours in dealing with your children in this metropolitan area. And, you are doing it alone; your father had the support and reinforcement of your mother."

"Yes, that's all true," the client agreed. It was a lot easier in those days."

"Add to that something else. Your father did not discuss things with you. He required unquestioning obedience. He valued having children accept whatever their parents or other adult authorities told them. But you have tried to teach your children to think for themselves. And one of the results of teaching our children to think for themselves is that they ask questions and that includes questioning their parents."

More work of this type eventuated in some changes in the woman's conflicted feelings about being disloyal and a failure because she was not rearing her children as her parents did. Eventually she recognized that doing the best that she could under different and trying circumstances did not constitute failure or disloyalty.

There is some research to support the idea that social support and education provide resources that are beneficial to parents experiencing the stress of childrearing (Koeske & Koeske, 1990).

The Marital Development Perspective and Marital Tasks

The marital development perspective has firmly demonstrated its worth and utility. Treatment that ignores the marital tasks that are required at given stages of the marital relationship may be limited in its effectiveness. Some illustrative uses (adapted from Nichols & Pace-Nichols, 1993) are described in this section.

Assessment

The constructs of the marital life cycle and marital tasks (see Table 7.2) are useful both in the initial and ongoing assessment of clients and their problems and in determining their readiness for termination of therapy. How well are the partners succeeding in performing the marital tasks of their stage of marriage? What kinds of marital task deficiencies and conflict are found in the assessment with new marital therapy clients?

Balance and Perspective

Familiarity with the marital tasks may help clients to form a more balanced perspective regarding their marriage and relationship. The knowledge that they are on track and moving together as they successfully cope with at least some the tasks of their present marital life cycle stage is helpful. After a few sessions in which they have come to perceive their marriage in terms of its wholeness, as a gestalt, some clients begin to see their problems in perspective. "On the whole, we're doing pretty well, except for this (or these) problem(s)." Many clients feel it is significant that they are doing the best that they can with their problems at that particular stage of their life and relationship (Nichols, 1988). When they begin to feel that there is good faith effort and improvement in some of their joint efforts, there is a "haloing" or carryover effect so that success in those areas makes less satisfactory performance in other areas more acceptable.

A Process Orientation

Use of a marital life cycle viewpoint, with core and specific tasks, underlines for clients the fact that marriage is a process. It is not static. Adaptation to new phases and new situations is a normative part of marriage. This view can be quite helpful in sensitizing spouses to the normality of examining their marriage periodically and working at changing their current behaviors and interactions. It is reassuring to recognize that the tasks do not have to be accomplished at the beginning of their relationship, all at one time, once and for all but are to be addressed across a long period of time. Such reexamination and recognition that some potential problems can be predicted also can help clients to avoid crises. For example, Levinson et al.'s (1978) finding that men's marital problems peak around age 30, clinical observations supporting the notion of a marital "seven year itch" (Berman, Miller, Vines, & Lief, 1977), and Carl Whitaker's description of a problem point after 10 years or so of marriage (Neill & Kniskern, 1982) all indicate potential crises that may be avoided or their impact moderated if the spouses are helped to recognize the normality and necessity of periodic reexamination and reworking of their commitment.

"Teachable Moments"

The marital life cycle provides baselines and general guidelines for ascertaining readiness to learn about the next stage in the partners' development as a couple. Once clients reach a discernible and stage-appropriate point in their relationship, the therapist has the opportunity to try to guide them to the next level. Their individual and marital development are merged in this process as such teachable moments are used.

Reframing and Reinterpretation

Along with other approaches, the marital development perspective offers the possibility of reframing or reinterpreting problems so that they become more manageable. "Care" or "caring" can be used instead of "love" or "loving," for example. This shifting over to whether and how they care about the mate often gives clients a new freedom to consider how they feel and what they think they have in the relationship rather than to flounder in how they think they ought to feel (e.g., romantically "in love with"). The focus on the marital life cycle also emphasizes that the marital relationship is valuable in its own right. This provides a better model than the idea that becoming a parent is equivalent to becoming an adult, which prevails among some teenagers.

Therapy Implications

The marital development perspective provides a logical and strategic starting point for therapeutic exploration. When couples bring in complaints about the marriage, the therapist is in a position to explore with them how and where they are succeeding or failing in discharging the marital tasks for their present stage. One can work with them directly on the pertinent marital tasks (e.g., the general tasks of "settling into" the marriage, working out new relationships with their parents, and taking a new place in the extended family networks as a couple; or the core tasks relating to commitment, caring, communication, conflict/compromise, and contract).

Therapeutic interventions can involve education, reeducation, or direct intervention into the marital partners' interaction. Exploration of their communication, for example, may include helping them to understand that they can communicate clearly and disagree profoundly. Dispelling the erroneous idea that good communication means agreement can help clients comprehend that they verbally maneuver to avoid being clear, and thus avoid exposing differences. Therapeutic efforts can be directed toward helping them to modify their anxiety or fear of disagreement and to become more comfortable with the exposure of differences (Nichols, 1988).

The therapist can also "work backward" from a marital focus to concentrating on individual issues that hinder the individuals from accomplishing the stage-appropriate marital task or tasks. It makes sense to many couples to move from the joint failure to accomplish marital tasks to looking at individual factors that contribute to the failure. This sets the stage for exploring object relations issues, questions about individual life cycle accomplishments and developmental lag, and lingering family-of-origin problems.

Family Interrelationship Issues

With the marriage serving as the nexus of the family relationships, the therapist and the clients are in a position to focus on both the prior and the succeeding generations. That is, one can work with the effects of the partners on their offspring as well as the effects of their families of origin on them. There are enough instances of successive children behaving symptomatically to suggest that any time there are serious child behavior problems the marriage should be closely scrutinized and carefully assessed (Nichols & Everett, 1986). Adult clients may be aided in recognizing that some of their troublesome actions and attitudes—such as being scapegoated, parentified, "sent on a mission" by their parents (Stierlin, 1974, 1977), or otherwise triangulated (Bowen, 1978)—began when they were children and resulted from their becoming involved in problems extruded from their parents' marital relationship. Such therapeutic work often lifts burdens of powerful but inappropriate guilt feelings and helps to change problematic behaviors.

A DIFFERENTIATING COUPLE: THE BROWNS

Many of the issues encountered with individuals, couples, and families in Stage 2 of the family life cycle are found in the Brown case, which has been described in terms of therapy with a differentiating couple (Nichols, 1985a).

Description and Background

Attractive, well-educated, and articulate, the Browns resembled many other white, middle-class couples that therapists encounter. Paul, 28, was dark-haired, bearded, slim in build, and average in height. Carol, a year younger, was a tall, slender blonde. He was a graduate engineer. She had taught school briefly before becoming a homemaker. Married nearly 6 years, they had two daughters, ages 4 years and 18 months. Carol and Paul both were in excellent physical health. Both were the second of three children, each having an opposite sex older and a same sex younger sibling. They lived near both of their families of origin and had weekly and often daily contact with them. Carol was manifesting the more overt pain. In contrast to Paul's pleasant, rather bland demeanor, she obviously was tense, occasionally flashing a stricken look that was one of her characteristic responses whenever she felt pressure.

Assessment

Presenting Problems

In response to the standard question, "What brings you in?" the Browns initially said, "Communication and relating to each other." They added that they had been in therapy previously and had worked on these issues in conjoint sessions without much success. They had decided to give therapy another try at the urging of their clergyman. Both voiced a need to feel that things were going to go differently than during their previous attempt to get help.

Carol explicitly indicated that she wanted to get some relief and improvement in both her marital and personal situations. She acknowledged significant dependency needs on Paul. Gradually, her fearfulness was delineated as a long-term and pressing problem. Paul, obviously threatened by his wife's complaints and demands, was a somewhat reluctant participant in the assessment process. His immediate needs included a desire to avoid feeling blamed for what was going on in the marriage.

The partners moved a little closer together as they described how they were trying to cope with the task of leaving their respective families of origin and beginning to form a marital dyad and family of their own.

Developmental Issues

The assessment disclosed that the Browns were having trouble with some of their stage-appropriate individual, marital and parental, and family life cycle tasks. These included the following:

- Reworking the authority relationship with parents. Each partner needed to become an "orphan." That is, they needed to become differentiated so that each was able to take his or her place in the world as a responsible adult relating to their parents and family-of-origin members as an adult and no longer as a "child" of the parents.
- Affiliating satisfactorily with the extended family. Learning to fulfill parental roles as a couple. There were indications that the Brown's older child was being scapegoated by Carol, while Paul remained on the periphery of the childrearing.

With respect to the core tasks of the marital life cycle, the picture was as follows:

- *Commitment*: Carol was ambivalent toward commitment to Paul and confused about his role in her life. She had experienced doubts about his ability to meet her needs during courtship but when she had attempted to withdraw from the relationship on two occasions, he had become so depressed that she became frightened and relented. Paul seemed to be clearly committed to the marriage, but admittedly was bewildered by Carol's expectations of him and her negative reactions when he did not meet her expectations. When faced with her expressions of ambivalence and dissatisfaction, he would withdraw.
- *Caring*: Here, again, Carol was uncertain about her feelings for Paul and his for her. Paul was certain that he cared deeply for Carol, but he was hurt whenever she tried to lean on him strongly and expressed her disappointment that he was not available to support her.
- *Communication*: They were as honest as they could be in their attempts to communicate and generally came through as trustworthy and as persons of integrity. The problems were not so much with what they were able to express about what they felt as with their ability to comprehend what the other wanted and to feel they could deliver what was desired. Paul, for example, could hear Carol saying that he was "like a

third child" when he was at home but seemed unable to make any of the changes she requested.

• *Conflict/compromise*: The Browns were in disagreement about roles, especially Paul's role within the family, but their efforts to effect change characteristically ended in varying combinations of criticism, hurt feelings, and withdrawal.

• *Contract*: Carol expected Paul to meet her emotional needs, to release her from the enervating tensions that had long gripped her. She felt that he was not holding up his end of the bargain when this did not occur. Paul expected a traditional relationship in which Carol would care for the home and children. He expected to work hard outside the home but to do very little at home and to provide little in the way of companionship for wife or children. Her strong dependency on him was somewhat overwhelming at times, and Paul felt that she was not doing her part.

Individual Diagnoses

Carol's conditions met the criteria for the DSM-III-R diagnosis of 301.90, Personality Disorder Not Otherwise Specified, with particular emphasis on her fears, fearfulness, anxiety, and occasional depression. Paul had features meeting the 301.60, Dependent Personality Disorder diagnosis, along with some compulsive features. He acknowledged an inability to make decisions, whether at home or at work. Reluctant to take a stand in any situation, he admitted fearing that others would not like him or would disapprove of his answer or decision. "Only if I get angry enough can I make a decision," he said.

Families of Origin

Both Carol and Paul came from "mid-range" families (Beavers & Hampson, 1990), that is, families that tend to hold on to their children and produce neurotic offspring. Indications of appreciable amounts of unconsciously determined behavior prevailed with both young persons. Both had been parentified by their parents to some extent. Comparatively, the "centripetal" dimension (Beavers & Hampson, 1990) was more pronounced in Carol's family. Paul's family could be located more closely to the mixed stylistic dimension and a little more closely to the healthy family range of the scale than Carol's family.

Deeply enmeshed in her family of origin, Carol was continuing to strive desperately to get outside of it although she was terribly frightened of leaving or offending her parents or siblings. More individuated than Carol, Paul tried to stand outside of his family of origin and protect himself by ignoring his parents and tacitly freezing them out. Nevertheless, the ties were still strong and he was still not adequately separated out and established as an adult.

Differentiation Difficulties

Carol's problems in differentiating from her family of origin came through in several ways. For example, her mother was constantly on the telephone with "helpful suggestions" about childrearing, which Carol experienced as criticism and interference. Paul confirmed that his wife's mother did tend to be intrusive and did provide Carol with reasons for being upset.

The strength of Paul's ties with his family of origin did not come through so clearly. That there was a need to work on differentiation was evident, but the extent to which he had to struggle in order to become more appropriately individuated emerged only later in treatment. His family of origin would permit him to marry and have a family of his own in a much more free fashion than would his wife's family. Unlike Carol's family, which did not wish her to go away at all, his would let him separate but would call him back periodically to exercise what emerged as his role as parentified offspring. For example, his mother called him once in the early morning hours because his father had not returned from a trip as expected, even though Paul's grown younger brother was at home and had made the only telephone calls to the state highway police that were indicated under the circumstances.

Goals for Therapy

At the outset, goals were established for Carol and for the marriage. The immediate goals for working with her were reduction of her fear and anxiety, moderation of her depression, and expansion of her coping abilities. Outcome goals included helping her to become essentially dependency free, so that she no longer needed to latch on to others in the ways that she currently did, and helping her to become reasonably fear free. These were seen as necessary achievements in order to help her separate from her family of origin in a fitting manner and to function adequately as a married adult.

The immediate goals with regard to the marriage were to stabilize the marital interaction and to discover whether there were qualities within the relationship that could be developed so as to sustain both Carol and Paul and provide adequate satisfactions for them. Once the commitment of both partners to being married to the other was clearly established—

and this happened with Carol only after a clarification of her distortions and confusions surrounding the relationship, and a recognition of the fact that Paul really was committed to her—setting an outcome goal for the marriage was possible. In the broadest sense, the outcome goal finally set was an improved marriage that would provide room and opportunity for fulfillment of the classic "two irreducible functions of the nuclear family," stabilization of adult personalities and primary socialization of the young (Parsons & Bales, 1955).

Treatment Procedures

Initially the therapy involved individual sessions with Carol, interspersed with periodic conjoint sessions. Then there was a brief period of individual sessions with Paul, followed finally by conjoint marital sessions. Two family-of-origin sessions were held with Carol and her parents and siblings. It would prove possible to accomplish the necessary tasks that Paul had to perform with his family of origin by exploring issues with him in therapy and coaching him on learning to deal in new ways with his family on his own.

Individual Sessions

The immediate aim with Carol was to help her learn how to reality-test different sets of circumstances while supporting her to try to take steps that would enable her to cope more adequately with the situations that she was encountering. Such a stance was quite different from what she had experienced in her family of origin. Even the basic idea that one could examine what was happening and being said and take a proactive, rather than a reactive, defensive position was new to Carol. From her mother she typically met denial that there was any difficulty in any situation that she faced. The mother glossed over problematic situations in such a way that Carol ended up feeling either guilty for internally disagreeing with her mother or demeaned and helpless because she had given in to someone else, or else feeling both ways at once.

There was a movement back and forth in the sessions between the present and the past and between a focus on Carol as an individual and on the marital and family systems in which she was located. Attention was given to loyalty conflicts when she was being encouraged to follow a different route than her mother would choose, for example. Also, real neighborhood circumstances (in which she had been scapegoated by another woman in social situations) were dealt with in the conjoint sessions, and Paul's help was enlisted whenever possible.

Obtaining relief from the fear that had long gripped her and spread throughout her life was a major key to Carol's improvement as an individual, marital partner, and parent. Family photograph albums helped to provide some understanding of family events and processes during Carol's early and middle childhood. In the photographs it was possible, for example, to spot the period in her life in which her tensions first became evident. Subsequent exploration of that period helped her to recall some important events that previously had been outside her awareness.

Then Paul was seen individually for several sessions, primarily to work on his own family-of-origin issues. He talked about how he had spent as much time as possible outside the home when he was growing up. Much of that consisted of "playing and sometimes eating and staying overnight" with a neighbor family. Subsequently, we were able to tie some of what we learned here to his early attempts to avoid being parentified and to use it in helping him to break some current patterns with both his own and his wife's families of origin.

Conjoint Marital Sessions

Due to improvement in his wife, the positive results of the periodic conjoint sessions, and a few individual sessions, Paul came to trust therapy and to believe that it was helpful. Then it was possible to give some attention to his limited involvement in marital and family life. Paul's involvement in the therapy process was facilitated by looking at things in tailored "structural" terms that were compatible with his "structural" engineering approach to the world and using diagrams where possible in explanations.

Helping both Paul and Carol to rework their family-of-origin relationships and to differentiate themselves more appropriately was made an explicit therapy goal with them at this juncture. A significant part of this endeavor involved encouraging each spouse to support the differentiation efforts of the other. Just as Paul was enlisted to help Carol in restructuring relations with her parents, so her assistance was sought in several of his endeavors with his family.

The primary issue with Paul was establishing a workable relationship with his parents, that is, keeping some contact while avoiding their triangulation efforts. Over the years he had gradually pulled away, starting with his elementary and junior high school years when he had spent large amounts of time with the neighbor family previously mentioned. Having incurred expressions of disapproval from his parents because he had been "away from home so much," and "had preferred being with the neighbor's family," he subsequently had used a variety of more "acceptable reasons" for avoiding contact, including college, marriage, work, and his recreational running activities.

With Carol's support, Paul began to reestablish a structured relationship with his family. For example, the couple scheduled some contacts with his family of origin on a family-to-family basis in which he and Carol and their children would visit on an occasional Sunday or have his family over for a meal. Paul did not go to his parents' home alone to "solve their problems," as they were likely to call on him to do. Also, feeling that he had succeeded in breaking his father's assumptions that he "owned" Paul on Saturdays through a lengthy period of avoiding contact with his family prior to entering therapy, Paul arranged to spend a part of a Saturday with his father and brother in recreational or work pursuits every couple of months.

The partners were coached to take some stands on behalf of their own family unit against Carol's mother's efforts to get everybody within the family of origin's orbit to conform to whatever norm the mother deemed appropriate to the occasion. Instead of spending a "mandatory" 2-week vacation helping Carol's parents and siblings build a vacation cottage, for example, the Browns were assisted in maintaining the separateness of their own family unit by renting a separate cottage across the lake and going over to help part of the time while withdrawing with their children for meals and nap times and for some personal marital and family time.

Exploration of "models of relationships" (Skynner, 1981) from their family of origin that were influencing their current marital and family action proved helpful. They noted similarities and differences between the families they grew up in and their current nuclear family. Paul came to understand how he had been pulled into a spousal surrogate role in the past, how he had come to feel disloyal to his father because of loyalty to his mother in triangular situations, and how he was currently attempting to be loyal to his father by repeating essential elements of his father's patterns. Consciously, he had not wished to model after either the parental marriage or his father's role.

Paul's indecisive tendencies were related to the triangle position that he had occupied between his parents over the years. His life had involved a continual need to "walk the line" between his parents and not take sides in their disagreements. Placed very much in the middle, he had felt that there was no way that he could win. Currently, he was not caught in a bind between his wife and some other person, as he had been when trapped between his parents. Rather, he was entangled in fears that if he did what his wife wished him to do, either as a husband or as a father, he would be disliked or disapproved of by "some vague force." Similarly, in the work world and in social situations he was vaguely uneasy. He caught on rather quickly during therapy that it was the "ghosts looking over his shoulder," the internalized perceptions of how others would react and the unaltered patterns of relationships that he had carried into adulthood from his past, that were hampering him.

We used role play to anticipate and rehearse how he could deal with predictable issues at work and in social and family situations. As with Carol, we worked on "building up behavioral muscles." Once Paul was able to be proactive and successful in the easier situations, he was ready to begin working on the more sensitive relationships in his family of origin and current nuclear family life.

The Scapegoated Child

Dealing with the effects of marital and individual conflicts on the oldest child in particular was also a focus of therapy. Ambivalent toward her oldest daughter, Carol frequently treated her as a scapegoat when tensions got high in the marriage. Although in some pain because of what she was doing, she often would become angry at the 4-year-old and yell at her. Eventually, she recognized that the child was not readily accepting the role and was yelling back at her in an angry, defiant, and nasty way. At that point, not only did Carol recognize that her daughter was bearing the brunt of extruded marital tensions but also that the scapegoating behaviors had a transgenerational flavor: The interaction was part of her conflict with her own mother. The child was responding to Carol as Carol had wished to respond to her own mother, but Carol had been—and still was—afraid to react. Vicariously Carol was expressing her rebellion against her mother's controlling, rejecting behavior. The cycle became clear: Carol would induce the behavior and then punish the child for misbehaving. Punishing the daughter enabled her to identify with her mother—as a "good" mother who did not permit "bad" behavior—by carrying out her mother's patterns of childrearing and being loyal to Mother and, at the same time, to struggle with and punish a mother substitute with some degree of impunity.

Carol and Paul were "spiraling" each other's concerns about the older child by this point, frightened at thoughts of having "messed up" their child and uncertain about how to try to relate to her. For a variety of reasons, the partners were referred to a child psychologist who had a strong background in family work. Finding the child essentially normal and free of psychopathology, the psychologist used several sessions to calm the parents' fears and help them to learn about normal child development and parenting. She described the couple as "starved for information and help around normal childrearing." Subsequently, some of the conjoint sessions focused on the transgenerational aspects of childrearing in relation to the partners' backgrounds. Their efforts to put into practice what they had learned were strongly reinforced.

Family-of-Origin Sessions

As noted, two sessions were held with Carol and her parents and siblings. Prior to those meetings, Carol wrestled with the questions, What do you wish to learn? What do you wish to accomplish in the meetings? Essentially, she determined that she wished (1) to obtain information and understanding about certain times and events that she could not remember from her childhood, and (2) to change her relationship with her parents and one of the siblings.

The major origins of the centripetal nature of Carol's family of origin stood out starkly. Her parents protected themselves from a repeat of earlier losses by trying to make certain that their own children did not separate from them. In some ways, they appeared to be trying to recreate the lost families of their own childhood and to get their children to serve as parents for them. (Not only had the father lost his family at an early age, but also the mother had lost three brothers by death during her childhood and gone through several years in her early teens in which her father was hospitalized with a series of disabling physical and emotional problems.) Carol's father made it clear in one session that it was painful even to think about the children separating from the family. He cried as he said, "I don't want to lose you. I don't want you to move away and not be close." The tentacles of guilt induction reached almost visibly toward all three children during this activity.

Carol learned that it was not her mother she feared so much as her mother's feelings about her father. The mother was communicating with her behaviors, "Don't leave me alone with this man. I can't supply all his emotional demands or meet all of his dependency needs." At the same time, the mother's denial was apparent. She had established a family rule for the children: "Don't criticize. Don't talk about anything in the family in negative terms." Carol realized for the first time the lengths to which her mother went in protecting herself from being left alone with the care of her husband, assuming the role of protecting his emotional fragility by trying to make the children responsible for him. The father had already made his son into a father figure for himself, and Carol's apprehension was that her mother's denial concealed an attempt to unload more of her father's massive dependency needs on her.

The sessions were partly successful, primarily in changing the relationship between Carol and her sibling, the other parentified child. She decided that the chances of her parents changing to any appreciable degree were practically nonexistent. They would not let her go; she would have to differentiate herself. When she discussed this with Paul, he supported her conclusions and worked to help her distance herself from the family's centripetal forces.

Subsequent to the family-of-origin sessions and the lessening of her fears through significant work in individual and conjoint sessions, Carol had two interrelated and liberating "Aha!" experiences. In the first, she formed the idea that she was "passing through her family" rather than being destined to be a permanent resident in it, controlled continually by her mother and, indirectly, by her father's needs for protection. She came up with feelings of an integrity of her own, which were supported as being appropriate to her individual and family life cycle stages. Her "body feeling like steel," which could be traced back to age 4 when she had feared losing her mother, was related to defending herself primarily from invasive actions, attitudes, and feelings that threatened her from outside herself but inside the family, threats that came after her basic personality strengths had been established. Family photos also were helpful in establishing that she had been given early nurturance by her mother and her maternal grandmother.

A simultaneous "Aha!" experience was the release from certain attitudes toward her own children. She was able to perceive her children as passing through their family of origin. This lessened her fears for them and helped her feel accountable for them in a different way than previously. As she put it, "I can see myself as responsible for teaching them the best that I could and for launching them. I didn't have to take care of them all their lives. It was all right for them to leave me eventually. Somehow, it was all right for them to leave me temporarily, going to school, going to play. That was training for leaving me totally to be on their own eventually."

Outcomes

Clearing away unresolved family-of-origin issues and assisting the Browns to begin to function more cleanly in the present made it possible to get their basic commitment and caring established solidly between them, to work with them in effecting clear communication about their wishes and feelings, to develop better conflict resolution skills, and to clarify and rework their marital contract. Part of this change was related to Carol's recognition that "I had projected my feelings onto Paul. I realized that I didn't know him. This lifted the blame off him and off our relationship." Additionally, it was associated with Paul's growing ability to come out of his own shell and to be more giving and fully participant in the marital and family life.

8

THERAPY WITH
CONTRACTING FAMILIES

The family is born dying . . . and being reborn, again and again.

Arguably, this is the most complex and dynamic of the stages of the family life cycle. The greatest number of cycles and persons typically are involved in the family relationships and interaction at this stage. At no place in the family life cycle does the cogwheeling of generations become more evident and the tasks for the generations more numerous and complicated than at the launching and contraction period of the nuclear family. A three-generational perspective is important in many therapy situations if the therapist is to deal intelligently and effectively with the issues that are presented but possibly nowhere more than at this stage of the family life cycle (see Table 8.1).

Recent decades have brought forth a three-generational situation that is unprecedented. A major factor in the emergence of the new situation has been the increased longevity of the population. That is, large numbers of persons are living into their 60s and beyond, as contrasted to earlier generations when it was rare for both of the marital partners to live through their 40s and 50s. As recently as three or four generations ago—couples marrying around 1890—the odds were approximately 50–50 that one of the partners would have died before the launching stage was reached. Today, both partners typically are living at the time that the children are launched from the home. The expectation of life at birth reached a new record high of 75.7 years in 1992 (National Center for Health Statistics, 1993).

This increase means, in brief, that the grandparents—the parents of the parents doing the launching—are likely to be present and to live for many years after the youngsters have been launched. Frequently, this faces the "middle generation" with the task of dealing with important dependency needs and support issues of both their offspring and their parents, causing them to be a "caught generation" (C. E. Vincent, 1972).

Although it is not universal, this three-generational situation is common enough so that it must be regarded as the typical picture today. (It may be complicated further by disruptions in the family life cycle such as those brought about by divorce and remarriage, but the concern in this chapter is with uninterrupted family development.)

During this stage of the family life cycle, the husband and wife, who are simultaneously parents and the children of their own parents, are involved in perhaps the most trying and complicated set of tasks and relationships of their lifetime. Daily they are occupied in dealing with life in the nuclear family they have formed. Stretching and adapting their changing relationship with growing, beginning-to-differentiate, and differentiating offspring; coping with changes in their individual lives and often careers; keeping the marriage going and growing; and continuing their lifelong relationship with their own parents and families of origin all

TABLE 8.1. The Family Life Cycle, Stage 3—Contraction: Individuation and Eventual Separation of Youth

Family life cycle developmental tasks

1. Releasing family members appropriately (see also the parental tasks associated with the marital life cycle, Table 8.4) and incorporating new members by marriage.

2. Providing for the physical and economic needs of family members.

3. Balancing adolescents' growing need for freedom and relative independence with appropriate assumption of personal responsibility en route to their departure from the home and adjusting parents' corresponding relinquishment of total responsibility, including the continuing evolution of communication to deal with changing relations between generations.

4. Providing for the socialization of children into more mature roles within the family and for socialization of adults into roles as parents of individuating and differentiating offspring.

5. Affiliating satisfactorily with the extended family and the kinship and friendship networks.

face them with a elaborate and often intricately intertwined juggling task (see Table 8.2).

Not the least of the tasks of the middle generation is the need to deal with their own parents, the grandparental generation. The grandparental generation faces impending decline in physical abilities and health and the eventual death of first one spouse and then the other. Retirement and financial security are issues for most older couples. If appropriate patterns of dealing with the spouse have not been formed previously, retirement may bring problems in terms of how they relate to each other and how they use their newly gained leisure time. These and other changes may result in shifts in the dependence–independence relationship between the grandparents and their own children. The loss of autonomy may become a significant issue for the older couple and the question of how much and what kinds of responsibility to take with regard to them may become a matter of major concern for their children (the middle generation). The familiar "reversal of the generations" in which adult parents assume roles vis-à-vis their parents that the older generation formerly occupied in relation to them most frequently occurs during the launching/contraction stage of the family life cycle, although there may be intimations of such changes earlier.

At the same time, the middle generation is faced with the need to work out new patterns of relatedness with their departing and departed children. The younger generation (the children/grandchildren) simultaneously

---

TABLE 8.2. The Individual Life Cycle–Middle Adulthood

The major task of middle adulthood is concerned with restabilizing one's life, reordering priorities, and preparing for the later years.

Tasks

1. Reexamining changing relationship with family of origin and with one's parents, including dealing with the possibility of assuming responsibility for parents' emotional, physical, and economic dependency.
2. Evaluating one's aspirations and vocational and economic achievements, reordering priorities, and seeking an appropriate balance for present and future, including preparing for possible retirement.
3. Adjusting to changing physical and sexual abilities, requirements, and expectations while maintaining satisfactory functioning and identity.
4. Maintaining appropriate and adequate social and personal relationships.
5. Demonstrating the continuing ability to function interdependently and in a socially responsible manner, while manifesting a firm sense of personal and social identity.

has the task of implementing educational, vocational, and friend-ship/marital goals of their own while appropriately detaching and rerelat-ing to their parents and family of origin. For most of the younger generation, the task involves learning to relate to their parents on an adult-to-adult basis first as a single person and subsequently as a young married person.

There is no easy dividing line between the launching stage and the postparental stage. Some families have a period in which there are four living generations, whereas others lose the grandparents early and may not go through a period in which three generations of a family are living simultaneously.

Losses tend to be comparatively high in this stage of the family life cycle, particularly in comparison to the expanding stage. Children are leaving home, the parents are reaching middle-age and grappling with its accompanying transitional issues, their parents may be facing declining physical and other abilities, and death may be beginning to intrude in the extended family. In a genuine sense, the family is born dying. Subsequently, it is reborn as succeeding generations develop.

INDIVIDUATION AND SEPARATION ISSUES

When the contracting stage of the family life cycle is reached, the young are beginning to individuate and separate themselves from their family of origin. Neither the beginning nor the ending of this stage is clearly marked, however. Even the commonly agreed upon criterion of the departure of the last child from home—for good—is becoming less clear-cut as a starting point. The departure of the children from home and the recasting of the parent–child relationship is complicated in the case of those who are subsidized while pursuing graduate or professional education, buying a home, or beginning a business. Additionally, some offspring return home, often with children, following their separation or divorce from their mate. These factors make it even less evident when the contraction stage starts. In a sense, it "starts before it starts." That is, preparation for launching the young into the outside world to live their own lives begins long before the actual departure occurs.

Parents are working themselves out of a job from the beginning of their days as parents. Otherwise, the normal processes of development are disrupted. Healthy childrearing consists of a continual and often tenuous balancing of the dependency scales, providing the child with adequate amounts of support while simultaneously encouraging appropriate autonomous and independent functioning. To use a homey metaphor, the parent strives to provide youngsters with sufficient slackness in the halter that attaches them to permit healthy exploration and growth, while holding firmly enough to the rope to protect the offspring and to rein them in if they begin to exceed safe limits and to risk danger.

A major goal in healthy childrearing in a democratic society is to produce young adults who are capable of mature interdependence in their lives. The idea that complete independence ever occurs on the part of either parent or child is generally erroneous. Most adults will continue to be related to their parents, although in different ways than during their formative years, as well as being related to a peer in a couple and marriage relationship for much of their lives, and to a child or children of their own. That is, in healthy growth and development those who follow the path of marriage and family formation move from total dependence to mutual interdependency with a peer, and to being the source of total dependence for their own children. It is with these roles and relationships in mind that one refers to the marriage as the nexus of the family.

By the time that the young man or woman leaves home, whether to go to school or to work and to a separate residence, he or she has had several years of experience in orienting toward the world outside the family. Both the psychophysiological push of adolescence and the structure of the society, which groups teenagers in age peer groups largely isolated from mainstream society, have facilitated movement away from parents (see Table 8.3).

As noted, at the same time that this development is occurring with the adolescent/teenager, the parents often are struggling with their own midlife or middle-age difficulties. The individual midlife transition for the male, sometimes popularly and somewhat incorrectly referred to as a midlife crisis, typically comes around age 40 (Levinson, Darrow, Klein, Levinson, & McKee, 1978). At that juncture, he may be involved in a significant struggle to come to grips with where he is in relation to where he would like to be in fulfilling his aspirations. Research indicates that for some men this period involves withdrawing not only from the spouse but also from the family and engaging in erratic patterns of behavior including moodiness, outbursts of temper, and other actions that have not been typical of them (Levinson et al., 1978).

The significant struggles of women constitute one of the critical phenomena of our times. For many of today's women who have become conscious of their traditional "place" and who struggle for change, the issues of "Who am I?" and "Is this all there is?" come before middle age. Often, for some of those who start out with an essentially traditional wife/mother orientation, the dissatisfaction and questioning begins at the stage in the family life cycle in which their children get ready for kindergarten and school.

Faced with changes in themselves that include the passing of their youthfulness at the same time that their children are beginning to move toward physical maturity and departure from the home, the parents invariably have to cope with loss. For adults who are discouraged and deeply concerned about their own future, the loss that they face may be experienced as unbearable. The power relationship between child and parent shifts in terms of who is needed by whom as the movement toward relatively mutual individuation continues (Stierlin, 1974).

Patterns of Family Process

Family therapists have depicted several patterns of family interaction and process that influence how the offspring may be attached to and affected by their family of origin. These patterns are described below.

Enmeshing–Disengaging Action

The concepts of "enmeshment" and "disengagement" were introduced to family therapy initially by Minuchin, Montalvo, Guerney, Rosman, and Schumer (1967). They used them as descriptors in their early work in identifying parent–child dynamics among low-income families with delinquent children. However, the concepts have become generic to the family

---

TABLE 8.3. The Child Individual Life Cycle–Adolescence

The adolescent's major task is to learn to deal with rapid and extensive physical and social life alterations and attempting to secure a firm sense of identity and direction while navigating the ambiguous course between a starting point of total dependency and an eventual launching on a life of relative independence.

Tasks

1. Demonstrating appropriate steps toward individuation and differentiation from family emotionally and taking an eventual role as a self-responsible young adult.
2. Making preliminary decisions about vocational choice and economic future and developing the requisite intellectual and other skills to pursue those goals.
3. Achieving comfort with one's changing body, channeling sexual drives, and establishing gender identity.
4. Establishing appropriate and adequate social and personal relationships with peers and members of one's own generation.
5. Demonstrating a growing ability to function relatively independently in a socially responsible manner and an evolving emergence of a sense of personal and social identity.

---

therapy field as a classification continuum regarding a family's interactional processes.

Enmeshing and disengaging behaviors refer to an emotional level of interactive functioning within families. The enmeshing patterns involve an identifiable emotional intensity among family members in terms of attachment, frequency of interaction, and reciprocal dependency. The individual members of the system will share a common, although not always explicit, personal survival need to maintain the family process. In an enmeshing system, external or internal events reverberate quickly and profusely throughout the entire system. One member may speak as if he or she were speaking on behalf of another member(s). Toward the extreme of the continuum, the highly enmeshing family may display either (1) closed and rigid external boundaries that isolate the system from external influences or (2) diffuse external boundaries that allow the enmeshment to spread unchecked across several generations. Whatever the nature of the external boundaries in such families, the internal subsystem boundaries are diffuse and poorly defined, allowing many intrusions to occur, such as that of a child into the spousal subsystem.

Enmeshing actions should not be confused with emotional closeness, intimacy, or issues of communication. The intensity of the enmeshing actually may create emotional withdrawal on the part of certain members of the family as a protective defense of their autonomy and individuation. Adults coming from enmeshing families of origin may limit their capacity for interpersonal intimacy as a result of being fearful of replicating enmeshing patterns and thus losing autonomy. Overall, members of enmeshing families have experienced close affective attachment and carry into mate selection and their adult relationships both the result of such attachments and the expectation that relationships should be of that nature. The cost of such enmeshing patterns often is limited individuation and difficulties with separation from one's family of origin.

The disengaging patterns of family process are characterized by a remarkable absence of affective intensity in family attachments. Relationships throughout the family subsystems are marked by emotional distance, lack of sensitivity to individual needs, and a high frequency of independent activities. Families falling toward the extreme end of the continuum lack cohesion, something that is reflected in rather diffuse external boundaries. Internal boundaries in such families may be either (1) rigidly set with little relationship to other internal subsystems or (2) completely diffuse with individual family members each going in their own separate direction. Individuals in such systems become independent and autonomous early but often at the cost of experiencing emotional loss or severely limiting personal affective ties with parents and siblings.

Minuchin's enmeshment and disengagement concepts have been criticized as being more "linear" than "circular" and are all too easily reified and regarded as if they were entities in themselves. Nevertheless, they offer the family therapist an important descriptive mechanism for use in assessing and understanding the quality of a family's interactive process.

Centripetal and Centrifugal

Stierlin (1974) has described "centripetal" and "centrifugal" separation patterns in families with adolescents. Centripetal families orient the children toward the inside, toward staying in the family, whereas centrifugal families do not serve as such a magnet. In extreme form, centrifugal families are underorganized and have a minimum of relatedness prevailing among members. Parents in centripetal families adapt a "binding" mode of dealing with adolescents. In centrifugal families they use an expelling mode of relating (Stierlin, 1981). Beavers (Beavers & Hampson, 1990), as noted in Chapter 5, also has used the terms in his model of family functioning. His description of the types of problems often found in the offspring of midrange, borderline, and severely dysfunctional centripetal and centrifugal families can be particularly helpful in providing suggestions for assessment and treatment placement of such families and their children.

Stierlin (1981) has described a third pattern in which the parents react with ambivalence and continuing conflict to their own developmental crises. Rather than simply holding on to their child or letting him or her go, they do both. They make the child a "delegate," an extension of themself, sending him or her on a "mission." Stierlin uses psychoanalytic concepts in describing the major missions of delegates as serving the parent's affective, ego, and superego needs (p. 55). Two kinds of conflicts arise for the delegate: loyalty conflicts and mission conflicts. Loyalty conflicts develop when a delegate is in conflict with one parent when trying to be loyal to the other (e.g., the Hamlet paradigm). Mission conflicts arise when the delegate attempts to execute two incompatible missions.

Other Descriptive Concepts

Other authors have used different terms in referring to similar processes. Aponte (1976), in discussing low-income families, has described the "underorganized family." Hoffman, borrowing from Ashby (1952), has talked about the "too richly cross-joined system" (1975) and the "too poorly cross-joined family" (1981).

Effects on Parents

Drawing on his clinical work, Stierlin (1974) has delineated three ways in which the forthcoming departure of the offspring affects parents. He found them either denying that the departure was coming by refusing to talk or think about the matter, reacting with feelings of gloom and deep depression, or anticipating being lonely and depressed when the children left but indicating that they could cope with the situation.

Parents send out messages to their offspring with varying degrees of clarity that contribute either to a relatively easy separation or to hard and difficult struggles. When the messages indicate that the parents can live without the child, and how they will live without him or her, it is difficult for the child to depart without fear. Messages that convey that the parents will not be able to live when the child is gone make it difficult, of course, for the youngster to leave without undue guilt feelings.

For their own good, the husband and wife need to recognize and deal as appropriately as possible with the loss that they sustain as a child leaves home. There are guidelines for predicting the severity of the loss of a person from the family and from one's own life. Among those are recency of the loss. That is, the passage of time does help diminish the pain of a loss, unless there is active blocking of the mourning process so that the grief work cannot be completed. Previous experiences with losses, their number, their severity, and how well they have been faced and dealt with also provide indications of the probable severity of present or forthcoming losses. The smaller the family and the greater the imbalance in the family resulting from the loss, the more severe it is likely to be (Toman, 1993).

For the marital couple, the task is to work through the feelings of loss and to detach sufficiently from the departing and departed child so that appropriate amounts of emotion invested there can be reinvested in the marriage or in other pursuits and interests. Just as the individual task for middle adulthood involves restabilizing, so a major marital task at this stage has to do with stabilizing the marriage for "the long haul" (Berman & Lief, 1975).

How do the partners handle the vacuum left by the departure of their children? Intimacy may increase or it may decrease, depending in large measure on the foundations built prior to the launching time. Similarly, conflicts may increase or decrease when there is no longer the buffering or instigating presence of a child or children. Marital partners may find the "empty nest" stage a depressing, threatening, and nonfulfilling time of their life, or it may be a time of significant activity for mutual enjoyment and fulfillment with the spouse.

TYPICAL FORMS OF THERAPY

The complexity in the contraction stage of the family life cycle results in a corresponding complexity in the selection of therapeutic focus. Among the questions affecting the choice of treatment emphasis are the following: How well is the family discharging its developmental tasks? How well are the spouses discharging their developmental tasks as a marital couple, as well as their respective individual developmental tasks? How well are the children (as adolescents and/or young adults) discharging their own developmental tasks?

Therapy in this stage can focus on the total family, the adult parents/spouses as individuals or as a marital subsystem, the children (adolescents and/or young adults) as individuals or as a sibling subsystem, the parent–child subsystem, and on the family-of-origin relationships. The contraction stage of the family life cycle is probably the phase in which conjoint family therapy occurs most commonly. A large amount, perhaps the majority, of the family therapy that occurs in connection with this stage consists at least initially of complaints involving the children. The rudiments of a decision tree approach are described below.

Decision Tree Suggestions

It is not possible at this stage in the development of integrative family therapy to provide precise and firm indicators for the type of interviewing focus and treatment interventions to be used with specific problems. Therefore, the descriptive schema that follows should be regarded as partial in coverage, tentative rather than definitive, and in need of a considerable amount of refinement.

What is the starting point?

When the Problems Involve a Child

When the complaint from the family refers to difficulties associated with a child, the preference in integrative family therapy is, of course, to treat the problems in a family context. Therapists vary in terms of whether they see the total family first or see the parents initially and then the total family. Satir (1964) established early in the family therapy movement the practice of seeing the parents separately for a couple of sessions before bringing in the remainder of the family. Bell (1975) similarly saw the parents first for an orientation phase. Therapy then typically proceeded through a child-centered phase, a parent-centered phase, and, finally, a family-centered phase.

Although some family therapists have agreed with Bell's (1975) early decision to exclude children under 9 years of age, others have concluded that with slight modifications the entire family can be included. Young children down to age 4 and perhaps younger can be incorporated without being treated like miniature adults if play activity is used (Zilbach, Bergel, & Gass, 1972). Young children often communicate their feelings and thoughts by actions, specifically through their play activities, rather than by verbal statements. The younger the child, therefore, the greater the desirability of a playroom setting or the inclusion in the therapist's office of the standard play materials used in child guidance clinics (Orgun, 1973).

Play activity enables young children to avoid restlessness and to be more comfortable with being in the room while threatening material is explored with the parents and older family members. Additionally, the younger child's presence and play often can point to underlying family feelings and issues that otherwise might be overlooked (Zilbach et al., 1972).

Some problems can be handled effectively by working directly with the couple. One of the findings in working with family systems has been that certain forms and instances of child misbehavior actually are symptomatic of problems in the marriage. Difficulties sometimes get extruded from the couple interaction and find an outlet in problematic behavior in one or more of the children. A primary treatment decision often is whether or not the child or children should be seen at all or whether the therapist should work directly with the parents from the outset. There is controversy in this area.

One of the best indicators for deciding to work directly with the parents on behalf of the children and not include the children seems to be the clinician's perception that the children's symptoms are primarily reactive to parental attitudes and action. Another important indicator is how deeply the symptoms or maladaptive patterns are ingrained in the child. How is he or she handling the developmental tasks appropriate to that stage of life? One must make a judgment as to whether removing external pressures will enable the child to recover and to get back on his or her appropriate developmental track. Or will the youngster require direct therapeutic attention either in family, individual, or sibling subsystem sessions in order to recover?

The assessment process needs to include an awareness on the part of the clinician that a disruptive or "disturbed" child's actions and attitudes may be the source of marital disruption as well as the result of marital disharmony. This is not a one-way street; the effects can go both ways. Children can be upset by parents. Parents can be upset by children. Symptomatology can emerge on either side of the fence.

The general tendencies of therapists have been summarized as follows: The younger the child, the greater the emphasis placed on working with the parental subsystem. With preadolescent clients and their families, the primary focus is likely to be on strengthening the parental coalition and increasing parental effectiveness. Such treatment starts with conjoint family sessions, although in some instances the parents may be seen prior to the initial family session. Typically, the focus shifts to sessions with only the parental subsystem present (Rosman, 1986).

When the Problems Involve an Adolescent

With older adolescents and young adults, the major goal generally is to facilitate appropriate separation of the young person from the family, that is, to prepare for and assist with the launching process (Rosman, 1986). As stated in the family life cycle description (Table 8.1), the family's task is: "Balancing adolescents' growing need for freedom and relative independence with appropriate assumption of personal responsibility en route to their departure from the home and adjusting parents' corresponding relinquishment of total responsibility, including the continuing evolution of communication to deal with changing relations between generations."

Hence, the initial conjoint family sessions often are followed rather quickly by individual sessions for the adolescent/young person, sometimes by sibling subsystem sessions, and by couple sessions for the parents for the purpose of promoting the disengagement process.

When the Problems Involve an Adult (Spouse/Parent)

Although certain individually diagnosed conditions (e.g., agoraphobia, depression, alcoholism, narcissistic disorders, eating disorders [Jacobson & Gurman, 1986]) can be treated successfully through marital therapy, the view here is that the more conservative approach of starting first with the individual client generally is preferable. This allows the therapist more freedom to focus specifically on the diagnosed individual and his or her physical and biological conditions, as well as on his or her contextual background prior to entry into the marriage. Seeing the diagnosed person apart from the spouse at the outset does not mean that a systems framework is not used.

Provided certain conditions are met by the marriage and the spouse of the affected person, the treatment may soon be shifted to the context of the marriage. If the marriage is clearly at the point of dissolution or if its future is uncertain, the choice is to continue therapy with the affected individual without involvement of the partner. If the couple's handling of the major marital tasks—commitment, caring, communication, conflict/compromise, and contract—indicate that the marriage is strong, efforts will be made to involve the spouse in the treatment at appropriate points (Nichols, 1992b).

Some of this treatment includes using the assistance of the so-called "nonproblematic" spouse (i.e., the spouse who is not the identified patient) as a helper in the treatment process, as well as working with both spouses to incorporate the changes made by the identified patient into the couple's marriage, family, and daily life. A basic question is whether or not the spouse can be helped to gain adequate understanding and acceptance of the affected mate's difficulties so that he or she can be supportive of therapy and the mate's efforts to cope with and master the condition. Sometimes a few sessions with the spouse that focus on education, the spouse's ideology about the condition, and clarification of feelings can be sufficient to make possible the enlistment of the spouse as a helper in the therapeutic process (Nichols, 1992b).

Two other questions need to be monitored constantly as the spouse is involved in dealing with the affected mate's condition and therapy: (1) Is the spouse continuing to be adequately understanding and supportive? If so, treatment in the marital context and with the assistance of the spouse can be continued. (2) Is the spouse becoming threatened and acting in ways that undermine progress? If so, the affected person may need to be seen in individual therapy, at least for a time (Nichols, 1992b).

Seeing one spouse in individual therapy does not mean that the other spouse should be excluded entirely from contact with the therapist. Many individually oriented therapists today still try to ignore the marriage and deal with their client as if his or her private, personal issues are all that matter, as if the client is an isolated, independent entity. At the extreme end of this approach, some therapists still refuse to meet with the other spouse or even talk to him or her by telephone. It has not been difficult to collect a considerable amount of clinical evidence over the years that the individually oriented therapist who ignores marriage or tries to treat a couple without understanding marital dynamics and having training in marital therapy can be very dangerous to marital health. Official neutrality by the therapist regarding the marriage when treating a married person in an individual format often results in damage by default, in other words. The result frequently can be described as "The [individual] therapy was a success, the marriage died." Certainly there are ethical issues involved in seeing one spouse alone and excluding the other.

A brief description follows of the course I take when I see a married person individually. I tell the client that I need to see the spouse for two reasons. First, I wish to learn what I can from the spouse in order to help the client. I point out that over the years I have found it quite helpful to get the spouse's perspective, that the spouse typically can provide understanding of my client that no one else can. Second, I wish to do this in order to help ensure that the therapy does not needlessly threaten the spouse or damage the marriage. To this I add whatever is pertinent in particular cases.

I will offer to talk with or even in some instances to call the spouse after my client indicates to them that I would like to see them for one session, if the spouse has any questions. I typically see the spouse alone but may, depending on the circumstances, see him or her in a conjoint interview with my client. When they do come in—and this happens in the vast majority of cases of intact marriages and sometimes in cases of separation or divorce (when I see a former spouse, of course)—I make the agenda clear at the outset, that is, I want their help to better understand the client and that is the sole purpose of the interview.

On the rare occasions in which the spouse seeks to bring up personal issues and to make the session into a personal interview, I point out what is happening. I make it explicit again that I did not ask them to come in for that purpose and that I will keep faith with them and stay on the subject of understanding their mate. If the nonclient husband or wife who has come in for the single interview then makes an explicit request for help with their personal concerns, I have to decide whether to take a bit of time to do that, whether to refer them to somebody else, or whether to consider the appropriateness of recontracting with my client for marital therapy.

When the Problems Involve the Marriage

When the presenting complaints or the problems uncovered during the initial assessment pertain to the marital relationship and marital interaction, conjoint marital therapy is indicated. The marital relationship may be mildly disturbed or it may be severely pathologic and problematic. Some difficulties lie in the object relations attachments. Henry V. Dicks's 1967 book, *Marital Tensions*, is still one of the best sources for good examples of couples whose disturbed object relations capacities fit together in "cat and dog" fashion. These are couples who "cannot live with" and "cannot live without" the person with whom they are united in unholy deadlock. There are other couples who can form a good second marriage, who are capable of living in a healthy relationship with another person, although not with the present partner.

Among the reasons for choosing marital therapy as the first form of treatment are the couple's indications of awareness that they have problems in the marriage and a willingness on the part of both to maintain the marriage; an indication that a situation exists in which disruptive symptoms of one or both partners maintain or exacerbate those symptoms (Sager, 1976); individual therapy has failed or cannot be used; indications that improvement in one individual will result in the appearance of symptoms in the other partner or in divorce (Haley, 1963); and existence of a fragile marital relationship, immaturity, interlocking pathology, or paranoid trends that may be increased by separate meetings of the therapist and the nonparanoid spouse (Whitaker, 1958a, 1958b).

When the Problems Involve the Family of Origin

Family-of-origin issues are always involved in some sense. Here the reference is to problems that explicitly require attention to a client's family of origin in order to effectively alter maladaptive patterns. Some attention is given to family-of-origin relationships in the section "A Chronically Problem-Laden Marriage: The Values" later in this chapter.

Conjoint Family Therapy Sessions

The presumption from the beginning of the family therapy movement has been that working with the family system is central. There is still a preference for having conjoint family sessions at the outset unless there are indications to the contrary, as illustrated in the preceding sections. Getting the family together, particularly involving the father, is not always an easy task (L'Abate, 1975; Shapiro & Budman, 1973; Slipp, Ellis, & Kressel, 1974).

Some family therapists insist on having all family members present before proceeding with treatment because they believe that the failure to secure the participation of some members significantly negates therapeutic efforts. Napier and Whitaker (1978; Napier, 1976; Whitaker & Bumberry, 1988), for example, consider it exceedingly important for the therapist to win the "battle for structure" or the "battle for initiative" at the outset. However, research has indicated that few therapists are likely to be so insistent on total family attendance as to refuse to begin unless that condition is met (Berg & Rosenblum, 1977).

Most therapists appear to grapple at times with the issue of helping potential clients to redefine the therapeutic focus from an individual to a family systems perspective. A common obstacle to gathering the entire family for the initial assessment and treatment stages, for example, is the parental perception that the problems reside in the child (or adolescent or young adult). "The kid is giving us fits. He won't do his homework. He cuts classes. We think he may be using drugs. We want him straightened out." That's the kind of message that comes across implicitly and often explicitly and blatantly, frequently accompanied by rationalizations such as the following: "We never had any trouble with his sister. She was raised in the same family. There's nothing wrong with the family. We need this kid fixed. That's why we called you."

Convening Issues and Strategies

The belief that the problems exist within a given individual and the accompanying insistence on individual therapy is not the only factor that contributes to difficulties in convening the entire family. General anxiety, denial of problems, covert maneuvering of family members to exclude a given family member, the threat that total family involvement poses to existing family homeostasis and alliances, and lack of effort on the part of the family and the therapist also have been depicted as contributing to failure to convene (Teismann, 1980).

Although suggesting that convening is more properly the task of the family with the support of the therapist, Teismann (1980) has presented several useful strategies for convening families. He describes one set of strategies under the heading of an enabling stance. These involve efforts to increase the attractiveness of attending (e.g., suggesting to a reluctant father that his son needs a man's example that only the father can provide or offering a [safe] consultant's role to the unwilling family member until he or she is ready to become a full participant) or efforts to decrease the attractiveness of not attending (e.g., stating therapist confusion over what benefit the hesitant person seeks for him- or herself by not attending therapy). The other set of strategies fall under the stance of enforcing. This involves the mobilization of referring and other networks to bring pressure on the family to convene itself (e.g., therapist enlistment of schools, physicians, clergy, and others to join in the convening endeavor).

Clinical experience indicates that parents' fears of being blamed sometimes contribute to their reluctance to get involved in family therapy with their offspring and that getting past the blame issue in some instances is critical to securing total family participation. With respect to the husband/father, L'Abate (1975) has suggested that apprehensions about being blamed and having their role undercut may cause those with rigid role orientations to decline to participate. Explanations that the family is the unit of therapy can carry the clear message that no individual is to be made the focus of blame. This can include the statements that a child's behavior (or symptoms) generally reflects family processes, disruptions in family communication and relationships, and that working with the family and having its support is essential in helping the child to change.

The therapist is well advised to regard his or her task first as a matter of reeducation of the parents to the systemic nature of problems and symptoms and only secondarily, if at all, as the need to deal with client "resistance." Bell (1975) has indicated his experience that it has never been necessary to refuse to make an appointment in order to compel both parents to attend. Rather, "quiet insistence that it is necessary to see both parents" (Bell, 1975, p. 25) generally has been sufficient to ensure full participation.

Starting with the Family

Making the initial contacts with clients were described in earlier chapters. It should suffice here merely to point out that making initial connections with the family as a whole and with the individual members is both a delicate and a critical process. Aiding the members in "settling into" therapy can be expedited by a variety of approaches. Whether the therapist does so primarily as a "conductor" in the manner of a Virginia Satir, John Elderkin Bell, or Salvador Minuchin, or as a "reactor/analyst" following Ivan Boszormenyi-Nagy or James Framo (Beels & Ferber, 1972), for example, depends on the orientation and preference of the clinician.

The role of the therapist in conjoint family therapy with families with adolescents certainly is more demanding and trying than with younger children. The struggle between the adolescent striving for more self-determination and often lack of restraint and the parents holding on and trying to maintain control puts the therapist much more "in the middle" than in many other kinds of therapeutic undertakings. To be challenged by a suspicious and distrustful teenager is not an unknown experience for therapists, some of whom periodically engage in dialogue similar to the following:

TEENAGER: This is not fair. You're on their side.

THERAPIST: How do you mean?

TEENAGER: You're all grownups.

THERAPIST: I'm not on their side, and I'm not on your side either.

TEENAGER: What do you mean?

THERAPIST: I'm on my side. I'm here to do the best job that I can in working with all of you.

At the same time that family work with families with adolescents challenges the therapist, the developmental status of the adolescent and his or her ability to participate at times in the therapy interaction in at least quasi-adult ways provides new opportunities for therapeutic intervention. Humor can be an effective intervention and tension reduction device with many families with adolescents. For example, with some families that are caught in a struggle over the teenager's room, the suggestion that they adopt the rule "Nothing growing there that shouldn't be" may strike a responsive chord with both parents and teenager and help to open up workable dialogue. Good judgment has to be exercised, of course, regarding the particular clients and times when humor can be used.

Adolescent–Parent Conflict

Reestablishment of the parents as the executive unit, the authority, in the family is an important and common issue with families that have adolescents. Although the therapist needs to take charge of the therapy from the beginning, efforts to do so should not undercut the parents. Just as parents should be working themselves out of a job from the beginning, so should the therapist. There is a need in many instances to help parents develop or restore an appropriate intergenerational hierarchy (much as Minuchin, 1974, emphasizes in his structural family therapy) and to develop effective problem-solving skills with their offspring.

In one common pattern that presents in therapy, one parent is over involved in an antagonistic relationship with the adolescent and the other feels caught in the middle between the two antagonists. In reality, the adolescent–parent conflict may represent parent–parent conflict that has been deflected to the adolescent who has been triangulated into the parental relationship and interaction. However, efforts to intervene by identifying the underlying parental conflict and recommending that the adults deal with it directly or by moving the peripheral parent into the primary disciplinary role have proven unsatisfactory (C. F. Johnson, 1993).

Uncovering the parental conflict typically resulted either in the adolescent increasing the problem behavior or in the family stopping treatment. Putting the peripheral parent in charge of discipline resulted in a cessation of the problem behavior and the predicted (Minuchin, 1974) emergence of marital conflict, but all too often in subsequent marital breakup. The second approach did not adequately deal with the parental split, thus leaving the marriage vulnerable to the emerging conflict.

In response to these findings, Johnson (1993) developed a new model that has proven effective in preventing and resolving adolescent–parent conflict, which is intended to achieve the following:

- Strengthen the parents' position at the top of the family hierarchy while allowing the adolescent some voice in decisions that involve him or her.
- Expedite "detriangulation" of the adolescent and parents but without confronting the marital conflicts directly or perpetuating the parental split. Instead, the therapist intends to move the parents toward each other and to encourage them to work together while

simultaneously inculcating and nurturing in them the skills necessary to resolve conflicts as they emerge.

- Assist the adolescent in his or her developmental task of acquiring
  the skills necessary to live independently.
- Be ingenuous enough to be readily understood and put into practice
  by families with differing levels of intellectual and verbal comprehension.

The model, briefly described, has three steps: The adolescent makes
a proposal or suggestion to the parents, outlining what he or she believes
to be a fair and workable resolution of the issues. (It should be noted that
a wide variety of conflicts can be approached this way.) Next, the parents
discuss the proposal, negotiate with each other over it. Last, they inform
the adolescent of their decision.

Johnson (1993) describes several guidelines and issues that need to be
taken into account by the therapist and outlines the kind of guidance the
therapist should provide to the adolescent and the parents. The approach
involves the recognition that autonomy develops best when adolescent
participation in decision making is encouraged but parents make the final
decision. Adaptations to remarried family and single-parent situations are
described.

Sibling Subsystem Sessions

Sibling rivalry is probably the first association many people have to the
term "sibling." Where this situation prevails, it often can be linked to
parentification, indulgence, or infantilization of one child. The parentified
child is pulled inappropriately into the parental relationship and frequently is given excessive responsibility for taking care of the parents, the
household, and the siblings. Along with the inappropriate responsibility,
the child gains great amounts of favors and attention. This establishes
interactive patterns between that child and the siblings that are basically
confrontational. The other children cannot compete for attention with
that child and feel left out, hurt, and often angry.

Therapy with the sibling subsystem typically is not undertaken only
because of concerns over sibling rivalry as such. It is also indicated where
there are concerns about boundaries between generations, a need to
separate children's roles from those of parents, and a desire to reestablish
and reinforce an appropriate hierarchy of authority in the nuclear family.
Additionally, therapy with the sibling subsystem can be effectively used to
help the siblings provide support for one another when parental conflict
is strong or emotional neglect of the children is evident. Bell's (1975) lower

limit of 9 years of age for children to participate in family group therapy appears to be a good guideline for determining whether or not children are suitable for sibling subsystem therapy. I have found the sibling subsystem therapy approach to be particularly effective with adolescent and adult siblings.

In the midst of conjoint family therapy in which the children are not participating freely, I frequently find it helpful to arrange for two or three sessions with the siblings without the parents being present. As Bank and Kahn (1982) point out, once the parents are not present, a group of "impassive, truculent, resistant, nonverbal siblings" can come alive and be wonderfully frank with the therapist (p. 306).

The therapist generally needs to prepare the parents carefully for the fact that he or she wishes to see the children as a group, apart from the parents. An explanation along the line of, "We have found that children can help each other and that it usually is helpful to the parents as well for an outside professional person to meet with the children and explore what bothers them," accompanied by candid responses to questions about procedures and so forth, normally is sufficient to gain parental permission and cooperation for the therapist to meet with the children.

Careful and honest explanations to the children regarding their parents' concerns for them and the purposes of the meeting are crucial when the therapist does meet with the youngsters. "What do you see as the problems in the family [or at home]?" "What would you like to see changed?" may be questions that have already been addressed to the children in conjoint family therapy. If not, they can be raised in sibling sessions, but with particular care and concern for causing potential loyalty conflicts for the children vis-à-vis their absent parents. Additionally, the question, "How can you help each other [meaning the siblings] deal with the troubles at home?" needs to be raised and explored.

"Is there anything that you would wish to say as a group to your parents?" This last query tends to produce a number of responses and concerns over how the response(s) will be relayed to the parents. Sometimes, the children wish to have the question addressed to each of them by the therapist in the next conjoint family session and to speak for themselves individually. On other occasions, they express a desire for the therapist to speak for them in the conjoint family session. Either of these approaches seems preferable to having one of the children serve as a spokesperson for the group. The message(s) may be as simple and bland as a statement that the children found it helpful to talk among themselves with an interested and impartial professional and they appreciate the fact that their parents made it possible for them to do so, that the talk cleared the air and lowered tension. With other groups, there may be one or more explicit statements or requests that the children wish to direct to their parents.

A Clinical Example

Two sibling sessions were used early in treament with the Stamps family in a effort to get the therapeutic process moving when it appeared that an impasse was developing. The Stamps had sought help to get a difficult teenager "fixed up." Betsy, 17, was doing poorly in academics, had a boyfriend that the parents disapproved of, and had a "don't care and rebellious attitude." Following some exploration, they agreed to try family therapy and came in with Betsy and her older sister, both of whom were living at home.

Observation of how the family arranged itself in sessions provided mute indications of generational division: The parents were side-by-side on one side of the room and the daughters—Betsy and Anna, 19—were together opposite the parents. Despite efforts to involve all four family members, the parents did most of the talking. They contrasted Betsy with Anna, who was on the dean's list at the local community college, had a boyfriend whom they liked, and was "responsible and cooperative, easy to get along with." "She comes in on time, while Betsy is always late," they reported. They quickly sketched a fairly classic pattern in which the older daughter played a "good child" role and the younger, a "rebel" role.

Wishing to move the focus off Betsy as the identified patient and to break the developing impasse, I soon suggested the use of a few sibling subsystem sessions. Although I did not mention the fact, it appeared to me that Anna was quietly uncomfortable with the family patterns and might be a good resource in forming a working relationships with Betsy. Bank and Kahn (1982) have written that the therapist has the challenge of discovering the nature of the bond between siblings, learning how the bond was forged, and determining how responsive it will be in therapy (p. 296). I had formed the impression that there was a fairly strong and viable bond between Betsy and Anna. It developed subsequently in the sibling sessions that there were feelings of similarity between the sisters but also feelings of difference in how they reacted to parental expectations and pressures. Anna was also "rebellious" but in much less overt ways than Betsy, outwardly complying but quietly going her own way and doing what she wished to do whenever she could do so without engendering conflict.

In introducing the idea of sibling sessions to the family, I specifically noted the difficulty in communication that was prevailing in my office as well as in the Stamps' home. "You obviously have been trying hard here and have made it clear that you are not happy with how things are at home, but talking about what needs to be changed and how this could be done seems to be very difficult. Sometimes it is helpful to see part of the family apart from the whole family. It is sometimes easier for the children to get started talking that way. We will come back together and see if we can open up the communication so that you can talk better and more comfortably." Once this was followed by the explanation mentioned above, the family agreed to the suggestion.

The three sessions with the daughters dealt initially with their desires to have their parents cease comparing them because they felt driven apart by the comparisons and with their concerns about their parents "hanging onto" them. They were able to articulate apprehensions regarding how their parents would fare when they left home. "What do you think you could do to help the home situation?" was the question that I explored with them after the complaints had been laid out and their feelings vented. We also discussed what they wished to say to their parents and how they could say it in ways that the parents could understand and accept.

I did some interpreting of their parents' anxieties, normalizing the parental concerns as accurately and honestly as I could. It helped to make statements and suggestions such as "Your parents have had children around for 19 years and now they're facing the possibility very soon of having both of you leave home. That's something they haven't been through before. Perhaps it's scary for them. Do you think it would be helpful to ask them how they feel about your leaving home?" Anna and Betsy seemed to catch on for the first time to the idea that their parents might be facing some uncertainty. Parental rigidity took on new meanings, especially when we looked at it in terms of the parents' evident desires to try to make certain that their daughters were prepared to handle life on their own.

When we resumed conjoint family sessions, the daughters were able, on the basis of some coaching, to express their concerns rather directly to their parents and to listen to what the parents said to them. We began to deal with the concerns of all four family members regarding the transitions that were beginning to occur as the family contracted. This evolved into family problem solving in which all participants and both subsystems— parental/marital and sibling—began to assume responsibility for making the transitions work effectively. For example, Anna took some responsibility for double-dating with Betsy and for introducing her to some more acceptable young men. Some negotiation of hours and curfew times followed, made easier for the parents by the fact that both daughters were involved. Following through on the start made in therapy, the Stamps family began to report more effective communication at home.

The final phase of therapy involved marital therapy for the partners to help them adjust to the coming life together without children at home. Although this was not a family troubled with serious pathology, it seems evident that the use of the three sibling subsystem sessions greatly facilitated a therapy process that was threatening to become stymied. Similarly, a fourth sibling session at the time the daughters left therapy was useful in consolidating their gains and in leaving a clean field in which their parents could continue their marital work.

The Stamps were an example of parents who were bound to their own parents. Their concerns about their children dealt not only with what would happen when the children left home but also with whether they were rearing children whose behaviors would be approved by their own parents (the grandparents). Working with them included taking up the question of "Who is (figuratively or literally) looking over your shoulder as you do your parenting?" Thus the liberation of the teenagers and the liberation of Mr. and Mrs. Stamps were connected and took place concurrently.

Sibling Sessions with Adult Clients

When the client is an adult, the family therapist may wish at times to consider involving siblings in the therapy experience instead of or in addition to only working with the parents from the family of origin. Many clients harbor strong fears about bringing their parents into therapy, and recreating the sibling subsystem may be more acceptable and less threatening. Many of the same family-of-origin data that generally are obtained from parents can be relived and worked through just as easily and effectively with siblings. Sibling sessions may also have long-lasting effects by improving formerly poor sibling relations. The sharing of early experiences and perceptions among siblings engenders a useful bonding among them despite the differences that they experienced growing up in their family of origin.

Sometimes all of the siblings may be experiencing the same kinds of problems. For example, all may be struggling with unresolved grief over the loss of a parent. In one case, three adult siblings, all of whom were in individual psychotherapy, were assembled together with their mother in order to deal with the residual effects from the sudden death of their father 20 years earlier. Sharing their experiences for the first time, giving each other support, and, very importantly, getting "permission" from their mother to let their father "be dead" enabled them to let their truncated grief process open up and flow appropriately. Subsequent to the sibling sessions, they were able to maintain regular contact and to form ongoing relationships that had not been possible earlier.

Marital Therapy

This section includes material that is primarily illustrative of some common and difficult kinds of cases and situations that present to the therapist.
Conjoint marital therapy frequently is aimed at restoring or establishing a workable complementarity between the spouses. I find it helpful
to focus initially how on the "C's" of commitment, caring, communication, conflict/compromise, and contract appear and the part they play in
the marriage and marital interaction (see Table 8.4), as well as on any
individual pathology that prevails. Typically, much marital therapy moves
back and forth between interventions with individual concerns and interventions with relationship and interactive issues (see, e.g., "A Differentiating Couple: The Browns," in Chapter 7).

Chronically Problem-Laden Marriages

Among the most difficult to understand and treat of the confusing and
frustrating cases that come to the therapist is the chronically problem-

TABLE 8.4. The Marital Life Cycle

Affirming the integrity of the relationship and preparing for the remaining years.

Core tasks

Commitment
Maintaining a solid couple boundary and internal bond.

Caring
Maintaining closeness and caring in spite of the possibility of divergent
   interests, individual development, or sameness and boredom threatening
   marital satisfaction.

Communication
Attending to maintenance of intellectual and emotional sharing.
Reexamining assumptions about communication and presumed shared
   meanings.

Conflict/compromise
Reconciling personal and marital needs and desires.

Contract
Reworking the expectations and "bargains" of the couple relationship.

Parental tasks

(As related to or influencing marital life cycle)

Childrearing
Coping with the tasks of rearing adolescents.
Letting go of children.
Dealing with the "empty nest" period.

laden marriage that lasts for years in varying states of disharmony. Such cases typically appear when the couple is in this stage of the family life cycle or in the next stage. The partners seemingly cannot live together in peace and cannot sever their relationship. Such marriages have been described as "cat and dog" marriages (Dicks, 1967) and as conflict-habituated marriages (Cuber & Harroff, 1966). When the tensions in the relationship are elevated above tolerance levels for the partners, neurotic or psychotic reactions emerge that may be handled within the marital dyad (Stewart, Peters, Marsh, & Peters, 1975). Some of these cases come to the attention of therapists and other professionals, but the mates do not necessarily make much progress in treatment.

Dicks's (1967) adaptation of Fairbairn's (1952, 1963) object relations theory to marital interaction provides a helpful description and explanation of such relationships. A useful summary of Dicks's concepts of splitting, projective identification, idealization, and collusion has been provided by Stewart and associates (1975). Dicks attempts to account for enduring but mutually provocative marriage relationships by viewing marriage as involving a latent transaction process between the spouses' hidden subidentities. In such relationships, the spouses invest each other with qualities derived from past psychological objects, particularly parents. Each spouse perceives the other as possessing some kind of shared internal object problem that complements with their own. The mate is idealized in either negative or positive terms to fit the other's needs, as both partners hope unconsciously to obtain integration of their own personality by finding lost parts in their mate. Dicks describes mate selection as involving the recognition of a "fitness" in the other for mutual working through or repeating of unresolved conflicts or splits in each personality. At the same time, each mate senses a guarantee that the problem will not be worked through with that person. The resulting marital collusion, an unconscious agreement and patterns of interaction aimed at keeping things as they are, makes therapy exceedingly difficult and problematic with such cases. Those marriages continue because of the persons' real need for growth and integration; each partner represents part of the total personality that is found in the marriage, neither feels that they can be a total personality on their own. A healthy marriage, on the other hand, involves complementary growth in the direction of individual completeness and enhancement (Dicks, 1963, 1967). Willi (1982) has added some recent work on marital collusion.

Many of these chronically problem-laden marriages do not, as I have indicated, lend themselves to therapeutic progress to any significant degree. There are some indications from clinical observation that family-of-origin sessions may be much more efficacious than working on these cases from a transference perspective.

A CHRONICALLY PROBLEM-LADEN MARRIAGE: THE VALUES

An example of a marriage in which marital collusion played a significant role and transgenerational issues were evident is provided by Jack and Sandra Value. The collusive process was not nearly as virulent as some of the cases described by Dicks, but it nevertheless was effective in maintaining a long-term marriage with chronic problems.

In terms of the marital tasks, the C's, the commitment and caring parts were well established. Briefly, the Values were both committed to the marriage. Neither gave any indications that they had serious questions about continuing in the relationship or that they could conceive of being married to anyone else. Their commitment to changing the relationship was not so obvious, particularly on the part of Sandra. Although frustrated with the attitudes and actions of the other from time to time, each claimed to love the other and manifested signs of caring.

Work with them focused on their communication, intertwined with dealing with their conflicts and helping them to improve their conflict resolution skills, for an eventual outcome of altering their marital contract in a healthier direction. As with many couples, skill development was encouraged and instituted where indicated. Again, in a typical fashion, as blocks were removed and the communication improved, the underlying anxieties, fears, and conflicts emerged. Their uncomfortable complementarity was strongly related to their largely unconscious implementation of models of relationship that they had internalized in their respective families of origin.

How some of these issues were played out and dealt with in a conjoint interview is summarized below. Various tasks related to the individual, as well as the marital, life cycle tasks can been found. For example, Jack was concerned with evaluating his aspirations and vocational and economic achievements—frequently negatively—and grappling with the effects of adjusting to changing physical abilities.

The session described here was the sixth with the couple and reflected a greater initiative on Jack's part in comparison to Sandra, something that was rather unusual. She was more reactive than was generally the case. Jack opened the appointment by relating an incident that had occurred earlier that day. He discussed it as an illustration of their ongoing interaction. Examination of the interaction and the use of some reality testing in the session elucidated several salient patterns in the marriage and their association to parental models of relationship from both families of origin. Jack's initial attempts to gain the support of the therapist against what he perceived as Sandra's insensitivity were dealt with by a tacit acknowledgment of his pain and a concentration on the couple's communication and interaction in the incident. The partners were essentially redirected to addressing their concerns to each other, rather than to or through the therapist.

The incident was as follows. Jack's superior at the nonprofit foundation where he worked had charged another nonprofit organization for the use of a meeting room for a holiday event. Jack told Sandra about the matter when he got home. Both Jack and Sandra were outraged at the superior's actions, feeling that charging another nonprofit group was against the policies of the board of directors of the foundation and that the superior had wrongly acted as if he were representing the policy of the board in making the charge. Understanding his wife to say that he ought to go directly to the board about the matter, Jack felt "put down," that he was not a success, and that he was considered a failure once again by his wife. Ordinarily the next step for him after feeling that way and thinking that it was unfair of her would not be to discuss his reactions but to get angry and brood, building a second layer of resentment and estrangement. This time, however, he brought the fresh event and his resultant feelings into the therapy session.

Surprised to learn that her husband felt as he did, Sandra reported that she had said something essentially as follows, "If I were Jane Doe, I would go to the head of the board of directors and say, 'Thus and so' about this matter." She then had spelled out in brief detail what she would do in those circumstances as a means of correcting what both she and her husband considered wrong in the superior's behavior. She had gone on to say, however, "If I were not Sandra Value, I would not know about it," meaning that she knew about what had happened because of her husband. Jack agreed that those were the words that had been spoken earlier in the day.

During the exploration of the incident, it became evident that Sandra had in fact given indications that she recognized the bind that it would put her husband in if he were to go directly to the chair of the board and that she was neither saying directly nor implying that her husband should go over his superior's head with the matter. As the therapist helped them to clarify what actually had transpired in the incident, Jack pointed out that he still had difficulty in believing that his wife was not saying or implying that he should have done something. "I know that's what she said, but I still have a hard time feeling that she is not telling me that I'm wrong," he insisted.

"Have there been other times that you have felt this way?" asked the therapist. "How far back can you take these feelings?"

"Uh, as far back as I can remember. My mother was never wrong. Gee, she especially never told a lie! Never in her life [in her view]! Whenever we disagreed or something went wrong, I was wrong."

This link with his family-of-origin experiences led to some delineation of how his mother had externalized and denied her responsibility for error or for anything being wrong, and, in turn, to a brief discussion of how this must have felt to him when he was growing up. It emerged that it was only after he had become an adult that he had really become aware of how his mother externalized. The residual effect of living in relationship to such a pattern in a powerful parent was noted and reflected on briefly.

During the discussion, the clients mentioned some patterns that had prevailed in Sandra's family of origin. Subsequently, Jack pointed out, "Sandra tries to put me down, but not all the time. Sometimes she tries to protect me. Her mother did that, too, tried to protect her father."

Quickly, Sandra exclaimed, "She did but because he wanted her to. He would ask her to back him up and to protect him, as you call it." Later in the session, Sandra said that she was glad that her (deceased) father was not around to know about the present behavior of the Values' oldest child, because "it would kill him." Jack noted that she was again protecting her father. Sandra was not able to deny that this was the case because it was evident from her explicit statement that she felt that her mother was handling the disappointment over the youngster very well.

The theme of failure recurred when Jack mentioned his recent awareness that his athletic prowess—specifically his ability to keep pace with men 20 years his junior in racquetball and volleyball—involved identification with his father's athletic successes. Athletics had been the only area in which his father had been successful in his life, according to Jack. Portions of the tie between father and son were confirmed by Sandra when she noted that currently her father-in-law was being stressed by a recent decrease in his physical abilities that would not permit him to maintain his former level of performance in tennis.

The therapist made an attempt to provide some relief for Jack and to help him rationalize feeling good about his own athletic ability. This included pointing out that there were other reasons that one might feel elated at being able to perform better than younger persons besides issues related to one's father. These other reasons included, for example, "normal" competitive striving and some zestful feelings about being able to perform despite one's middle-age status.

"Yeah, you know I actually enjoy being the underdog more than being at the top," responded Jack. Asked to expand on those feelings, he continued, "If you lose, it's okay. You weren't expected to win anyway. You can kind of be successful without having to do better than the other guy, just do better than you were supposed to."

This brought back the subject of success, which had been a theme in earlier appointments with the couple. Moving from relating Jack's difficulties with experiencing and enjoying success to his perceptions about his father's lack of success, the therapy returned to how the success theme was handled in the Values' marriage. Jack complained to Sandra, "You don't appreciate it when I am successful. You obviously don't enjoy it. And you never have."

Sandra rejoined, "I feel like I have to downplay anything that I do that I feel good about. I may enjoy it, but I can't act like it or let my feelings show. Because from the way you act, it's very clear that you don't enjoy the things that I do, my little triumphs and achievements." They were in agreement that he did not seem to get any enjoyment out of his own successes either, even when he could admit that he had been successful in an endeavor.

It was possible to elucidate some of the meanings of the "protect husband" theme that appeared in this pattern in which Sandra held back mention and enjoyment of her achievements. The therapist pointed out to the couple how they had been "unconsciously colluding" to produce a pattern in which Jack was protected from having to deal directly with feeling successful by feeling unsuccessful and by being helped to feel unsuccessful. Jack's role in presenting himself in the marital relationship as unsuccessful and unable to acknowledge and enjoy his own successes was a largely unconscious pattern, now emerging into awareness, in which he virtually invited his wife to protect him by neither acknowledging nor appreciating her successes or his own.

By returning to an examination of the kind of process that was involved in the incident with which the hour was opened, it was possible to elucidate some of the mechanics of how the Values kept the collusive process operating. To the extent that Sandra was ambiguous in her statements and communications to her husband about significant matters, he was able (and was enabled) to distort things very easily.

The actions and dynamics of each partner could be related to their families of origin. Sandra's need to protect Jack and her attempts to do so by ambiguity actually made her behaviors reminiscent for him of the behaviors that he had witnessed in his own parents' marriage. Jack's invitations to Sandra to protect him actually made his behaviors reminiscent for her of the behaviors that she had witnessed in her parents' marriage. The Values, in other words, had partially reproduced models of relationships witnessed in the marriages of their own parents. Jack's mother had always been "the right one" and continued to play that role in the family. She evaded and "never" admitted responsibility. Jack's father was "unsuccessful." By his wife's implicit definition and externalization of responsibility, he had taken on the role of being blamed and considered responsible for whatever went wrong in the work and family worlds in which he lived. He cooperated by accepting the externalizations. Compounding the difficulty was the fact that Jack's grandfather, a prominent Western attorney, had been "super successful." In Sandra's family, her mother was "the strong one. She can take it." The mother had protected her husband because, as noted, he had requested it, according to Sandra. Her father had been "a good man." Sandra identified with him in some ways and "practically worshipped him."

In the Values' own marriage, Jack felt responsible for whatever went wrong and felt that his wife always put him in that position, that she put him down continually. Sandra was "strong" and "self-sufficient," and felt that her husband requested that she protect him. (In a sense she was correct, although she evaded responsibility in a manner somewhat reminiscent of how Jack's mother had evaded responsibility for her attitudes and actions.) Sandra felt scornful of her husband at times and expressed some deprecatory feelings, for example, about how he handled anxiety by "worrying out loud."

In brief, Sandra helped Jack in his need to be protected by being strong, by being scornful of his "weakness," and by being ambiguous. The latter permitted him to convert things into a relationship or situation similar to that in which he grew up, that is, one in which, if there were anything wrong, it had to be the responsibility of husband, children, or anyone other than the wife/mother. Jack colluded in the transactional process by presenting himself as unsuccessful and blameworthy and by a tendency to convert ambiguous conditions into situations in which he felt that he was being blamed and considered inadequate. Thus, as noted, the Values not only reproduced some of the models of relationship seen in their parents' marriages but also manifested in a relatively mild fashion a complementarity of the kind discussed by Dicks (1963, 1967).

A brief summary of some of the major actions and dynamics of the session with the Values includes the following:

1. An initial examination of the incident that Jack brought up at the outset as being indicative of the couple's ongoing interactions included some reality testing and clarification of what had transpired in the incident. Although the indications were that he had reacted somewhat inappropriately and had distorted the meanings of his wife's statements in the incident, exploration led to a more in-depth probing into their patterns of interaction, including some discussions of times in which there was evident ambiguity in her statements and communications to him.

2. An elucidation of their interaction included outlining the major features of their salient patterns, such as the "protect husband" and "avoid success" themes.

3. An examination of patterns in the parental marriages led to further understanding of how models of relationship from those marriages were being reproduced in their own marriage.

4. Some interpretation of the unconscious collusive process by which the patterns were being manifested in their marital interaction was begun in the session.

5. Some ways in which the partners could begin to alter the patterns of transactions in their marriage were delineated as follows:

- Pointing out that one first step toward securing some change was increasing awareness of how they interacted.
- Emphasizing the important and practical value of reality testing, including some specific examples of how they could try to make observations and ask questions about what was happening or what was meant by the other partner without being accusatory or blaming, that is, as nondefensively as they could. Also, guidance was offered on how to respond more openly and less defensively when asked to do something by their mate.
- Emphasizing the value of being as clear and consistent as possible in their efforts to avoid ambiguity and distortion. This included some illustrations of clear communication, building on what had been done in earlier sessions.
- Emphasizing the importance and benefits of continued efforts to understand what happened in their parental marriages and how those things were appearing in their own marriage, and emphasizing the importance of increasing their awareness and understanding of their families of origin, so that they could continue the process of differentiation of selves.
- Examining and beginning to interpret some of the transgenerational aspects of the relationships with one of their children, a situation in which Sandra really brought the lineage and "nongenetic transmission" of family issues into explicit focus. This portion of the session served in large measure to confirm much that had gone on in the early part of the hour.

In the next conjoint session following the one described, an examination was undertaken of the context in which Jack's father's failures had occurred in the Great Depression of the 1930s. The events were to some extent reframed and the failures redefined. The goal was to let the client realistically view his father as being more successful than he had perceived him previously, thus beginning to open the door for Jack to let himself consider being more successful without encountering transgenerational loyalty conflicts and fears. Jack emerged from that session noting that previously he had always accepted his father's own definition of his failure without question. All of this was done with an awareness on the part of the therapist that Jack was making a bid for the therapist's support.

There were some things that were not handled as explicitly as they could have been in the session. One that was touched on slightly, for example, was the matter of family loyalty conflicts. Rather than being brought into the open and dealt with explicitly in this session, the issues inherent in making changes from patterns followed by parents were dealt with rather indirectly. This session should be viewed in the larger context of ongoing therapy. Several of the matters that stood out clearly here had emerged in a less clear form in earlier appointments. Although this couple made some progress, they did not remain in treatment long enough to deal adequately with some of the long-term difficulties in their relationship, stopping at the end of the 3 months established by the wife as the length of her participation prior to beginning with the therapist. Additional therapy would have involved more family-of-origin work, possibly including bringing the surviving parents into family-of-origin sessions.

9

THERAPY WITH POSTPARENTAL COUPLES

If you like it, tell a grandparent.
—Sign in the window
of a children's store

Of all the things that move man,
one of the principal ones is the terror of death.
—ERNEST BECKER, *The Denial Of Death*

There is no easily discernible line, no discrete and disjunctive break between the launching stage of the nuclear family and the postparental stage. The departure of the last child from home has been chosen as an arbitrary marker for the dividing line between stages. This departure process and the recasting of the parent–child relationship, however, is complicated when the adult children are subsidized while pursuing graduate or professional education, buying a home, or beginning a business. Active parenting behavior may continue for some years after the last child has left home and there may be reversals of the launching process when a child later returns home for a period of time or permanent stay, for example, following a divorce. The complexity of the intergenerational interaction varies. Some families have a period in which there are four living generations, whereas others lose the grandparents early and may not go through a period in which three generations of a family are living simultaneously.

TABLE 9.1. The Family Life Cycle

Family developmental tasks

1. Incorporating new members by birth (grandchildren), dealing appropriately with loss of members of the older generation (parents of the spouses) and preparing for eventual loss of the parents (who have or will become the older generation).
2. Providing for the physical and economic needs of family members, including possibly closing the family home or preparing it for occupancy as older adults and adjusting to living on reduced income.
3. Establishing and maintaining satisfactory patterns of affection and communication among the generations in the family while continuing to balance the developmental needs of family members in different stages.
4. Providing for the socialization of the members into their new family roles (adult children into changing roles with parents and parents into grandparent and aging roles).
5. Affiliating satisfactorily with the extended family and the kinship and friendship networks, including realigning relationships to deal with gains and losses in the networks.

The major focus in this chapter is on the middle generation as it becomes the grandparental generation and moves into its final years. As the younger or child generation produces offspring, there is a shifting of generations. The middle generation moves into the position formerly occupied by the older generation and the younger enters the place formerly held by the middle generation (see Table 6.1). Typically, this final stage begins when the middle generation partners are in their 40s or 50s. With the eventual death of their own parents, of course, they become the oldest unit of the family.

AGING ISSUES

This final stage of the family life cycle involves a continuation of tasks that began in the launching stage (see Table 9.1). The parents have the dual tasks of reintegrating the marriage following the departure of the children and of coping with loss (see Tables 9.2 and 9.3). Some of the important parts of this stage were anticipated in the reference to the cogwheeling of generations in Chapter 8. Much of the activity discussed under that rubric continues into this stage.

Four significant issues associated with the tasks for the stage are concerns with the following:

• Changing dependency roles including, in some instances, the possibility of coming full cycle and again becoming dependent on others. Members of the middle generation who only years earlier may have engaged in a "reversal of generations" and taken over major responsibility from their own parents now may find themselves moving back into a dependency relationship in which they lean on their own children. They find themselves grappling with the things that their parents faced "only yesterday."

• Declining physical abilities and possible serious illnesses. The increased prevalence of physical problems associated with aging and disease require both the older person and the therapist to pay particular heed to the impact of organic factors on normal and pathological emotional development (Colarusso & Nemiroff, 1987). Although it is important to possess information on the client's general physical condition with all age groups—for example, the background form I use with all clients (Figure 5.1) seeks information on the client's last physical examination, health and illnesses, and any prescription medication being used—attention to physical condition and possible organic difficulties is especially important with elderly persons.

• Increasing losses including eventually the loss of one's own life. The individual life cycle involves a series of psychological and physical losses that may also include social and economic losses. Losses in any one of these areas can affect other areas in a truly systemic manner. As the

TABLE 9.2. The Individual Life Cycle–Aging

The major task of the older years is dealing effectively with the aging processes, possible illness, and eventual death while seeking to maintain a sense of purpose, meaning, and fulfillment in the face of one's losses and eventual demise.

Tasks

1. Reexamining changing relationships with one's family and accepting where applicable the necessity of altering dependency relationships to receive assistance from others graciously.

2. Employing resources wisely and selecting and maintaining social activities appropriate to current interests and abilities.

3. Adjusting effectively to changing physical abilities and altering sexual activity and identity as appropriate.

4. Coping with loss of friends and family members and in some instances learning to live alone or to seek to form new social relationships.

5. Finding as much meaning in one's life and place in the universe as possible and preparing for one's eventual death.

individual moves through old age, shifts involving both somatic (e.g., vision, hearing, and perhaps chronic disease) and psychological functioning occur. Reactions to loss of functioning may include loss of self-esteem, depression, or grief. Chronic disease may bring increased dependency on others, accompanied by hostility (Broden, 1970). Loss once again is a major issue for the original marital couple during this portion of the family life cycle. It is to be presumed that the loss of the children from the home during the launching stage generally has been faced and managed, for better or worse, by the parents. The death of the partners' own parents faces them with another kind of loss, carrying with it as concomitants the necessity of recognizing that they, the survivors, are truly orphans, and aging orphans who are themselves mortal. As they, the parental generation now becoming a grandparental generation, cope with such strong emo-

TABLE 9.3. The Marital Life Cycle

Achieving balance in life between achieved and potential satisfactions and forthcoming losses, including for some, making a transition into retirement, and preparing gracefully for the ending years.

Core tasks

Commitment
Supporting each other in finding and celebrating meaning.

Caring
Maintaining a satisfactory degree of closeness in the remaining years, including manifestations of caring and appreciation for past sharing, as well as manifestations of continuing affection and concern.

Communication
Deepening communication to provide for examination and sharing of the positive meanings achieved in the marriage, as well as preparing for potential loss and living without the spouse.

Conflict/compromise
Developing adequate patience and skill to deal as a couple with fears of loss of productivity and the possible meanings of the loss.

Contract
Supporting each other in attempts to find and celebrate meaning and cumulative achievements, in joint fulfillment of current potential for satisfaction, and in joint grief work where losses occur.

Parental tasks

(As related to or influencing marital life cycle)

Childrearing
Realigning relationships to include in-laws of children and trigenerational or quadgenerational family network.

tional realities, they also find themselves facing forthcoming retirement, health changes, declining physical strength and ability, and other issues that their own parents encountered some 25–30 years earlier. This familiar cycle keeps repeating itself.

• Meaning in the face of change. During the latter part of this stage in particular, couples reorganize their marital relationship around age-related factors such as illness, retirement, interpersonal or shared loss, widowhood, and death (Carni, 1989).

The major clinical concern in this chapter will be with loss and death. Many of the issues dealt with by the couple in their marital and parental interaction are similar to those of earlier stages, and thus do not warrant separate treatment in this chapter. Some unique features, either have been addressed earlier or typically are not encountered as significant clinical problems, such as the attainment of grandparenthood.

THERAPY AND OLDER PERSONS

Although there are some indications to the contrary, therapy practice in general does not appear to have kept pace with changes in life expectancy. Although significantly larger proportions of the population of the United States and other countries are now living into their 60s, 70s, and beyond, therapists do not appear eager to engage in treatment with older persons. When they do, they do not necessarily do so with optimism. Typically the assumptions of therapists do not seem to have changed dramatically from the pessimistic perspective enunciated by Sigmund Freud early in this century. Freud (1906/1959) declared that near or around the 50s the elasticity of the mental process, on which the therapist depends, is as a rule lacking, and that older people consequently are no longer educable. Among the signs that change is occurring are statements from some therapists who provide long-term individual therapy that older persons need not be treated superficially (Colarusso & Nemiroff, 1987).

Therapist Concerns

Therapists' biases and anxieties may be the major factor in their failure to engage in effective therapeutic work with older persons. Therapist avoidance of older clients is related to a variety of factors, but particularly to the therapist's reactions to aging. Older clients may stimulate the clinician's fears about his or her own age and aging, may evoke reactions about conflicts and difficulties with one's parents who may be about the same age as the client, may bring forth anticipation of therapeutic impotence and failure because of a belief in the omnipresence of untreatable organic states in older persons, and may embody a fear of colleagues' negative comments regarding working with the elderly (Butler & Lewis, 1977). Other issues grappled with (or avoided) by both therapist and client include changes in sexual drive and activity; the assessment of career accomplishment and the recognition that not all personal goals will be achieved; planning for and/or adjusting to retirement; thoughts about one's own death; and altered relations with one's adult children, parents, and maturing/aging spouse (Colarusso & Nemiroff, 1987).

Client Concerns

The concerns manifested by clients vary somewhat according to whether the client is in the early part of the postparental stage (typically age 45 and older) or has moved into late (ages 65–80) or late-late (80 and older) adulthood. Concerns about loss of effectiveness in the work situation, career assessment, and forthcoming retirement (King, 1980) tend to come in the earlier parts of the stage, for example. Increased awareness of one's own death and the limited time remaining in one's life typically emerge as major concerns in the later years.

There are exceptions regarding when the concerns emerge. This is illustrated by the statement of a highly active and productive professional:

"I became acutely aware of my physical limitations and, more importantly, my mortality in my middle fifties. For a couple of years, thoughts would come into my awareness periodically of my mortality, that I was not going to live forever. Interestingly enough, they eventually passed, and I came to peace with the fact that I had to pace myself differently and be more discriminating in deciding what I would try to do with the rest of my life. I don't look forward to dying, but I'm not as anxious about it as I was for a time. I recognize that it makes sense to make choices and to take care of myself physically."

Fears regarding diminishing sexual interest and ability may appear at any time during the postparental stage. Contrary to popular views regarding elderly persons, sexual feelings and activity remain powerful, dynamic issues for many persons until death. The limitations on the sexual life of older persons are more likely to be imposed by the environment than by physical decline (Broden, 1970). Unfortunately, some therapists do not handle the sexuality of older clients well and may

react with surprise and anxiety when it appears in the interview (Colarusso & Nemiroff, 1987).

Clinical Issues

Some of the clinical issues in dealing with problems of this part of the
family life cycle are similar to those in therapy in other stages and some
are unique. Among the common features are the need to normalize the
problems faced by clients wherever and whenever appropriate. With older
clients, it is particularly helpful with those who have not completed the
requisite developmental tasks for making the transition into later adulthood to help them identify specific areas as normal developmental concerns, rather than indications of pathology. This can lower anxiety, elevate
hope, reinforce ego strengths, and encourage alternative, adaptive functioning (Baker, 1984).

Older Parents of Adult Clients

There often is a need to reach out therapeutically to older parents of adult
clients. It should not be uncommon for therapists to seek to work with
the parents of their adult clients, not solely in order to help their clients
to differentiate from their family of origin, but also for the purpose of
facilitating the maintenance of good, contemporary adult-to-adult relationships.

Adult Children of Older Clients

It is not uncommon today for parents who are in their late 60s and 70s
to need help in dealing with their married children. Sometimes they ask
for an older therapist who "can understand us." Among the unique
features of therapy in this stage is the need in many instances to intervene
with the children of the older person to help them to understand the needs
and behaviors of their parents. In contrast to working with parents to help
them understand the needs and behaviors of minor children, this part of
the life cycle deals with issues and developmental tasks that the adult
children have not experienced. Interventions that successfully influence
the attitudes of the adult children can significantly alter the environment
in which the elderly clients live and function (Broden, 1970). Sometimes
there may be a need to address the practical concerns of the elderly parents
of the adult child, as well as to work with the two generations therapeutically. Augustus Y. Napier (personal communication, February 2, 1995),
for example, has explored a pattern of sending therapeutic and practical

support into the home of elderly parents. He then meets with them and their adult children with the assistance of the support person, a social worker colleague.

Older Adults and Marital Therapy

Older adults occasionally seek a therapist because of conflict in their marriage. One common presenting problem is conflict created as a result of the departure from home of children who formerly played key roles in stabilizing a long-term, unhappy marriage. When children who serve as buffers between their conflicted parents leave home, there are at least five paths commonly followed by the parents. Parents may (1) seek to recapture the children and press them back into their former buffering role, (2) secure a divorce, (3) continue their conflict, (4) eventually "cool out" the conflict and continue residing together but pursue separate lives within the shell of a desiccated marriage, or (5) seek therapy.

Concerns about the marital relationship that surface in relation to the departure of the children from home (King, 1980) may become the impetus for seeking therapy at any time, prior to such departure, soon afterward, or several years later. My experience with those older persons seeking therapy in such instances has been that many of them do not make a contact immediately after their children leave home. Rather, there typically is a lag time before the postdeparture conflict escalates and reaches proportions that result in calling for therapeutic help. The contact comes after the couple has been unsuccessful in breaching the boundaries established by their departed children around the children's new life and relationships so as to continue old patterns of involving the children in their marriage.

Although some older couples present marital complaints at the outset, others present the problem as conflict with the younger generation. Not infrequently, the in-law is referred to initially as the source of the difficulties: "We would like to see our son and our grandson more often [etc.], but she [the daughter-in-law] won't do it, and she gives him [the son] fits if he insists on coming over." Or, "He [the son-in-law] doesn't want anything to do with us."

My initial task with such couples is to try to assess the importance of the conflict they describe with their married child and his or her spouse. If my clinical judgment indicates that there is a possibility of enabling the couple to deal with the situation with some coaching, I will use that approach. If the assessment indicates otherwise (e.g., that the parents are attempting to recapture their child and bind him or her to them and their own needs, or that the child has not adequately individuated), other steps are taken. If it seems that the adult child has individuated adequately, I likely will invite the young couple into sessions as the initial intervention of choice. Unlike family-of-origin sessions in which a client meets with his or her family of origin without his or her spouse being present, these sessions are couple–couple meetings. It seems vitally important to maintain the integrity of the relationship and life of the child and his or her spouse in such instances, symbolically emphasizing that the child has left home. If the adult child has not adequately individuated, it may be necessary to try family-of-origin sessions in order to help him or her reach the point of separating from the parents.

Simultaneously with working with the cross-generational issues, this approach reinforces the responsibility of the parents to deal with their own marital issues between themselves. After dealing with the initial complaints as appropriately and effectively as possible, I attempt to move into working with the older couple's marital relationship. Even minor amounts of probing into their relationship while working with the problems with their adult child are likely to uncover the parents' own marital conflict. Observation of the older couple as they make such complaints, for example, generally discloses that they are not in agreement about the problems.

When it has been established that the older couple do have some marital conflicts, the approach I typically use is to engage with them in a process of exploration, similar to that used with younger couples. This involves exploring with them how they met, how they were initially attracted, how they decided to get married, and how their relationship developed across the years. Beyond this general history of the relationship, I have specific questions for us to explore together: How did the marriage and the partner change? How has each of them changed? What were the disappointments with the marriage and with the partner? Each of these is examined and interpreted in relation to relevant family, marital, and life cycle issues. I give particular attention to feelings of blame and to modifying such feelings, normalizing what has occurred as honestly and realistically as I can.

"Midwiving" the relationship while trying to ascertain what positive forces are available for the couple's use becomes an important mode of intervention. Is there anything worth salvaging? My task is to help the couple make this discovery and to make their own decisions not only about the viability of the marriage but also about what they wish to do. I consider it important to help them determine whether they have given themselves a chance to make the transition to a workable couple relationship following the departure of children. At this stage, interventions and therapeutic concerns are essentially the same as with other couples experiencing conflict and considering divorce.

Concerns with Suicide

The older adult's stage of the life cycle has in common with adolescence a high incidence of suicide. Death is often selected by the elderly as a solution to problems stemming from physical illness, loneliness, general feelings of uselessness, economic exigency, and a desire to join a deceased spouse in death (Broden, 1970). Suicide by "giving up" and dying as a result of self-starvation and loss of the desire to live is not uncommon, although not necessarily labeled as suicide. The clinician or other professional person who queries the client and his or her family about suicide thoughts and possibilities may find these queries helpful in cutting into debilitating feelings of hopelessness and helplessness on the part of the client. Clients may be more willing and able to talk about their concerns than family members or therapists have assumed.

Concerns with Death and Dying

More so than with any other age group, the therapist treating the elderly is likely to deal with clients who are dying. At different phases in the process of dying, the client's needs differ. In the instance of a fatal illness, Schoenberg and Senescu (1970) have divided the initial stages of illness into detection, diagnosis, intervention, remission, progression, and the terminal stage. The final or terminal stage is further broken down by Glaser and Straus (1968) into several critical points that may occur: the person is dying; the person, the family, and the hospital staff prepare for death; the point is reached where there is nothing more to do; the final descent; the last hours; the death watch; and death itself.

A critical issue is whether or not individuals who are facing certain death wish to know they are dying. Denial, to a greater or lesser degree, is a common defense in persons with a fatal illness, according to Schoenberg and Senescu (1970). They prudently recommend that such defenses be respected "unless there is clear evidence that the advantages of breaking down a patient's defenses outweigh the advantages of maintaining them" (p. 231). Some research has long shown that the majority of persons wish to be told of their potentially fatal illness (Schoenberg & Senescu, 1970).

LOSS: BEREAVEMENT AND GRIEF

A comprehension of loss, bereavement, grief, and the entire mourning process is essential to dealing with this stage of the family life cycle. "Loss" pertains to being deprived of or being without something one has had (Peretz, 1970a). "Bereavement" refers to the loss itself, to being robbed, as it were, of something valuable to oneself, and to being left sad and lonely. "Grief" applies to the feelings engendered by the loss, the emotional reactions of the bereft person, including anger, hostility, fear, depression, despair, and others. Grief is used here as part of the larger process of mourning, which includes not only the emotional reactions of the person to the loss but also the total behavioral pattern exhibited by the survivor from the time of the loss onward (Bowlby, 1969). Mourning processes may be considered essentially concluded when the survivor has accepted the loss and reinvested emotions in new objects and pursuits and is restructuring his or her life in a reasonably stable and functional manner.

What constitutes a loss for one person may or may not be experienced as a loss by another individual because loss is at the same time a real event and a perception in which one confers personal or symbolic meaning on the event. For example, the loss or diminishing of physical abilities may be experienced as a demeaning experience by some and as a normal and inevitable part of aging by another. One significant aspect of loss by the elderly often is the threat of further loss; for instance, the loss of physical skills may threaten the loss of a job and a consequent loss of pride, as well, for some persons (Peretz, 1970a).

Individual Loss

The losses of the elderly person are multiple and varied. Not all losses in this period are object losses (loss of a person or object in which one is deeply emotionally invested). Some obviously stem from changes associated with the biological processes of aging, that is, changes in one's body and physical functioning. Peretz (1970a) has described the individual's losses as taking the following different forms:

- The loss of a significant loved or valued person (through death, separation, divorce, or acute or chronic illness).
- The loss of some significant aspect of the self (including positive self attitudes, health, bodily functions, and social roles and status).
- Loss of external objects (such as money, home, or homeland).
- Developmental loss (meaning loss that occurs in the process of human growth and development).

Reactions to Loss

How does the bereaved person react to the loss of persons from his or her life? What determines how he or she reacts? Bugen (1977) has proposed a model with two dimensions: centrality–peripherality and preventability–nonpreventability. "Centrality" refers to the major meaning the person holds for the mourner. This ranges from being so strong that there is "no life without" him or her; to a needed element in one's own life such that the loss is felt deeply and constantly; to a person to whom one was behaviorally committed through daily activities; to a person whose existence was a reminder and symbol of one's hopes and beliefs (such as President John F. Kennedy). "Peripherality" refers to the situation in which the person who has been lost is not experienced as irreplaceable or one's rewards and pleasures are not contingent upon the deceased.

"Preventability" refers to the general belief that the death might have been prevented or that the survivor directly or indirectly contributed to the death. "Nonpreventability," of course, refers to the belief that nothing could have been done by anybody to prevent the death; or that everything was done that was possible to prevent the death; or that the death can be attributed to fate, God, misfortune, or inevitability.

Bugen's model includes the following four major grief reactions:

- Central relationship—Preventable death: Intensive and prolonged.
- Central relationship—Unpreventable death: Intensive and brief.
- Peripheral relationship—Preventable death: Mild and prolonged.
- Peripheral relationship—Unpreventable death: Mild and brief.

Following this model, with a mourner who considered the deceased a central person in his or her life and also believed that the death was preventable, one would expect an intense and prolonged grieving process.

My suggestion is that Bugen's model is helpful but does not provide a complete approach for dealing with grief reactions. It is indeed important to know the specific ways in which the lost person was important to the mourner, and whether the areas of dependency between them were acknowledged without shame, guilt, or resentment and if not, how the areas of dependency and reactions to loss were expressed and resolved. However, the therapist also needs to understand the typical coping patterns of the mourner, the social and cultural milieu and their attitudes toward loss and death, and the special resources the individual and family have for coping with loss (Peretz, 1970a).

Lengthy lists of bereavement reactions have been compiled by others. These include, for example: "normal" grief; anticipatory grief; inhibited, delayed, and absent grief; chronic grief (perpetual mourning); depression; hypochondriasis and exacerbation of preexistent somatic conditions; development of medical symptoms and illness; psychophysiological reactions such as hypertension and ulcerative colitis; acting out (psychopathic behavior, drugs, promiscuity); and specific neurotic and psychotic states such as anxiety, phobic, hysterical, depressive, and schizophrenic reactions (Peretz, 1970b).

Loss of the Spouse

The most significant loss in the typical family life cycle as it moves onward toward the eventual disappearance of the middle generation is the loss of one's spouse. Although the loss of a parent or child by death may be exceedingly painful and personally disruptive and leave a residue from which one never totally recovers, it typically does not produce the disjunctive practical outcomes that accompany the death of one's marital partner and does not require the same rearrangement and restructuring of one's life.

The following discussion will deal with the reaction of a spouse on an individual basis, partly because that is where it is experienced most and partly because very little that is clinically helpful is known about systemic response to the death of a spouse. Only recently, for example, has the family therapy literature included a book dealing specifically and generally with the topic of death in the family (Walsh & McGoldrick, 1991). Families generally do not consciously prepare their members for dealing with death. The discussion that follows does not deal in any detail with situations in which there is a high degree of ambivalence and even relief at the death of a spouse, deaths in which there was something unsavory or shameful involved, or situations in which a family loses a member to homicide (Burgess, 1975). Those situations pose challenges for the individual and for the family system that require even greater sensitivity than normal on the part of the clinician. Most of the emotional reactions discussed below would be found in relation to any important loss, particularly loss resulting from the death of a close love object.

Loss of a loved one by death typically produces a crisis in a marriage and a family. As one works with the surviving partner, crisis-intervention and stress understandings and techniques typically are part of an appropriate background for dealing with loss of a spouse by death (Hill, 1949, 1958; McCubbin & McCubbin, 1989).

There are several good studies of the reactions of survivors to loss. The pioneering work in this regard was done by Lindemann (1944), who worked, in the 1940s, with 101 recently bereaved survivors of a nightclub fire tragedy. Lindemann described both psychological and somatic symptomatology and both normal and morbid grief reactions. Realistic acceptance of a new role, coping with guilt feelings, and acceptance of the mourning process all were identified as important elements in the resolution of grief.

Other studies have been provided by Kübler-Ross (1969) and Parkes (1973). Kübler-Ross suggested that there are five stages of adjustment: denial, anger, guilt, preparatory grief, and the "good-bye" stage. She also indicated that there is a separate set of stages for the dying persons themselves in mourning their own forthcoming loss.

Acute Grief Reactions

A useful formula for understanding acute grief reactions can be constructed from the available empirical research reports and clinical observations. Lindemann's work is the primary guide in the following description, but the work of Oates (1955) and my own observations and experiences with bereft individuals and families also are included.

1. The initial reaction to the loss or to being informed of the loss is shock, followed by numbness. Going numb appears to be nature's way of providing for protection against the pain. The person may not be able to discuss the loss or to accept support and comfort. Family members who wish to be supportive may be able to help simply by sitting quietly with the person at such times, rather than attempting to talk or to "do something."

This initial reaction may last from a day to several days, depending on the circumstances of the loss (whether expected or unexpected) the psychodynamics of the bereaved person, the nature of the relationship with the dead person, and a number of other issues.

2. A period of denial typically is evident. Expressions such as the following are frequently heard, "I don't believe it. It can't be true." The denial of the mental pain generally is accompanied by a range of agitated behaviors, including difficulties in settling down physically and problems in sleeping. Other physical reactions in an intense grief reaction often include tightness in the throat, decreased appetite, sighing, feelings of exhaustion, weakness, emptiness, and emotional waves lasting from 20 minutes to an hour (Lindemann, 1944; Peretz, 1970b). These reactions may or may not include outbursts of tearfulness and crying. For some persons, most of the crying comes later, after the original walls of disbelief and defenses of denial have been breached.

3. Surprising emotional reactions may be forthcoming as the denial breaks down and the next stage begins. Not only the survivor but also others around that person may be shocked and upset by the emotional reactions that erupt. Anger, rage, and bitterness all may pour out in alternating patterns that seem beyond the boundaries of reason.

Guilt reactions are prevalent. They may stem from the recall of ways in which one has failed the deceased person, including negligence, infidelity, quarrels, impatience, and others. "Survivor guilt" feelings, guilty reactions because one is still alive when the other person is dead, may be present. These may be expressed in the refusal to allow oneself to feel better or to anticipate going on living. Guilt feelings because one is feeling angry toward the deceased are quite common. Angry outcries against others and the Deity may be forthcoming, followed by reactions of guilt or bitterness over the loss.

Ambivalence may lie behind both guilt and anger feelings. The family of the dead person, for example, may be relieved that a prolonged illness and its accompanying stress have ended, but feels guilty at being relieved. The mixture of disappointment and anger with love and affection may be expressed in irrational anger at the deceased person for leaving, depriving the survivors of their presence, and leaving a burden for the survivors (Peretz, 1970b). "Why did he have to go and get himself killed? Why did he go to that football game? If he had stayed at home, he wouldn't have been in any accident!" "Why wouldn't she stop smoking? We told her it would kill her, we begged her to stop, but she wouldn't. Damn her, she was so selfish!"

The commonly experienced feelings of unreality may include illusory phenomena. One may believe that they hear the dead person's footsteps or, at least momentarily, that they are experiencing their presence. "I'm going crazy!" is a common fear and feeling. Eventually, most persons come to feel that they are not crazy. If they are able to accept the fact that a loss has occurred and that it is all right for them to have strong emotional reactions to the death and departure of the spouse, they move into the next stage.

4. When the breaching of the walls of denial has occurred and the initial irrational reactions have passed, painful feelings of emptiness and yearning for the lost object typically become prominent. Although this stage does not take place in the same way for all survivors, it is common for the person to think about and talk about the events of the death over and over. Sometimes even those who have not blamed themselves come to spend a considerable amount of time trying to determine whether they could have done anything to prevent the death, or make the deceased more comfortable, and so on. "Was it my fault? Could I have done anything?" These and similar questions may be voiced as the survivor turns over and over the memories of the death and last day. Many survivors repeat such questions internally, struggling with them without voicing them aloud or sharing their concerns with others.

5. Eventually, with most survivors, there comes a time in which the loss has been accepted and much of their living is done in the present. At odd moments and at unpredictable times, when they are reminded by circumstances that they formerly had a mate present but do not any longer,

there will be a return of the pain. This has been called poetically and accurately "selective memory and stabbing pain" (Oates, 1955). By this phase of the reaction, the survivor typically has withdrawn most of the emotional investment in the deceased spouse and has begun to invest in other pursuits and other persons. In pathological cases, individuals may continue to worship the deceased, to act as if he or she really has not died, or to take other paths that involve denial of the experience of loss and the nature of the relationship with the deceased partner.

Throughout the period of mourning, the survivor's abilities to function may vary widely. Endeavors that were routine in preloss days may take a significant amount of effort to accomplish. Sticking with a task may be difficult and sometimes impossible for the grieving individual. Talking may be done compulsively. Aimless behavior may mark the days of individuals who improve, and would be expected to improve, as the grief work is accomplished. New patterns of organization may evolve over a period of time, patterns that do not involve interaction with a mate who is no longer present.

Attention to clients' general functioning and dream life can be exceedingly beneficial in helping them to recognize their progress in coping with their loss and grief. A woman who had sought by various kinds of denial to avoid the pain that acknowledging the loss of her husband would bring experienced nightmares during the first few weeks. With strong therapeutic support, she gradually began to settle down. She reported a dream in which she was sitting on a sofa on which her husband was reclining with his feet in her lap. His feet were cold. Asked for associations to "cold," she responded, "Dead, death." "What do you think that means?" she was asked after some further exploration and discussion. "I'm accepting that Henry is gone. I'm letting go, gradually, but I'm letting go. It's going to be all right," she responded. This was confirmed by her subsequent behavior.

Support for the Bereaved

During the acute reaction phase, when the bereaved spouse is struggling to cope and keep functioning, social supports and rituals can be exceptionally helpful in maintaining balance for both that individual and the family. Making arrangements for the funeral, as painful as it may be, provides structure in a time of dimmed reality, for example. Condolence observances such as visits and other contacts by clergy, relatives, and friends provide a clear role for the bereaved with definite expectations, timetables, and practices, and also encourage open expression of grief (Peretz, 1970a).

Experience indicates that this is a rather crucial time in the bereavement process for the surviving spouse. The recommendation here is that the surviving spouse be as involved as he or she desires and is able in the activities and decision making around funeral arrangements and subsequent plans. Appropriate encouragement to take a role needs to be balanced with an expressed willingness to handle the things that the person does not feel up to facing.

Adult children of the surviving spouse can unwittingly retard their parent's progress in beginning to move through the grief process by taking over and making decisions that the person is capable of making. On the other hand, there may be legitimate reasons for the adult children to intervene in instances in which the parent's grief reactions are resulting in obviously unwise decisions and actions. Preplanning for contingencies by the spouses and their adult children can, of course, help to avoid some hasty and unwise behaviors and potential misunderstandings and arguments.

"When I walked in the bathroom at home and saw her shower cap, I lost it," said a 61-year-old man, describing his reaction on returning home from the hospital where his wife had just died. "I cried like a baby." Later that day he asked his daughters and a friend to remove his deceased spouse's personal possessions from the house. In making the request, he said,

> "I'm not talking about the photographs or books or things like that—leave those where they are—but her personal things, her clothes, her cosmetics, her jewelry. Give anybody what she had said she wanted them to have and divide and dispose of the rest as you think appropriate."

Privately, apart from their father, the daughters questioned whether he was moving too impulsively. Fortunately, a son was present to say accurately, "No, it's okay. Dad knows what he's doing. He told me a couple or 3 years ago that if anything like this ever happened, if Mom should go first, he would move her personal things out. He said that keeping them around would be too painful and slow down his grieving."

Behind the decision was the knowledge that one can prolong the grief reaction by maintaining a relationship with memorabilia associated with the death or dead person. These may include preserving the deceased person's room "as it was" and perhaps even spending daily time there, retaining their clothing, and needing to visit the grave frequently (Bugen, 1977). For that man and family the bereaved surviving spouse's involvement and the support provided by the family meshed effectively.

Duration and Handling of Grief

The mourning period varies in length for different individuals and circumstances. In normal reactions, the grief process should be essentially completed in 6 months to 1 year, and the shorter period appears to be the more typical pattern. Some clinicians hold that it is necessary to go through a full year of activities following the loss in order to complete the grieving process. They regard birthdays and certain holidays as necessary transition periods (Bugen, 1977). This "once around the calendar" idea, however, seems to be based more on theoretical and a priori considerations than on empirical grounds. The meaning of birthdays and holidays varies widely among survivors. The grieving process of the individual is likely to be more affected by the personal significance of dates and occasions than by what they mean to others, even to other family members. One's wedding anniversary may be highly meaningful to a surviving spouse and bring painful reminders of the loss, while the deceased person's birthday may have the greatest salience for a sibling of that person, for example.

The acute phase of the grief reaction typically is completed within 1–2 months (Lindemann, 1944; Peretz, 1970b; Bugen, 1977). For some persons, the ending of this phase is clearly marked. Some typical descriptions of how the transition out of the acute grieving process was experienced are given below. A 61-year-old male said,

> "It was like I was walking in molasses. By 4 or 5 o'clock every day, I was totally exhausted. I would work as hard as I could and accomplish almost nothing. My body was so heavy, it was like I had to order it to move. One day, about 2½ months after my wife died, I realized that the heaviness was gone. I was moving like I always had. I thought, 'I'm on the way out of the woods.' "

Another man described the experience as finding that "Suddenly, one day I was walking in the sunshine again." A woman who was unexpectedly widowed, agreed, "That's what it was like, starting to live in the sunshine again. One day, I decided, 'I've cried enough,' and that was it. I began to live again."

Abnormal and exaggerated reactions may last for many months or for years. The bereft person for various reasons is not able to cope with the loss and thus does not move directly toward recovery. Given the absence of cultural support for such reactions, a woman who jumped into the grave when her husband's casket was lowered into the ground obviously was manifesting an abnormal reaction. Two years later she was still hospitalized with a diagnosis of schizophrenia and was still unable to cope with her feelings of guilt and self-imposed need for punishment because of her earlier mistreatment of her husband.

Dealing effectively and successfully with the loss of their wife by death is exceedingly important for older men. These men are particularly high risks for death and suicide during the first year after the loss. McGoldrick and Walsh (1991) attribute the risk to the men's initial feelings of loss, disorientation, and loneliness and to the loss of the wife's services as a caretaker. They point out that socialization of males leads them to minimize their awareness of how dependent they are on their wife. Also, because men typically do not outlive their wives, they are not well prepared for the eventuality of doing so.

Widows, on the average, can expect to outlive their deceased husbands by approximately 7 years. The majority of older women who are widowed will not marry again because of either lack of opportunity or lack of desire to remarry, or both. Aside from the probability that they will continue to live as widows and not remarry, older women's adjustment processes are similar to other surviving spouses: accepting the death, grieving, learning to live alone, and investing in future functioning (Lopata, 1973).

The bereaved family must accomplish two major tasks in order to deal effectively with the loss and to acquire needed strength as a functional unit, according to Walsh and McGoldrick (1991). These are the attainment of (1) a shared acknowledgment of the reality of death and shared experience of loss, and (2) reorganization of the family system and reinvestment in other relationships and life pursuits.

The loss of a loved one by death brings a crisis that needs to be met with reorganization as the survivor works through the grief and begins to complete the process of mourning. Family relationships are altered by the death, and additional accommodations and alterations are required in response to the loss. This is particularly true when an older person loses his or her spouse. What kinds of living arrangements have to be made? Can the survivor live alone? Should he or she move in with one of the children, rotate living with several of the children, or get a live-in companion, if that is economically feasible? Should the survivor move into a nursing home? What about remarriage for the survivor? These and many other predictable questions are raised as the loss is faced and the need for reorganization of life without the deceased becomes part of the life cycle.

The Intervention Process

Dealing with the bereaved person can be done in two major ways, through work with the person individually and through interventions with the family. Some instances of approaches through both channels have already been mentioned.

Comprehending What Is Happening in the Grief Process

Helping the person(s) to comprehend what is happening to them in the process of grief facilitates recovery. An exceedingly effective part of an approach used over several decades has been to provide information to the bereaved person or persons on the stages that one may go through in reacting to the loss (described above as stages in the acute phase of grief). The following points are made:

- Grief is a process with a beginning and an ending. The acute phase does pass and things do get better. Unless we retard or block the process, there is light at the end of the tunnel.
- Knowing and understanding the typical stages does not erase the pain, but the knowledge can keep us from making matters worse because we understand something about what we are experiencing and the fact that it is a process.

This information and understanding, provided in the context of a supportive therapeutic relationship, generally helps to begin eradicating the client's feelings of helplessness and, sometimes, hopelessness.

Letting Go of the Lost Object

Traditional methods of grief work with individuals and families usually include physical presence, empathic listening, acceptance, and reassurance. Helping the mourner(s) to talk about the pain and hurt as this is possible, to review the life with the lost loved one, and to "say good-bye" are difficult tasks, but they are essential in therapy with bereaved and grieving persons. The purpose, in Bugen's (1977) terms, is to help shift a relationship with the deceased from centrality to peripherality. This often includes making it clear that it is all right, proper, and appropriate to go on living and to find new meaning in life. The assistance of others such as other family members, friends, and clergy may be helpful in persuading the mourner(s) that he or she can let go of feelings of hesitancy and guilt (Bugen, 1977).

Changing Important Cognitive Structures/Beliefs

A third element in effective therapeutic work with grieving persons may consist of changing certain cognitive structures, particularly those supporting an unrealistic client belief in responsibility for the death. An early task in dealing with grieving persons is to assess their capacity for hope (Peretz, 1970a). Bugen (1977) has described mourning as partly a belief that things are hopeless and that one is helpless. The longer such a belief in one's helplessness persists, the longer the grieving process lasts. Unchecked, feelings of helplessness can lead to a self-fulfilling prophecy in which the person progresses into a deep depression and, in some cases, into death (Seligman, 1975).

Feelings of helplessness can be spread or transferred to others (Seligman, 1975), for example, in group therapy. Hence, it is important to undercut beliefs about preventability and responsibility from the individual's perspective and/or the group's perspective.

The client needs help in altering the cognitive structure that supports the belief of preventability, especially when he or she feels personally responsible for the death. Every strategy that can appropriately contradict the belief of preventability should be used, according to Bugen (1977).

A CONCLUDING NOTE

This chapter emphasizes the kinds of issues that are likely to be encountered in therapy relationships with older adults. Hence, it presents a skewed picture. Missing are materials pertaining to the positive aspects of the postparental years. For many married persons, these are among the happiest and most fulfilling years of their lives. The omission of descriptions of the joys of being a grandparent and related experiences is deliberate because this is a book on working therapeutically with problems.

10

THERAPY WITH FAMILIES
IN TRANSITION: DIVORCE

*When I was growing up, I hardly knew anybody who was
divorced. Now, it's so common that if I haven't seen somebody I
know for 6 months or so, I don't ask, "How's your wife [or
husband]?" I may listen to see if they give me a clue [as to
whether they are still married] or, if they have kids, try to finesse
an answer by asking something like, "How's the family doing?"*
—Late-middle-aged professional man

No longer is divorce rare. On the contrary, marital dissolution by divorce
will be experienced by nearly half of the couples entering marriage in the
United States today, if current trends continue. After rising dramatically
during the 1960s and 1970s, the divorce rate leveled off during the 1980s
and has been steady in the 1990s. Divorce and remarriage statistics do not
appear to reflect disillusionment with marriage as such but rather a desire
to end the marital relationship with a particular mate. "Divorce is a
response to a failing marriage, not a failing institution," as Spanier and
Thompson (1984, p. 17) put it.

MARITAL DISSATISFACTION

The popularity of marriage continues unabated. Although marriage typically occurs later than it did a generation or two ago, the vast majority of

people continue to marry. And they continue to remarry. Whatever the age or stage of life at which they divorce, most divorced persons marry again. Most remarry within a few years. A sizable proportion—approximately one fourth—do so within a year of leaving the marriage. The median period of time between the divorce and remarriage is approximately 3 years (Spanier & Glick, 1980). Eventually, some four-fifths of all divorced persons remarry.

Expectations for marriage have risen dramatically over the past several generations. Concurrently, barriers against leaving a particular marriage have been lowered. Consequently, for many persons there is a reluctance to resign themselves to accepting disappointment and dissatisfaction with their current marriage. Instead, there is an openness toward leaving an unsatisfying marriage. One can continue to seek what is desired outside the marriage or in another marriage. Leaving the marriage, therefore, typically reflects a lack of personal commitment, disenchantment with one's partner, recognition that there was poor mate selection, or some other personal or social problem connected with a particular relationship (Spanier & Thompson, 1984). Nevertheless, the dream continues.

Marriages end in significantly different ways. Some short-term marriages may be ended rather soon, after one or both of the partners decide that their expectations are not being fulfilled. The process of dissolution is slower with longer-term marriages. Both clinical observation and some research show that the longer the marriage has lasted, the longer the participants may take to end it. Spanier and Thompson (1984), for example, found that "the longer the marriages endured, the more time was spent anticipating and moving toward the end of marriage" (p. 47).

TWO FORMS OF SHORT-TERM MARRIAGE

Although divorce occurs at all stages of the life cycle, it most frequently occurs among couples who have been married 3 years or less. Two types of these short-term marriages can be readily discerned: "starter" marriages and "bridging" marriages.

"Starter" Marriages

Because so many divorces occur among persons under age 30 who are married briefly and have no children, sociologist Constance Ahrons has used the term "starter" marriage (Schupack, 1994). Legally, ending such starter marriages is comparatively simple, as contrasted with unions in which there are children, custody concerns, and significant property to divide. The only major property issue for divorcing college students or other young adults, for example, may be the division of the stereo or compact disc player, the musical records, and the television. Possession of the couple's pet dog or cat was the focal point of emotional struggle in several cases I observed as director of a clinic serving a large number of college students in a state in which a no-fault divorce could be secured in approximately 3 weeks. This is not to imply that ending such marriages is painless, which certainly is not the case, but to note that terminating a starter marriage is relatively simple by comparison with a long-term marriage or a marriage with children and considerable property.

"Bridging" or "Sandwich" Marriages

Clinically, I have observed frequently over the past quarter century a three-marriage pattern, in which the middle marriage tends to be of brief duration. Whether the first marriage was long- or short-term, the divorced person quickly contracted a second marriage while he or she was in a "bridging" situation. Seeking to escape loneliness and repair damaged self-esteem, the emotionally blinded divorcee sailed uncritically into what appeared to be a safe haven, only to learn abruptly that the hasty second marriage was a mistake. Most of the persons I have observed or worked with have been much more deliberate in entering a third marriage. Typically, they sought professional help for preventive purposes fairly early during their third marriage in an effort to deal with problems before they were overwhelmed. The third marriage in most of the three-marriage patterns that I have observed and/or worked with has tended to be a long-term and rather stable relationship. The short-term second, or intervening, marriage thus can be described also as a "sandwich" marriage.

Some persons enter into nonmarital cohabitation arrangements that are intended to serve similar emotional purposes to the quick remarriage. That is, a nonmarital liaison is contracted, whether consciously or not, in an effort to avoid dealing with the pain, anxiety, and fear of again being single and not attached to a significant other person. Unfortunately, cohabitation arrangements may not serve the person any better than a hasty remarriage, and, consequently, may be terminated on the way to a second marriage.

The bridging or sandwich marriages described here should not be confused with patterns in which an individual continues to marry the same kind of personality in a string of marriages. Mate selection and marriage in the latter instances are symptomatic of underlying personal disorder, as described, for instance, by Bergler in *Divorce Won't Help* (1948). Clinicians do see some clients who are like those described by Bergler. Those persons do not learn from experience and persist in entering relationships and marrying under the impetus of neurotic needs. A middle-aged woman who was planning to marry for the fifth time and had selected a partner who was dynamically a replica of her first four spouses provides an illustration.

Such repetitive patterns, in which the same personality type is chosen several times, appear to be rare. Most persons do change and do seem to learn something from their earlier experiences. At any rate, escaping from or avoiding pain appears to be the major driving force in selecting a mate in a bridging marriage. This drive, which frequently blinds the driven individual to the characteristics of the chosen mate/haven, can be powerful enough to override other motivations. Solving old problems and conflicts from one's early life experiences and relationships thus takes a backseat to seeking relief from present anxieties and fears.

MARITAL DISSOLUTION

It is vitally important to recognize that while the marriage dissolves, the family system continues. "Marital breakup and family reorganization" is the most appropriate description of what occurs. The marriage is dissolved by the divorce, but the marital partners only cease to be spouses when they divorce. They do not stop being parents. For better or worse, and whatever the form of custody adopted for minor children, they are linked together through their children for the remainder of their lives. Similarly, their parents remain grandparents (although the in-law ties dissolve), and the transgenerational ties remain a part of the life of all three generations, even as other persons are brought into the enlarged and more complex family constellation when remarriage occurs. The family system and its adult members generally take from 1 to 4 years to undergo the divorce process, become stable, and resume a normal developmental course (R. S. Weiss, 1975; Peck & Manocherian, 1988).

Marital dissolution is part of a process that typically includes the following stages: marital discord, separation, divorce, single or single-parent living (for formerly married persons who have custody of a child or children), resocialization, dating/courtship, and remarriage. Cohabitation or "living together" sometimes is a part of the postdivorce process in lieu of the single or single-parent living stage.

The breakup of a marriage and the divorce process have been conceptualized in several different ways. A life cycle approach is taken by Carter and McGoldrick (1988). They depict a divorce phase (which includes deciding to divorce, planning the breakup, separating, and divorcing) and a postdivorce family phase (which may include single-parent custodial and single-parent noncustodial patterns). They also present a developmental outline for remarried family formation for those divorcing parents who remarry.

A model of family life cycle development based on the concepts of intimacy and identity is used by J. K. Rice and D. G. Rice (1986) in an explanation of the effects of divorce on both adults and children. The key task in securing intimacy is communion, whereas the key task in achieving identity is separation. The Rices describe the role of intimacy/communion and identity/separation in each of seven chronological periods beginning with birth and ending with senescence. They also attempt to depict the impact of divorce on each of those aspects of human development.

A four-stage model of predivorce decision making, divorce restructuring, postdivorce recovery, and remarriage was proposed by Piercy, Sprenkle, and Associates (1986). Six overlapping experiences for the divorcing spouses were outlined by Bohannon (1970) under the heading "stations of divorce." They are the emotional divorce, the legal divorce, the economic divorce, the coparental divorce, the community divorce, and the psychic divorce. Securing the psychic divorce is similar to the task of achieving a stable identity in my model of tasks for divorcing persons (see Table 10.1). R. S. Weiss (1975) describes divorcing adults as going through stages of transition and recovery. Transition begins with the separation and typically last from 8 months to 1 year, according to Weiss. By the time of recovery, 2 to 4 years after separation, the divorced person generally has attained a stable and strong identity and is living in a balanced and manageable manner.

Kaslow (1981; Kaslow & Schwartz, 1987) has advanced a "diaclectic" model of the divorce process that consists of three stages. These are predivorce (which involves deliberation and despair), during divorce (a period of legal involvement), and postdivorce (which is concerned with exploration and securing a new equilibrium). She correlates those broad stages with Bohannon's six stations of divorce and describes seven stages of feeling reactions for the participants. Actions and tasks of the divorcing persons and recommended forms of therapeutic intervention (e.g., marital therapy, couples group therapy, family therapy, child therapy, etc.) are also listed for each of the seven feeling reaction stages (Kaslow & Schwartz, 1987, pp. 30–31). These stages of divorce and reaction do not move forward in an inexorable and unvarying manner (Kaslow, 1981). Persons may change their minds, reconcile, and either continue the marriage or change their minds once again and resume the movement toward divorce.

There are many paths to marital dissolution by divorce. Couples vary widely in both the manner in which their marriage deteriorates and dissolves and the reasons that they decide to divorce. The latter range from cases in which the partners are undermined by parental interference to instances in which mismating has evolved through differential development between the partners. Martin (1976) has called subsequent mismating "the most common toxic process in marital disharmony" (p. 63). For the therapist, the most important concern appears to be the conditions that prevail when clients make their contact with the clinician. As noted elsewhere, "Therapists intervene in the divorcing process when and where they can. Most descriptions of 'divorce therapy' appear to be statements of what would be considered ideal rather than what typically occurs with divorcing couples" (Nichols, 1988, p. 239).

I hope that it is clear, in other words, that things do not necessarily evolve in a relatively positive direction in divorce and subsequent adjustment. Some couples continue their unhappy interaction long after the marriage has officially, legally ended. Marital breakup can be explosive and dangerous. One partner can become murderous ("If I can't have her

TABLE 10.1. Developmental Tasks for Divorcing Spouses

Tasks of the decision to divorce stage

1. Accepting the reality that a separation/divorce is occurring (regardless of why or by whom the decision is made).
2. Coping with initial emotional/psychological reactions.
3. Performing the initial planning of the contemplated actions.

Tasks of the separation/divorce stage

1. Making the necessary, practical living arrangements for oneself (and one's children), and practical arrangements for divorce and divorce settlement.
2. Informing pertinent parties (children, relatives, friends).
3. Restructuring relationship with spouse and children.
4. Adapting to new living patterns.
5. Seriously beginning the mourning process (bereavement and grief).
6. Coping with other emotional/psychological reactions to separation/divorce.

Tasks of the postdivorce stage

1. Completing the mourning process.
2. Achieving a stable identity as a single, formerly married person.
3. Achieving a new perspective on life and an appropriate orientation to the future.
4. Completing the restructuring of relationships with children, former spouse, and family.
5. Securing appropriate stabilization of one's social network.

Note. From Nichols (1988). Copyright 1988 by The Guilford Press. Reprinted by permission.

[or him], nobody can") or suicidal ("Life isn't worth living"). We have to be prepared to intervene quickly and forcefully if we sense that someone is in danger. We also need to be alert to the possibility of the abandonment of children by an upset or angry parent. Working with physicians, attorneys, and other professionals may be particularly important in preventing undesirable outcomes.

The descriptive approach that I am taking in this chapter considers the divorce process in three major stages: the decision to divorce stage, the separation/divorce stage, and the postdivorce stage. In therapeutic intervention, particular attention is given to the developmental tasks for divorcing spouses in the process of marital breakup and early postdivorce adjustment. These are described in Table 10.1. The form that such tasks take will be modified by other factors such as the individual, marital, and family life cycle stages of the divorcing partners.

THERAPIST STANCES

Therapist attitudes toward marriage and divorce have changed markedly over the past several decades.

Pro-Marriage

A generation or so ago it was widely assumed that the marital therapist or marriage counselor supported marriage. A popular mass media magazine began to publish a feature titled "Can this Marriage Be Saved?" During that period of "official" support of marriage, there was little question about the purpose of clinical work with married couples. It was to "save the marriage." Popular wisdom, and much professional opinion, held that couples should remain together "for the sake of the children."

An article in a professional journal by Aaron Rutledge (1963) three decades ago titled "Should the Marriage Counselor Ever Recommend Divorce?" was notable for its stance that there are reasons for recommending divorce in some instances. Rutledge gave two examples of cases in which he did not recommend divorce and the continuation of the marriage turned out to be very harmful for the wife. He implied that he probably should have recommended separation or divorce.

Official Neutrality

A period of "official neutrality" on the part of many therapists followed the pro-marriage period. Rejecting the "save the marriage" stance, those therapists ostensibly took no position on continuation or dissolution of the marriage. They defined the objective of their work as aiding and salvaging personalities. This stance often resulted in damage by default. Many individually oriented therapists today still try to ignore the marriage and deal with their client as if his or her private, personal issues were all that mattered, as if the client was an isolated, independent entity. It has not been difficult to collect a considerable amount of clinical evidence over the years that the individually oriented therapist who ignores marriage or tries to treat a couple without an understanding of marital dynamics and training in marital therapy can be very dangerous to marital health. As mentioned before, sometimes the verdict is, "The therapy was a success, the marriage died."

Anti-Marriage

As American culture began to feature a highly individualistic "do your own thing" component in the 1960s, some therapists began to demonstrate an active anti-marriage attitude. Paralleling this change in sentiment was an increasing consciousness of gender inequities in marriage. Marriage was described as being unfair to women. Sociologist Jessie Bernard (1972), for example, amassed data showing that there were "two marriages, his and hers, and hers makes her sick," as noted earlier.

Today, the pendulum is swinging back in the direction of therapists supporting marriage and trying first to salvage or improve it, rather than contributing to its demise by neglect or moving precipitously to encourage ending it. Michele Weiner-Davis's (1992) stance in *Divorce Busting: A Revolutionary and Rapid Program for "Staying Together"* illustrates such a movement. Examples of pro-marriage, anti-marriage, and official neutrality all can be found among contemporary therapists.

A Balanced Stance

Today, it appears clear that for a therapist to take the stance that marriage per se is undesirable is inappropriate. Similarly, marriage should not be approved uncritically and people encouraged to stay in obviously harmful relationships. A responsible therapist should not be an uncritical advocate of either marriage or divorce. Similarly, one cannot be neutral in the sense of adopting a laissez-faire attitude. To be neutral may mean to ignore inequities. The therapist's task is to approach each marriage on its own merits or demerits. One needs to help a couple assess their marriage and to draw their own conclusions as to whether it is harmful, dead, or salvageable.

In a balanced approach, therapists form opinions, working judgments, and evolving assumptions about whether a specific marriage, on balance, is helpful or harmful to the mates (and children if any), viable or moribund (dead), promising or hopeless. The conclusions that are reached and how the therapist reaches them are significantly affected by how one feels about marriage in general and the attitudes with which one approaches working with married persons.

When married persons come in for therapy, my motto with respect to the marriage as well as to the partners as individuals is, "First, do no harm." Unless the marriage is demonstrably harmful or is moribund, I am "for the marriage" as an entity in which the partners have made significant investment. This is particularly true if the partners wish to continue it and, especially, if it is life-enhancing or potentially fulfilling. Sidney Jourard gave a new interpretation to the point that "marriage is for life." Rather than referring to marriage as an automatic state that lasted for the lifetime of the spouses regardless, he described the purpose of marriage as being to enrich, to give life and joy to the partners (Jourard, 1975).

Being supportive both of an apparently healthy marriage and of the individual health of the partners is not the same as taking sides with one partner against the marriage or not taking a position at all. At the same time, it is difficult, if not impossible, for the family therapist to be responsibly neutral about some specific marital relationships. This is especially true if the relationship is harmful to participants and cannot be remedied. There are times, in other words, in which a therapist has to take a stance about whether or not a person should get out of a marriage.

A supervisee had the following experience. She saw a couple who had been married a short time. During the honeymoon the husband, John, became enraged and had attempted to strangle his wife. Ann, the wife, felt that it was a very close call for her. John apologized profusely and protested that nothing like that would ever happen again. However, his jealousy and anger would not stay under control for more than a short time. Ann was still scared of him and had separated from him when they saw the therapist.

The therapist determined that John, a highly successful business entrepreneur, was quite disturbed in his intimate relationships, especially in his dealings with women. She could not find any indications that he had any desire or ability to change. Furthermore, she picked up enough red flags so that when Ann called her, she ended up recommending, "Don't put yourself in a position where there could be any recurrences. Get out of there."

Several years later, the supervisee reported an additional contact with Ann in which she learned that Ann had divorced, and that John had continued to engage in similar abuse with his second wife and a girlfriend. From that contact the supervisee indicated, "I got all the confirmation I will ever need that following the data and following my instincts in telling Ann to 'get out of there' had been the appropriate course to take."

Being "for the marriage" in the sense used here means that the therapist does not bring in his or her own agenda of either saving or ending the marriage. The therapist needs to remember that he or she is an outsider and that the decisions—whether to continue in the marriage or to end it—are up to the clients. The therapist generally cannot want something more than the clients do—whether a good marriage, healthy living, or anything else—and still engage in helpful, successful treatment.

Guidelines for Therapeutic Work

The following guidelines for working with "the difficult divorce," which are virtually identical with those that I have developed in my own practice over several decades, have been described and illustrated by Isaacs and associates (Isaacs, Montalvo, & Abelsohn, 1986).

Family Reorganization

As noted above and elsewhere (Nichols, 1984, 1985a), the family system endures, even after divorce. There is need to shape the family relationships so that the developmental life cycle tasks of the members can be discharged as normally and effectively as possible. One important implication of this is that all family members who are old enough to benefit from therapy should be involved in therapeutic work dealing with divorce and postdivorce adjustment. When both parents are not available, the difficulty of the therapist's work is increased considerably (Isaacs et al., 1986).

Children's Needs

The needs of minor children, whose welfare is significantly dependent on the actions and attitudes of their parents, are explicitly given top priority. This does not mean that I become an advocate for the children and an adversary to the parents, but that I work on helping the parents recognize how and to what extent the children may be affected by what is happening. Part of this involves helping the parents to do the best that they can as parents in the midst of their own transitions. At the same time, I try to give them appropriate understanding and support for their own needs (Nichols, 1977, 1984, 1985b, 1986).

Subsystem Therapy

The fact that parents continue to be parents and will have to deal with one another, whether or not they are married, is emphasized with the adults and they are worked with as a parental unit whenever possible. I have found it possible even in some quite difficult cases (Nichols, 1988) to work with former spouses "for the good of the children" and "in order to help you handle your parental tasks" even when they actively dislike one other. It is useful to lay out clear expectations that they can and will work together in the sessions and to maintain clear guidelines for keeping to the childrearing topics.

Sibling system therapeutic work also may be effective even with difficult cases (Isaacs et al., 1986; Schibuk, 1989). My experience has been that it is particularly helpful with children in late elementary grades and older. I find it essential in most instances to spend some time dealing with potential loyalty conflicts, reassuring the children that they are not being asked to be disloyal to one or the other of their parents, but rather to help each other understand and deal with what they are experiencing as things change in their family.

As an attempt to counter what they call the "abdication dilemma," a pattern of working first with one household in a difficult divorce, then moving to the second household, and finally toward meeting with both households has been described by Isaacs and associates (1986). The abdication dilemma refers to the "almost complete failure" of parents to discharge the socialization tasks needed by their children (p. 182). The failure typically results from the stresses on the parents from their own emotional reactions (e.g., depression) and the battle that is going on between them as spouses.

When it is not possible to engage both of the divorcing persons in therapeutic work, the clinician may find that the only viable course of action is to work with the available parent. When one parent has abdicated and is engaging in actions that are harmful to the children, the therapist has the rather obvious task of supporting the other parent in his or her efforts to deal appropriately with the children's needs, as well as directly helping the children to cope with their bewilderment over the abdication. Children typically need firm but tender help in learning to accept the deficits in the parent as deficits in the parent, not in themselves.

THE DECISION TO DIVORCE STAGE

When individuals or couples present themselves to the therapist, it often is not clear what they wish to do regarding continuing or ending the relationship. Quite often, there is confusion without clear conclusion. "How did you decide to divorce?" "Can you help me to understand how it was determined that you would get a divorce?" These are appropriate questions when a couple or one of the partners discloses that a decision to divorce has been reached. Some probing typically is in order. Careful listening and observation of clients may indicate that there is some indecision regarding the matter, that things are not "set in concrete." These are instances in which it seems more appropriate to qualify the questions. One may say, for example, "It seems that you have thought of divorce, may be considering it as a possibility. Can we examine the picture, pro and con, so that you can be comfortable that you are not moving too fast and have made an appropriate decision?"

Sometimes, clients have jumped to the ostensible conclusion that they should divorce because they have not been able to solve some marital or family problems. A major task of therapy in such situations is to examine things carefully with the clients and to determine whether there are other alternatives. The clients have concluded that it is an either/or situation, either continue in an unsatisfying marriage or get a divorce. Coming to the therapist is a last-ditch effort by many of them to see if anything can be done to help the situation. In perceiving things in either/or terms, such clients are not markedly different from many others who cross the therapist's threshold. Is there a workable middle ground between the extremes of continuing the status quo without change or getting a divorce? Isaacs et al. (1986) have also concluded that determining whether a separation is inevitable or reconciliation is possible is the most critical issue with couples in this stage.

Exploring Commitment and Ambivalence

Exploration of their commitment along the lines of the preambivalent, ambivalent, or postambivalent dimensions of commitment described earlier (see Chapter 6) is indicated in such instances. "Preambivalent" is used to refer to individuals who have never seriously considered the possibility of ending the marriage. "Postambivalent–negative" refers to those persons who have decided that they wish to end the relationship and who give no indication that they would be seriously interested in reversing their position. (Postambivalent–positive individuals understandably would not be concerned with divorce.) It is, of course, the ambivalent clients who pose the challenge to the therapist of helping them decide what they wish to do.

Putting things in another way, when couples present to a therapist, the following patterns may be found:

1. Both partners wish to continue the marriage. Under this rubric there may be several variations:
    a. Both spouses wish to continue and the marriage is in relatively good condition. The spouses' emotional development and relationship patterns are basically functional. Of course, such couples rarely require therapeutic help.

b. Both partners wish to continue and the marriage is in relatively poor condition. The balance or complementarity in the relationship has shifted and perhaps one spouse has grown significantly or the other spouse has been clinically depressed.

c. Other combinations of the foregoing also may be seen.

2. One partner wishes to continue the marriage and the other does not. In this pattern, there may be concealment of the true intent on the part of one or both of the partners. For example, one spouse may have become emotionally invested in an external relationship or perhaps a spouse has simply "outgrown" the relationship and gradually withdrawn emotional attachment over the years. Discovering and elucidating the intent of the partners becomes the early task of the therapist in this situation.

Occasionally, one partner is "dumped" on the therapist's doorstep by the other. The departing spouse attempts to alleviate his or her guilt feelings or somehow to make it easier to break away by finding a therapist for the partner before the abandonment. Sometimes, the partner who intends to leave will attend one or two sessions before admitting his or her intentions. Others may inform the spouse of their intentions prior to the appointment. The appointment actually may have been made in reaction to the upset manifested by the rejected partner.

Finding a therapist for a rejected partner is one of four things that a departing spouse may do in an attempt to ease the way or assuage his or her guilt (Gardner, 1976). The others are to give the rejected partner money, send the partner back home, or to find the partner a lover.

Dumping actions can produce major crises for the rejected spouse and the family. The dumping process in which a partner goes to therapy with the spouse briefly and then abruptly discloses for the first time an intention to leave the marriage or reneges on a previously made promise to work on the marriage can be profoundly disturbing to the rejected spouse. Feelings of anger, betrayal, disappointment, and depression are common reactions. Dumping can produce some of the more difficult cases seen by therapists.

3. One partner wishes to continue the marriage and the other does not know whether he or she wishes to continue it. There may be ambivalence on the part of the undecided partner or simply a fear of the unknown that would cause the undecided spouse to oppose ending the marriage to some degree while not being sufficiently committed to it to wish to be involved in a viable relationship with his or her spouse.

4. Both partners are undecided about whether or not they wish to end or continue the marriage. Ambivalence is the hallmark of many individuals coming in for marital therapy. "Ambivalence" as used here refers to combinations of love and hate toward the spouse, with first one emotion and then the other predominating, resulting in a lack of consistency with regard to feelings about continuation or dissolution of the

relationship. The most difficult of all the patterns for the therapist is one in which one or both of the partners does not wish to stay in the marriage but does not wish to get out of it either. This is especially poignant when one or both wish to leave but lack the money or courage to do so.

5. Various combinations of these patterns appear in changing forms, one partner being undecided at one point and definite with regard to intention at another, both partners being definite at one time and undecided later, and others not knowing where they are at a given time, simply knowing that they are confused.

Clinical experience (Nichols & Everett, 1986) indicates that clients often see no need for additional therapeutic help once a decision has been made that the marriage is going to be ended. The addition of divorce mediation to the field a couple of decades ago has caused some couples to seek help in dividing property and working on custody decisions.

Checking the Commitment

When the clients are ambivalent and are not clear as to their stance and intentions, how does the therapist determine the level and kind of commitment to the marriage that exists? Several approaches that have been used successfully were described in Chapter 6. Because those clinical tactics are useful at this stage of a marriage, they are repeated here with slight adaptations:

1. Explore with them their feelings and assess their motivation regarding the marriage as well as possible from both what they say and what they do. (This involves assessing the object relations capacities of each partner, i.e., the emotional bases on which they need the other person, and the level of maturity in their object choice, including their ability to give emotionally to their mate.)

2. Ask them individually how they stand, feed back to them the therapist's impressions of where they seem to be at present in terms of their commitment and where they seem to be heading, and subsequently secure their reaction to those impressions.

3. Ask them together, in some instances, about their commitments. There are contraindications to this approach:

- The obvious inability of one partner to accept an ambivalent or postambivalent statement by the other,
- The therapist's need to strengthen the dependent partner, or
- The therapist's need for more complete and extensive examination of the stance of the partner who is considering leaving the relationship.

4. Share one's impressions with the partners together in some cases and get their reactions to the impressions and analysis of them and their situation. This can include as much straightforward explanation of an assessment on the matter of commitment as the marital partners seem to be able to absorb.

5. Observe what the partners do after an initial assessment has been made and they have been given whatever observations and recommendations regarding their needs and therapy that it has been possible to share with them. (Other actions include practical steps that may be indicated and/or recommended to them regarding children, seeking legal advice and help, and other matters.)

6. Push on the emotional boundaries of their relationship by raising in a casual and yet sensitive manner issues that would challenge or threaten the protective collusion between them: "In the midst of the problems and difficulties that you have described, have you seriously considered or talked about separation?" Observe how they respond to such questioning and pushing, and do whatever supportive work is necessary to cover the threat that such questioning may involve.

Certainly, there are clinical implications that stem from the manner in which the decision to divorce was made. Was it made by one spouse? If so, how did the other spouse learn about the decision? Was it reached by virtue of joint discussion and decision making? Was one of the spouses coerced into accepting something he or she did not wish to accept?

Joint Decision

For marital partners truly to make a joint decision to end the marriage evidently is rare. Clinical experience indicates that among those who seek therapy, the typical occurrence is for one to decide he or she wants out. The other may then be maneuvered into asking for a divorce. Or the rejected partner may be persuaded that he or she desires or would be better off with a divorce. Sometimes, the rejected partner may be coerced into reluctantly agreeing to a divorce because of a feeling that there is no option, that regardless of whether he or she desires it, a divorce is going to occur. In some instances, both realize that a divorce is going to occur, and one partner makes the move first. The other person may then feel profound rejection, even though he or she wished to end the marriage.

Unilateral Decision

Some of the more representative statements made by clients seeking therapeutic assistance in connection with a potential divorce include the following from three different cases: In one, Mary indicated, "John told me he wanted out. He said that he didn't love me anymore." In another, Hubert reported, "Sally said it was over. She told me, 'I love you, and I always will, but I don't want to be married any longer.'" In the third instance, Beverly said emphatically, "I decided it was over when I walked into a restaurant and there he was with his girlfriend. That was the last straw. Enough is enough." Sometimes the decision turns on a trivial event or argument.

Unilateral decisions to end a marriage evidently have always been possible, however, the power to make such decisions generally resided with males. Historically, males had much greater latitude and power than females in deciding to end a marriage. The paterfamilias (male head of a household) role in Roman law and the ability to "put away" one's wife by the thrice-stated "I divorce you" pattern of certain Middle Eastern cultures are but two examples of male domination.

Theoretically, it has long been possible for either partner to hamper or effectively end a marriage by refusal to participate cooperatively. However, circumstances traditionally made even desertion, the definitive version of unilateral "opting out," essentially a male prerogative. Women were quite limited in their ability to decide to leave marriage and in their options if they did decide to do so.

Beginning in the 1970s, clinicians observed a change in who sought assistance for marital problems. Prior to that time, approximately 90% of the initial requests I received for marital assistance came from the wife in the case. In the 1970s, this shifted to the extent that, with middle-class and upper-class clients, the initial telephone call was just about as likely to come from the husband as the wife. Now it was the male who was anxious and desirous to work on the marriage because of a threat of divorce. The "shoe was on the other foot" in that economically secure and confident women could—and were—wielding new power. Most of the divorce actions are filed by women.

The advent of the no-fault divorce doctrine in the United States a quarter-century ago has had many effects, some positive and some less positive. Eliminating the necessity of accusing the partner of some heinous offense in legal documents is a definite step toward civilized behavior. No-fault doctrines certainly have lowered the amount of unnecessary acrimony and character assassination that formerly prevailed in divorce actions. Unfortunately, such negative interchanges in property settlements and the displacement of property disputes into custody struggles, including in some instances false accusations of physical and sexual abuse of children, have not been eliminated by discontinuing the use of a dirty laundry list of "grounds" for divorce.

No-fault divorce has made unilateral decisions to end a marriage legally a much more common reality. Under the no-fault law it essentially takes only one partner to decide that "the objectives of matrimony no longer exist" or that "the marriage is moribund" and to open the way to a legal divorce. In effect, if one partner says the marriage is over, the marriage is over. Major emotional turmoil and titanic legal struggles over property and child custody may follow. Nevertheless, the marriage as a viable cooperative relationship is ended when one partner declares such is the case.

When Is the Marriage Over?

Obviously, there are instances in which it is difficult for the therapist to find much life in the relationship and to be able to predict that it has any potential for being healthy or functional in the future. This does not mean that the clients are ready to make a decision that the marriage is over and that they wish to secure a divorce. Regardless of the therapist's opinion, the decision is theirs to make even if they are not ready to make it at the time they consult a therapist.

When It Dies, Regardless of Burial

Sometimes, a marriage as a viable entity is moribund long before the partners can bring themselves to the point of giving it a formal burial.

What I think of as "The 6-Month Impasse Case" with the Samsons provides an example. The clients were decent people who genuinely cared for their children. Their request was to help them salvage their marriage if possible. For 6 months I worked with them as hard as I could work with anybody. Therapeutically "pulling out all the stops on the organ," I did everything I knew to help break the impasse. Unfortunately, neither of the partners would, or perhaps could, budge and deal with the other in a meaningful fashion. Consequently, the marriage did not appear viable. Rather, it seemed dead, a state of existence rather than a relationship with any health or life in it.

There did not appear to be much, if any, hope for that particular couple working out a satisfying relationship. From all indications, they had been mismatched from the beginning. They had conducted a long-distance courtship and had really not known each other very well. When they married and began to live together, the incompatibilities emerged almost immediately. They had stuck it out for 20 years or so.

Respectfully, I reviewed with them what we had done, pointing out that I felt all three of us had worked hard for 6 months, and that I did not know anything else to do. I suggested that we conclude that we had all tried and had not succeeded in improving the marriage. Hence, I felt in all honesty that we needed to terminate our work. They agreed, and we parted amiably and with evident respect for each other's efforts.

Eventually, some years after terminating therapy, the couple decided that their marriage was not viable and divorced. At the time of a follow-up report that I received some 4 years after the therapy terminated, postseparation and divorce living were going well for all concerned. Both former partners reportedly were much happier and were living much more productive lives than formerly. Additionally, some of the formerly poor parent–child relationships had improved dramatically once the parents parted company and the children were no longer caught in family triangles.

At the Time of Separation

For the majority of people, the physical separation symbolically, and perhaps emotionally, marks the end of their marriage. Research done as long ago as 1948 (Goode, 1956) found that separation was one of the most definitive and difficult points for persons who had divorced. Similar findings emerged in research several decades later. Spanier and Thompson (1984) also found physical separation signifying the end of marriage for most people. They noted that only a physical separation seemed to convince "those who were reluctant to admit the end of marriage based on its emotional climate" that the marriage actually was dead (p. 58).

When It Is Emotionally Dead

The emotional end of marriage seems to be symbolized by the diminution or ending of affection and sexual relations (Spanier & Thompson, 1984). As described in the 6-Month Impasse Case, however, some couples may continue to maintain the legal and external social form of marriage and not be able to bury the corpse until long after the marriage is effectively dead.

When One Partner "Crosses the Rubicon"

"Crossing the Rubicon" is a term for a decision that is final, even in instances in which long desired changes may subsequently occur. Clinically, one sees some couples in which one partner reached the point of no return long before the separation. Sometimes, such persons "cross the Rubicon" in terms of deciding that the marriage is over but determine that they will stay in it in order to protect their financial interests or for other reasons such as "for the sake of the children."

"When you finally stopped catting around and decided that you really wanted to be married to me, it was too late," one middle-aged woman told her husband. "Now, you say you want to try [to make the marriage work], but it's too little and too late. My feelings died a long time ago. There's nothing to work on."

Therapy Issues

Major guidelines for therapeutic interventions during the decision to divorce stage are provided by the tasks for the period set forth in Table 10.1. Beyond the initial work of determining what the partners actually intend to do with regard to staying married or divorcing, the predominant tasks for therapy are those discussed below.

Accepting the Reality

As it becomes clear that a separation or divorce is occurring (regardless of why or by whom the decision is made), clients need to be assisted in accepting the reality of what is occurring. Typically, it is not easy for clients to accept that a marriage is ending. Although some individuals enter marriage with the seemingly blithe attitude, "We can always get a divorce, if it doesn't work out," they do not seem to expect that divorce will occur—or that it is occurring *now*. Even those who are fearful that they cannot succeed at making a particular relationship work still give the impression that in another part of themselves they do not expect the marriage to fail.

Divorce is a time of pain and difficulty for the adults and children going through the experience. When the reality of the disruption hits, feelings of shock and numbness are typical. An appropriate guideline in helping clients at this point is the understanding that "even though it may not be a surprise, it is still a shock" to the person who is learning that a separation/divorce is occurring. Hence, the therapist needs to maintain a balance between sensitivity and representation of reality in such situations.

Coping with Loss and Grief

Understanding the emotional and psychological reactions of both partners in the dissolving marriage is essential to working effectively with them. As indicated elsewhere, separation and divorce produce some of the same kinds of grief reactions as other losses of significant love objects (Nichols, 1977). Comprehension of the processes of bereavement and grief described in Chapter 9, therefore, provides an appropriate background to working with clients during this stage.

Anxiety and specific fears about what lies ahead are to be expected.

Initially, they may be masked to some extent by the protective numbness that ensues after the disruptive reality of forthcoming separation/divorce appears. As the defenses begin to erode, however, there tends to be a return of anxious feelings and the emergence of specific fears about the future.

Planning Contemplated Actions

Having specific tasks that need to be undertaken can be exceedingly helpful during times of loss and grief. In the early stage of a loss by death, for example, planning the funeral arrangements and taking care of other essential details provides a pattern for coping and helps one to get through. Similarly, doing the initial planning to effect the separation, secure the divorce, care for children, and take care of other pertinent matters can provide significant assistance to divorcing clients in binding their anxiety and diminishing their fears.

"What do you need to do?" "What plans have you made for _____?" "What have you already done?" "Have you thought about _____?" "What are the pros and cons of doing _____?" "Are there other possibilities, other alternatives that you could consider?" These and similar questions can provide a framework for assisting clients in doing their preliminary planning.

The family therapist who is involved at this early stage often can assist the couple in working through leftover or latent marital disappointments and resentments. These issues would not only inhibit a couple's potential for working out a dissolution agreement but could potentially disrupt their postdivorce parental adjustment and responsibilities for years following the divorce.

THE SEPARATION/DIVORCE STAGE

For some persons, the departure of one of the partners from the home becomes, symbolically, the time at which the "real" divorce occurs. Will the partners struggle and engage in legal battles or work out the details in a reasonably cooperative fashion? If both come in together, there is the possibility for easing the transition and avoiding some unnecessarily painful experiences as they take steps to end the marriage.

Practical Arrangements

With or without joint preplanning, the splitting spouses make the necessary practical living arrangements, as well as contacting attorneys and taking other steps for ending a marriage. With attendant anxiety and pain, they deal with such things as dividing possessions, leasing an apartment for the departing spouse, and one partner moving out. Exploring with clients who have decided to divorce how to separate with as little acrimony and pain as possible can be worth all of the time it requires. Understandably, the more clear they are about practical matters and the stronger the agreement, the greater the possibility of minimizing conflict.

If the partners come to therapy together during this stage, it usually is possible to appeal successfully to both their self-interest and their altruism in order to secure cooperation between them. "It will be easier for you if the two of you can decide what you want and compromise where necessary, rather than having a judge decide things for you." Many parents seem to learn for the first time when they get into a divorce battle that the state has a major and basic stake in their marriage and childrearing. Things that they have considered rights such as custody of children turn out to be privileges that are contingent on their ability to stay out of court and perform their parental role within certain socially approved and legal parameters. Some gentle but firm education may be indicated.

Even parents who do a poor job of parenting generally care about their children, albeit sometimes "in their own way," and they want good things for their offspring. The altruistic appeal is primarily aimed at those concerns for their children. "It's clear from what you have said and how you have said it that both of you want the best for your children. But it's going to be necessary to work together, and perhaps to give up some of what you would like to have, in order to work things out so that the children are not caught in the middle between you. Let's see what can be done so that your concerns for your children are put into practice."

Therapists also must be clear about boundaries and must differentiate the role from the role and responsibilities of the attorney. It is important to be knowledgeable about legal proceedings, rather than to avoid or ignore those issues and dump their clients into the legal system. Therapists should always have available several legal colleagues who specialize in family law and who are supportive of spouses' ability to work out self-determined agreements with regard to custody and property. Many such attorneys may be eager to work with capable therapists.

Informing Pertinent Parties

If the children, families, and friends have not been informed of the forthcoming separation/divorce, the therapist can aid the clients to convey their intentions to those pertinent parties.

Telling the Children

"What do we tell the children?" and "How do we tell the children?" are questions frequently asked by clients. The response to the first is, "The truth." Examples include "Mommy and daddy have decided that they do not love each other any longer. You know how much arguing and unhappiness there has been at home. We think it best for Mommy and Daddy to live apart and to get a divorce. We think that it would be better for all of us." "Daddy has found somebody else that he loves rather than Mommy." The message needs to be delivered sensitively but honestly and in a form appropriate to the ages of the children. Parents may need education in child development regarding the abilities of children to comprehend what is being explained (Schwartz, 1992).

Frequently, parents also need to be coached to assure the children that they are loved and that their relationship with both parents will continue. Divorce of the parents does not mean divorce of parents and child. "Mommy and Daddy both love you very much. We will always love you, and we will always be your parents, although we won't be living together any longer."

Parents also need to be helped to recognize that children may be concerned about whether the divorce was their fault. Appropriate statements and assurances to the effect that "You had nothing to do with Mommy and Daddy breaking up. The problems are between us. We have worked hard but can't seem to solve them by staying together. It is not your fault that we are getting a divorce." The therapist can go through with the parents other possible questions that the children will raise, so that the parents can think them through and be prepared to respond forthrightly. "Where will we live?" "Do I have to leave my friends?" are among the obvious concerns of children.

Informing Families

The issues are quite different when clients are considering informing members of their families of origin. Client concerns about parental disapproval continue to be fairly common. One therapy issue may be the degree of differentiation of each spouse from his or her family of origin and thus how freely and comfortably parents and siblings can be informed. There are also issues regarding relationships with persons who will become "former in-laws." Unlike the situation with children, once the marriage is legally severed, one no longer has socially developed patterns and expectations for dealing with former in-laws. There may be some mourning of the loss of relationship with former in-laws of whom one was fond. The tendency, however, is for relationships between a divorcing spouse and his or her in-laws to deteriorate quickly after separation (Ambert, 1988).

The family therapist and the spouses can examine parental issues throughout the broader family network, such as problems with jealous or intrusive grandparents. Blaming and taking sides by the spouses' parents and/or siblings may be particularly virulent in some instances. Once again, it is important to help the adults to recognize that, whatever their feelings about other adults, the major victims of acrimony are the children. Occasionally, it may prove helpful for the therapist to secure the permission of the clients to meet separately with grandparents to hear and to help moderate their concerns.

Informing Friends

With friends, as well as with family of origin and children, it is essential for divorcing partners to recognize that the severing of the relationship is the privilege and concern of the married persons, not of other persons. One of the therapist's roles here is to help the partners work out how the message will be delivered. Friends may seek to effect reconciliation or may immediately begin to take sides. An important task for the therapist is sensitizing clients to the temptation to seek allies among their friends to support their individual "cause" and their disagreements with their spouse. Similarly, clients need to be helped in learning how to remind friends that while the clients appreciate the friends' concern and support, the decision has to be theirs. Clients also need to be prepared for a shifting in the relationships with those who have been mutual friends, recognizing that some couples will be likely to align with one or the other of them in social contacts following the divorce.

Restructuring Relationship with Spouse and Children

As the couple moves toward separation and divorce, the rudiments of their postdivorce relationship start to emerge. As a suggestion of the types of relationships that may develop, Ahrons (1981; Ahrons & Rodgers, 1987) described five relationship styles between former spouses: Perfect Pals, Cooperative Colleagues, Angry Associates, Fiery Foes, and Dissolved Duos. The final type, Dissolved Duos, may not have any contact after they divorce. This would seem to be characteristic of many of the "starter" marriage couples.

Briefly, the Perfect Pals continue to regard each other as good friends. Few in number, they seem likely to share parenting responsibilities in cooperative and effective ways. Cooperative Colleagues share a desire to minimize the trauma of postdivorce family living for their children and thus are able to work cooperatively as parents. They do not feel like good friends with each other. Angry Associates do not resolve their anger with each other, and it persists as an important part of their divorced relationship. Coparenting is hard but is possible for them. Their children may be trapped between them, however, and experience continuing loyalty conflicts. Fiery Foes exhibit an almost nonexistent coparenting ability. The children definitely get caught in the continuing power struggle. One of the parents, typically the father, tends to have decreasing contact with the children over the years.

Living Patterns

Recent research suggests that establishing a new lifestyle may be more difficult for the divorcing person than adjusting to the breakup of the marriage. There is a reciprocal connection between adjustment to a new lifestyle and adjustment to the separation, that is, adjustment to the separation tends to affect one's establishment of a new lifestyle, and establishment of a new lifestyle tends to help in resolving one's difficulties in dealing with marital dissolution. Those who are unable to form new relationships may continue to feel bitterness toward the former spouse or regret having separated/divorced (Spanier & Casto, 1979).

The departure of a spouse creates a vacuum in living and some degree of discomfort, even in cases in which the former spouse was an irritant. Coping with the absence is one of the many adjustment problems that need to be addressed by the separating and divorcing individuals. Such coping is not necessarily easy, even when one experiences some relief at not having to deal with the departed or ex-spouse on a daily basis. "I thought I wanted him out, gone, but I miss him" is a plaintive cry from some clients. Not infrequently, there may be more than one separation attempt.

For some persons, the "separation distress" described by Parkes (1973) may be caused primarily by the loss of attachment to the other person. Attachment may persist long after the erosion of love, according to R. S. Weiss (1975). "Separation distress" includes the focus of attention on the image of the lost figure; feelings of guilt for having caused the loss; and an "alarm reaction" composed of such feelings as fear or panic, restlessness, and extreme alertness to the possibilities of the return of the lost person, accompanied by sleeping and eating disorders (R. S. Weiss, 1975).

For others, the distress is less about attachment to the departed spouse than about the vacuum created by the loss of the person from one's environment. Careful exploration of the reactions of the "left" spouse (the one who remains in the couple's residence) may show that the alarming feelings stem not from a longing for the return of the departed but from discomfort with "the hole in the daily living and environment" that the departure has created. When this is the case, guidance in understanding our discomfort with change and our need to learn to adapt to a different environment can prove helpful to the client. Simple illustrations of the role of what Harriet Mowrer long ago labeled "interhabituation," such as the fact that we can miss even a piece of furniture that we disliked when it is gone, often provide a basis for clients to comprehend what they are experiencing. They begin to realize that with the passage of time, they will become more accustomed to the new living environment.

Mourning and Other Emotional/Psychological Reactions

During this stage, clients move into serious mourning as the reality of what is occurring becomes evident. The losses being suffered include not only the loss of the spouse and the marriage, but also loss of status and self-esteem. Emotional reactions of men and women may be both similar and dissimilar. Both need to mourn appropriately, even when they are convinced on objective grounds that ending the marriage was the best step to take. Mourning appropriately may be more difficult for men than for women, particularly if they have been socialized to hold back and deny their feelings and to negate their dependency needs. The suicide risk for men is much higher than for women. Only recently have we begun to recognize that the man who leaves his home may feel adrift, alone and lonely, and sometimes considerably more anxious and depressed than stereotypes of males would imply.

Status Loss

The status loss in separation/divorce generally is different for men and women. As noted above, women who have been reared in traditional ways have had more at stake economically and socially in being married than men. The male's social identity and much of his personal identity have been based primarily on his vocational role. The woman's social and personal identities have traditionally been based on her wife/mother role. Unfortunately, she has too often lived vicariously, in the reflected light of her husband's status and identity. Although there is change occurring with the rise of feminism and new economic and social opportunities for women, the traditional picture has not faded from the scene.

Clinical observations show some understandable differences in male–female reactions to loss of status. The loss of married status for the male may not make that much practical difference to him, because he still has his identity from his vocational role. Some females may feel quite helpless and exposed in a world in which they are not accustomed to coping alone. To the extent that she has been accustomed to being "the wife of" her husband, she finds that she is missing her identity as well as not possessing some of the coping mechanisms needed for everyday living as an autonomous person. She may grapple with the question of who she is now, whereas her former husband is still Jim Smith, computer technician. Again, this picture is changing, and the therapist needs to explore carefully what is occurring with each client, male or female.

Marital disruption in the form of separation/divorce is a stressful event (Bloom, White, & Asher, 1979). Whether it will continue to be a stressor of top magnitude as social attitudes regarding divorce become more permissive is not clear. At the present, however, the emotional impact of marital disruption and separation from one's spouse continues to be a major source of pain.

Support groups provide a much-needed service for many persons, particularly in the early stages when they are feeling cast adrift. Both men and women require assistance in many cases in learning about the resources that are available in the community for adjusting to divorce, in learning new behaviors, and in adapting to new roles. In cases in which there is a long waiting period, some of this assistance is needed during the period before the divorce is final. For those who do not get started on adaptation to postmarital life in such an anticipatory fashion, help may be needed after the divorce in locating community resources that will assist in the life transition that they are undergoing.

THE POSTDIVORCE STAGE

Therapy in the postdivorce stage, for the most part, tends to be a continuation of tasks and issues that began earlier. This is summarized briefly in this section under the headings of the tasks of the postdivorce stage. No separate discussion of the family problems of the single parent and single-parent living stage are included. Rather, the discussion in this section is limited to issues and problems of adults. Adjustment problems of children in the general postdivorce period are presented separately.

Mourning

Clients need to complete the mourning process. Mourning and the loss and grief process is considered complete when the client has reached the stage of essentially living in the present. One's emotional energy no longer is invested in past objects and relationships, but in current and future attachments. The marriage is primarily a memory. The former spouse is someone to whom one once was married. Ideally, the divorced persons can acknowledge the good that existed in the relationship and accept that as part of one's former life. Where there was little good, the ideal would be to accept that what occurred is history; painful, but completed to the extent possible.

Identity

Completion of the mourning process and reinvestment in the present comprises a significant amount of the task of achieving a stable identity as a single, formerly married person. For those who were enmeshed in stifling marital roles and derived their sense of selfhood from the marital status, successful achievement of this task involves reaching, perhaps for the first time, a stage of knowing who and what they are in their own right. Work with some clients toward achieving this task involves helping them to overcome deeply entrenched ideas of failure and stigma about being divorced. Exploration of the question, "What does it mean to you to be divorced?" needs to be accompanied by exploration into related areas such as those described below.

Life Perspective

Intertwined with completion of the mourning process and achieving a stable identity as a single, formerly married person is the achievement of a new perspective on life and a realistic, appropriate orientation to the future. The end of the marriage may or may not produce positive outcomes for the divorcing partners. For some individuals, divorce will bring a "new freedom" (E. O. Fisher, 1974). Some may turn it into a "creative divorce" (Krantzler, 1974), a "good divorce" (Ahrons, 1994), or a "healthy divorce" (Everett & Volgy, 1994) and a growth experience. Others will find it neither creative, good, growth producing, healthy, nor a desirable form of freedom.

What kind of meaning can divorced persons find for themselves? The therapist may need to help them do a kind of postmortem on the dead marriage. The purpose is to emerge with a balanced perspective on the pros and cons of what one has experienced. Clients may need help in avoiding a tendency to gloss over the negative effects. On the other hand, they may require support in acknowledging and accepting the gains made and the positive possibilities that lie ahead.

Relationships with Children, Family, and Friends

The restructuring of relationships with children, family, and friends, which began when divorce was first planned, persists into the postdivorce stage. One may be dealing with the children as a single parent with or without custody and with one's parents and friends as a single person again, but now with children and a dissolved marriage.

Social Network

Few persons maintain the same social network following divorce that obtained during marriage. They face myriad issues in maintaining some old friendships, establishing new friendships, and finding new sources of support to replace some of the underpinnings formerly provided by the marriage. Exploration of what the clients need and reality testing with them regarding available sources of support and the value to them of what they secure may occupy a fair amount of useful therapeutic time during this stage.

CHILDREN AND DIVORCE

The presence of children is no longer regarded as a virtually automatic bar to divorce. Large numbers of children are involved in divorce situations. Approximately three in five divorcing couples have at least one minor child. Two children typically are involved in each divorce in which there are any children under the age of 18 years (Spanier & Thompson, 1984).

Reactions to Divorce

Children's reactions to divorce are not necessarily the same thing as the effects of divorce on children (Nichols, 1984, 1986, 1989). Children react both to events in the process, such as the separation, and to the divorce process itself. Their reactions can be both short- and long-term in nature.

Elsewhere, I have related children's reactions to divorce to child development factors and to context factors pertaining to social change and the absence of social norms for dealing with divorce and remarriage (Nichols, 1989). Child development factors include the dependency factor, abandonment anxiety, and the contingency factor. Briefly, whatever threatens to disrupt the dependency supports of the child tends to produce abandonment anxiety. In its earliest form, this anxiety, which can become a specific fear, is that the child will not survive without the parents. The contingency factor pertains to the fact that a child's life during the divorce process is largely contingent upon the actions and attitudes of other people. How the parents handle the decision to divorce, the separation/divorce, and the postdivorce stages, and how they deal with their children inevitably affect the children.

Understandably, children's problematic reactions show up most markedly in emotional and educational difficulties. Rooted in complex family tangles such as troubled parent–child relationships, emotional disturbance in one or both parents, and continuing parental discord, these problems are evident before, during, and long after divorce (Wallerstein, 1991). The reactive nature of children's problems and symptoms implies that therapeutic work on their behalf frequently needs to be focused primarily on the context, rather than specifically on the child. This is particularly true when the problematic behavior or symptomatology was not evident prior to the emergence of marital discord and dissolution.

Effects of Divorce

Loss and parental discord constitute two major sources of postseparation/postdivorce stress for children (Nichols, 1984). Among the losses are not only the loss of one parent (most commonly the father) from the child's daily life, but also a decline in the family's living standard and deprivation of emotional supports for the child. Diminishing economic and social resources, in turn, may negatively affect the child's educational attainment, timing of marriage, and possibility of divorcing (Keith & Finlay, 1988). In a related vein, some research supports the socialization hypothesis that parental role models (e.g., single-parent living) and supervision are the major factors in determining the future family-formation behavior of offspring (McLanahan & Bumpass, 1988).

Ongoing conflict between separated or divorced parents typically has a negative impact on the child. Not only does it restrict his or her ability to cope with the situation but also it tends to damage the youngster's self-esteem (Berg & Kelly, 1979). Kalter (1987), drawing on clinical experience, emphasizes the long-term effects of divorce on children rather than the crisis event of separation. He suggests that such key developmental areas as handling anger and aggression, separation/individuation, and gender identity are affected by the divorce process. This process includes events that are set into motion by the divorce and unfold for years afterward. Potentially stressful circumstances include continued parental hostility, economic distress, multiple shifts in residence, the emotional loss of a nonresident parent, parental dating, and remarriage. Taken as a whole, these factors can be a source of developmental vulnerability or, in some instances, enhanced growth.

The diversity of children's responses over the long haul has been recognized by Hetherington and associates (Hetherington, Stanley-Hagan, & Anderson, 1989). They note that some children may be helped by coping with the marital transition, while others suffer developmental disruption or delay. Some children seem to cope well during the early phases but manifest delayed effects, particularly in adolescence. Rather than being related primarily to divorce and remarriage as such, the long-term effects are perceived by Hetherington and associates (1989) as being related more to the developmental status, sex, and temperament of the child; the quality of the home and parenting environments; and the resources and support systems available to the parents and child.

A recent comparison of research on the effects of five factors on children's adjustment to divorce found that one, the interpersonal conflict perspective, best explained children's adjustment (Amato, 1993). It was also noted that the other four—absence of the noncustodial parent, the adjustment of the custodial parent, economic hardship, and stressful life change—also had to be included in order to fully explain current research findings on children's adjustment to divorce. There are no simple answers to questions regarding children's postdivorce adjustment (Kelly, 1993). Clinicians, like researchers, need to be mindful of the effects of multiple factors on children in both their short- and long-term reactions to the effects of the divorce process.

Very little empirical evidence exists on the effects of divorce on young adults whose parents divorce. Exploratory research suggests that the breakup of the parental marriage can be a powerful experience in the lives of young adults (Cooney, Smyer, Hagestad, & Klock, 1986), affecting such factors as the subsequent ability to achieve the developmental tasks of young adulthood (Johnson, Wilkinson, & McNeil, 1995).

Psychological Tasks of the Child in Divorce

Wallerstein (1983) has discussed six psychological tasks of the child whose parents divorce: (1) acknowledging the reality of the marital breakup; (2) disengaging from parental conflict and getting on with their customary activities such as school; (3) resolving the loss that is occurring, such as the departure of a member from routine participation in the family life, and their concomitant feelings of rejection; (4) resolving anger and self-blame for the divorce; (5) accepting that the divorce is permanent; and (6) achieving realistic hope regarding their own future relationships. Some of these tasks deal with the divorce event and some with the divorce process. Failure to achieve them shows up in disruptions in the child's daily life, for example, in school performance (Nichols, 1989).

Postdivorce Living Tasks

For the period following divorce, Kalter, Pickar, and Lesowitz (1984) add five tasks to Wallerstein's six divorce-engendered tasks. As adapted, these are (1) coping with the parents' continuing disharmony, particularly regarding child support and visitation; (2) adapting to the repeated separations from each parent because of joint custody or visiting arrangements or, in the case of sole custody, the loss of regular contact with the noncustodial parent; (3) understanding realistically the options for (and limitations on) changes in custody and visitation; (4) coming to terms with reactions to the mother's dating, including conflicts over loyalty to father and competition for a secure relationship with mother; and (5) establishing a developmentally appropriate and adaptive relationship with the mother's new partner or spouse. Obviously, not all of these tasks would apply to all children. The last two would not be present for those whose mother did not enter a new relationship, for example.

Custody Questions

In the 1970s joint custody was widely hailed as the best arrangement for divorced parents and their children (Roman & Haddad, 1974; Arbarbanel, 1979; Greif, 1979). In one popular book, *Co-Parenting: Sharing Your Child Equally* (Galper, 1978), Bohannon's construct of coparenting was redefined as equally shared parenting. At least one state (California) revised its laws to make joint custody the presumption in divorce cases. By the early 1980s, provisions for joint custody as an option were written into the statutes of more than half of the states in the United States (Derdeyn & Scott, 1984).

More recent study has indicated that joint custody has its limitations and certainly is no panacea. Pearson and Thonennes (1990) found no association between children's adjustment and the form of custody. In a nationwide representative sample of children whose parents were divorced, Donnelly and Finkelhor (1992) found no evidence that joint custody made for better parent–child relations than sole custody. Johnston, Kline, and Tschann (1989) could find no evidence that the child's frequent access to both parents in joint custody arrangements ameliorated the child's distress. The reaction of children to joint custody is highly individual, and, as one might expect, the most crucial and beneficial factors have been found to be the attitudes, values, and behaviors of the parents (Steinman, 1981). Levels of conflict between joint custody parents and other parents have been found in one study (Maccoby, Depner, & Mnookin, 1990). Interestingly, the amount of conflict in parenting 18 months after separation was found in the same research to be positively related to the intensity of hostility between parents at an earlier time.

When one parent has sole custody, the conventional wisdom has been that children should live with the same-sex parent. Results from at least one recent, nationally based sample (Downey & Powell, 1993) call into question the notion that children fare better living with same-sex parents. Similarly, the research on contact with the absent or noncustodial parent has produced mixed results.

Mediation of Child Custody Disputes

This aspect of divorce mediation has emerged over the past decade or so. According to veteran therapists and mediators Everett and Volgy (1989), the child custody portion tends to be the major focus of emotional reactions in divorce mediation. It brings out latent disappointments and anger from the failed marital relationship. Accordingly, they start with the child custody dispute and then move to dealing with financial and property issues. Children as young as age 4 have been successfully involved in custody mediation. The final product of the process after some three to eight 1-hour sessions is a mediation agreement, signed by both parents. Copies are forwarded to the attorney of each, along with a cover memorandum of explanation. A provision is included for review of the custody access plan within a specified period in order to determine its continuing effectiveness (Everett & Volgy, 1989).

Needs of Children in Divorce

Generally speaking, children of divorcing parents need help and information that will enable them to develop as normally as possible. In addition to being informed at all stages of the process of what is transpiring and its meaning for him or her, the child specifically needs the following:

- *Clear intergenerational boundaries* so that a generational hierarchy is maintained and the child can be a child.
- *Adequate fulfillment of adult developmental tasks* by the parents so that the child can deal adequately with his or her own normal life cycle tasks and developmental tasks in relation to the divorce.
- *Good enough parenting* so that the child's age-appropriate dependency needs are upheld in an adequate state of dynamic balance.

- *Adequate support and sensitivity* to predictable "abandonment anxieties" so that they can be handled rapidly (Nichols, 1989, p. 73, adapted).

Therapy and Other Interventions

The theme of tailored treatment and intervention sounded throughout this book is certainly relevant to dealing with children of separating and divorced families. As noted above, most of the child's problems can be correctly perceived as reactive in nature. Because the reactions to the separating or divorced situations are disruptive of children's developmental needs, a major goal of therapy is to enable the child to get back on the appropriate developmental track.

Elsewhere, I have detailed some guidelines for providing therapeutic assistance to children during the various major stages of the divorce process (1984, 1985b). My preference is for indirect treatment of the child through effecting changes in the context wherever possible, particularly in the structure and nature of the parental handling of the situation. Group forms of intervention with the child also are preferred whenever possible, partly because they help to reassure the child that he or she is not at fault and that others share the same adjustment problems.

A considerable amount of attention has been given to research results in this chapter because (1) therapists need as much empirically based information as possible in an area in which "common-sense" guidance frequently is not trustworthy, and (2) intervention programs based on recent research findings have been successful in dealing with the needs of both parents and children in different segments of the divorced population (Wallerstein, 1991).

What are the contextual areas of concern and the support systems for children of separation and divorce?

Parent–Child Relationship

Whatever the therapist can do to help strengthen the parent–child relationship can be expected to contribute to the child's well-being.

Sibling Subsystem Therapy

Interventions with siblings as a group can be used as the major therapy focus or as an adjunct to total family therapy. Sibling subsystem therapy focuses on the family unit that generally remains intact during a time of family reorganization (Schibuk, 1989). It is most likely to be the major therapy focus in circumstances in which a parent will not participate in therapy but permits the children to get therapeutic help. Sibling subsystem therapy appears to be especially helpful in working out more realistic and appropriate expectations for dealing with the children's noncustodial parent (Nichols, 1986).

Contraindications to using sibling subsystem therapy as the sole mode of therapy include (1) the existence of sufficient animosity, hostility, or rivalry between siblings to make working with them unproductive; (2) the failure of the parents to permit the children to be in therapy without retaliating against them (Nichols, 1986); (3) the temporary absence of mentally ill siblings who are on medication; and (4) the potential development of adequate parenting, which would be hindered by the reinforcement of overly strong and rigid generational boundaries (Rosenberg, 1980).

Some therapists have suggested that a heterosexual cotherapy team be used with divorcing families, in order to help children develop an internalized family image (Sholevar & Sonne, 1979), and also in school groups (Kalter et al., 1984). I agree that using a heterosexual cotherapy team can be helpful in working with divorcing parents and possibly with the entire family. The role of the therapist with sibling subsystems is somewhat different. It is important to avoid assuming anything resembling a parental role with the sibling system because of the risk of creating unnecessary confusion and loyalty conflicts for the children. Hence, working alone and taking an avuncular approach in which one can be perceived as a professional "uncle" or "aunt" seems preferable (Nichols, 1986) to assuming a parental role.

Three outcomes have been notable in my work with sibling subsystems. First, the sessions involve exploration and clarification. The siblings typically emerge with a clearer comprehension of what is happening in the marital breakup and a more precise understanding of their own reactions. They may also get a better idea of how they can cope with the situation. Second, the youngsters may begin to establish better communication among themselves, and also better ideas of what they wish to communicate to or ask their parents. Third, exploration of the actual and potential sources of support for the children may result in the beginning of a plan for obtaining better support for them.

Extended Family

The extended family, particularly grandparents and aunts and uncles, may already be providing understanding and emotional and physical support for the children. Work with the sibling subsystem and with the parents may lead to effective involvement of extended family members as a resource.

Support Groups

A variety of models for group intervention with children of separation and divorce can be found in the literature. A six-session group program model has been developed in Toronto for use with preschoolers. Rossiter's (1988) report on it specifies goals, outlines the plan for each session, and offers preliminary observations regarding outcome. Farmer and Galaris (1993) describe another model for support groups for children of divorce, which was developed at the Marriage Council of Philadelphia.

Primary Prevention Groups

Some courts have mandated the establishment of early group intervention for children and adolescents whose parents have filed for divorce. Participation is voluntary. The approach described by Young (1989) involves a heavy use of topical, and occasionally didactic, methods. The purpose is to help the youngsters understand the nature of the forthcoming divorce in their family. The leader also serves as a communication analyst and therapist. Careful and explicit attention is given to prevent participants from labeling themselves "victims" and viewing themselves as being helpless. One major outcome is the participants' feeling that they are not alone. This is very similar to reactions long observed in educational groups for adults adjusting to divorce (Nichols, 1977).

Some schools also have devised a preventive approach to divorce counseling that fits the educational goals of the school. Typically, this approach follows a group counseling format. Such programs usually are provided by school counselors, psychologists, or social workers. The major focus has been on elementary age children because this is regarded as the largest category of children of divorce and research has labeled 9- to 10-year-olds as the most vulnerable age (Bernard, 1989). One such program that has been successfully implemented in elementary schools has been described by Pedro-Carroll and Cowen (1987).

There are times at which the family therapist working with a child of divorce may need to become involved with the school. When are the child's problems affecting his or her school performance and behavior to the extent that the therapist should become involved with the school? Some practical guidelines have been offered by DiCocco (1986). She describes four phases. Phase I involves mild problems that the school usually can handle (e.g., failure to turn in homework assignments, fighting on the school grounds). In Phase II the problems are more serious (e.g., extreme social withdrawal or excessive absenteeism) and the school contacts the parents. In Phase III things have hit a critical point (e.g., serious substance abuse, severe truancy). The school and parents may be blaming each other or the child. DiCocco recommends organizing both school and family into one adult ecosystem. The family therapist, as an outsider, is in a position to design an intervention for the entire ecosystem. Phase IV exists when the systems have not been successful and the child has been moved to a residential treatment center or some other external placement.

11

THERAPY WITH FAMILIES
IN TRANSITION: REMARRIAGE

*A basic difficulty for stepfamilies arises from the question
of what constitutes a family.*
—EMILY B. VISHER AND JOHN S. VISHER, *Stepfamilies*

Being single again after once being married is a transitory state for North
Americans. Most divorced and widowed persons, with the exception of
women in their 50s and older, will remarry within a few years. The
optimum time for remarriage is some 3 to 5 years after the initial
separation, according to some observers. The assessment of Sager and
colleagues (1983) is that such a period of time permits one to recover
from narcissistic injuries, complete the emotional divorce from the
former mate, and achieve other tasks that permit one to live again in a
marriage.

Historically, stepfamilies developed when a widowed parent remarried. Today's stepfamilies usually result from remarriage following divorce. This results in new sets of relationships and interactions that society
has not faced in such numbers in the past. Societal norms do not exist for
many of the situations faced by today's remarried families. These include
such everyday matters as how to define some relationships (e.g., those
with one's former in-laws) and even how to introduce persons to whom
one is related in the restructured family pattern (e.g., one's parent's new

spouse). The new type of remarried family living understandably poses a growing challenge to family therapists (Nichols, 1980).

Therapeutic efforts with remarrying couples and stepfamilies involve a considerable amount of educational work with the couples and children involved. All such clients need to be informed and sensitized regarding the issues of remarriage and remarried family living, as well as assisted therapeutically in dealing with their own feelings, conflicts, and problems.

REMARRIAGE

Even structurally, remarriage is a complex matter. The complexity and variety of patterns of remarriage make it impossible to construct a stage of the family life cycle that would be typical. Adults and children in one remarried family can come together at very different points in their life cycles than adults and children in another remarried family.

Patterns of Remarriage

Where only the adults are considered, there are eight possible patterns. The eight patterns are:

Divorced male—Single female
Divorced male—Widowed female
Divorced male—Divorced female
Single male—Divorced female
Widowed male—Divorced female
Widowed male—Single female
Widowed male—Widowed female
Single male—Widowed female

The majority of divorced parents remarry. The remarriage picture becomes even more complicated when children are considered. When gender, previous marital status of each partner, and the presence of custodial and/or noncustodial children are considered, 24 patterns of remarried couples are possible, according to the calculations of Sager and associates (Sager et al., 1983). Sager (Sager et al., 1983) perceives the remarried couple not only as a system in its own right but also as a subsystem of what he calls the "remarried family suprasystem." The larger network resulting from the divorce and remarriage includes not only the remarried couple but others such as the other biological parent of the child, grandparents, other relatives, and the child, who is the link between the stepfamily unit and the larger system.

Marital Issues in Remarriage

Adults who are remarrying commonly encounter three sets of problems affecting their relationship that are not present in a first marriage. Significant resolution of those problems is essential to the attainment of a strong and viable union between remarried spouses and the formation of a cohesive remarried unit.

"Ghosts from the Past"

First, the spouses need to deal with residues from the former marriage of either or both of them. Regardless of whether the former spouse is living or dead, such "ghosts from the past" may be present. If the former spouse is still alive, there may be unresolved feelings of anger, hatred, or continued attachment. Whatever the feelings toward a former mate, the present spouse may be fearful that some attraction still exists between the former partners. If the previous marriage was ended by death, the surviving and remarried spouse may idealize the deceased partner and former marriage.

Disillusionment with marriage, with risking oneself, or with making oneself vulnerable to commitment and hurt may last long after grief work connected with the loss of the former spouse as a person has been completed. That is, one may work through feelings of bereavement and grief and still be uncomfortable with the idea of being married. A fear of failure or of being rejected and left again sometimes crops up in remarriages. Also, there may be expectations that the present spouse will behave as the former spouse did and that some patterns followed in the first marriage may be repeated—for better or worse.

Discomfort may result from an attitude on the part of former in-laws that the remarried person is an interloper who has no business replacing a former son-in-law or daughter-in-law whom they liked. One's new spouse also may be uncomfortable with the fact that friendly relations are maintained with one's former in-laws. Whatever the form and quantity of such residues, they may pose major adaptive tasks for the remarrying adult.

The Presence of Children

The fact that there are children frequently makes a remarriage different from a first marriage. At least one of the adults tends to have children and thus to be involved in a parent–child relationship that predates his or her relationship with the new spouse. This tie may hinder in several ways the establishment of appropriate generational boundaries in the stepfamily. A considerable amount of time may be required for the stepparent and stepchild to work out adequate patterns of relating to each other. Unlike the first marriage, which can last for several years before children enter the picture, the spouses do not have adequate private time to adjust to one another.

Unresolved grief feelings on the part of children over the loss of the parent and the change in the family structure can affect not only remarriage but also the total functioning of the stepfamily. The temper tantrums of an elementary age child, for example, may signify his or her reactions against sharing a parent with a new spouse. The new spouse may be unable to share the mate with his or her children. Whatever the age of the children, from the very young to the adult years, their presence is a significant factor in the adjustment of the remarried couple. Powerful loyalty ties to the family of origin (Boszormenyi-Nagy & Spark, 1973) make it difficult for children to accept stepparents. One does not have to work with many such cases before hearing such reactions from children and adolescents as, "You're not my daddy!" Adult children may spit out, "I can't stand seeing that woman where my mother ought to be!" The therapist may find it even more difficult to work with loyalty ties that are not exposed so openly, with children who do not openly oppose the newcomer but engage in various kinds of withholding of cooperation or passive–aggressive behaviors, or who manifest depression.

Property, Money, and Inheritance Issues

Property, money, and, in some instances, explicit concerns over inheritance and estate affairs are typical issues in remarriage. Such matters generally are not present at the beginning of a first marriage. It is not uncommon for a remarried couple to have to deal with both spouses' preexisting financial obligations. As well as taking into account their assets and obligations, which often include child-support payments, the newly married couple also have to cope with their current financial needs. What tends to make this situation different from a first marriage is the greater amount of financial resources involved, as well as the fact that a third and perhaps a fourth person—one or more former spouses and children—have some stake in the resources. Children, for example, may object to a remarriage because of a fear of losing out on a portion of their inheritance or because of fears that their own children will be economically harmed by the remarriage.

Economic assets and obligations place not only an economic but also an emotional strain on many remarriages. How they are handled may be a barometer of the partners' anxiety about the new relationship and their level of trust of each other. Do I sign over my equity in the house and make it part of the common marital property? I have more savings than he or she does: What do we do about that? Some professionals dealing with remarriage recommend the use of a premarital agreement in which such issues are handled in a contractual fashion (Kaslow & Schwartz, 1987; Sager et al., 1983).

Adults and Satisfactory Remarried Family Adjustment

"As the adults go, so go the children" is as true for remarried families as it is for original nuclear families. Emily and John Visher (1990), pioneers in therapeutic and educational work with stepfamilies, have described six characteristics of remarried adults that they think are associated with satisfactory adjustment for stepfamilies. As adapted, these include the following:

1. *Completed mourning.* Both of the remarried persons have mourned their losses adequately.
2. *Realistic expectations.* Both adults in a satisfactorily adjusted remarried family expect realistically that their new family will be different from a first marriage family. The Vishers (1990) point to several reasons why the families are different. These include the facts that adults and children meet at different places in their life cycles and bring different ways of doing things from their past family patterns. Satisfactory adjustment requires that the need for accommodation of differences be recognized.
3. *Strong, unified couple.* Remarried parents know that children benefit from the sense of security provided by the presence of a stable couple and from assurance that the stepfamily unit will continue.
4. *Constructive rituals.* Recognizing that feelings of belonging and positive shared memories develop from familiar ways of doing things, the adults establish constructive rituals and traditions in the stepfamily. When possible, traditions from past family experiences are retained or combined in the new rituals.
5. *Satisfactory steprelationships.* The adults have taken adequate time and care to develop satisfactory and viable roles and relationships regarding their stepchildren. They have not attempted to move into parental roles or to take over discipline. Instead, they have allowed relationships to develop in a mutual fashion.
6. *Separate household cooperation.* This refers to the cooperation of adults from two households in rearing the children. Attaining cooperation

rather than competition is not possible in many situations, but when it is accomplished, the children are not caught in a crossfire and have fewer loyalty conflicts (Visher & Visher, 1990).

Each of these requirements faces the therapist with therapeutic and educational opportunities and challenges, which are illustrated below.

REMARRIED FAMILY LIVING

The stepfamily system displays features that are not found in an original nuclear family unit. An understanding of those unique and unusual features is vital to working in an effective way with such systems and their members.

Unusual Features of Remarried Families

The following major features of remarried families, compared to original nuclear families, all are associated with ambiguity.

1. *Lack of clear definition.* The absence of clear definition in the system can cause substantial problems for stepfamilies. It is difficult to determine what constitutes the system, who should be included in the concept of family, and how members should be addressed or how they should be classified. There is even a lack of consensus among professionals about what the family should be called: stepfamily, blended family, reconstituted family, or remarried family. This lack of definition extends to kinship definitions and terms. What are the parents-in-law of a newly married person in relation to his or her children? Who are the former parents-in-law in relation to the divorced spouse after he or she has married someone else? What is a stepparent?

2. *Absence of norms.* Stepfamily members are confronted at the outset with the absence of models and norms for playing their roles. What are the guides for being a stepparent? What are the responsibilities of a stepparent toward a stepchild? What is the role of the stepparent? What do stepchildren owe their stepparent? Vitally important here is an absence of the strong incest taboo that prevails in the original nuclear family and in the extended biological family.

3. *Ambiguity regarding authority and power.* Power and authority assume unusual forms in stepfamily organization. Power (the actual ability to do something) and authority (the legitimate right to do something) are divided among various adults. Typically they are split between

the biological parents and the stepparents. The boundaries of the family unit or subsystems within which the children reside may not be firm and fixed, preventing power and authority from flowing across them from the outside. The nonresident parent, for example, lives elsewhere but certainly has an effect on what transpires within the child's residential unit. Generally, the former spouse shares in both parental power and economic decisions regarding the children, particularly if he or she is providing economic support for the children. A custodial mother, for example, may not be completely free to make decisions about summer camp, school attendance at a private school, dental work, or other matters, because her former spouse either must be consulted or may manipulate the payment of child support. Similarly, a child may be permitted to do some things when visiting with the nonresidential parent that he or she is not allowed to do at home, thus creating struggles between the child and the residential parent when the youngster returns home.

Educational Interventions

Interventions with stepfamilies may, as noted above, involve some educational work. It is often necessary to identify difficulties that are stemming from unclear and unrealistic expectations. Lacking clear-cut definitions and clearly applicable norms and models, members of stepfamily systems often attempt to apply the same kinds of expectations and behaviors to stepfamily living that they learned either from their earlier nuclear system or from their family of origin. Some of the educational information that is useful to stepfamilies follows.

1. *A stepparent is someone who has married a parent.* It is not the same as being the biological parent of a child. There are no guidelines for being a stepparent. Stepparents do not have the same rights or privileges in relation to their stepchild as the child's natural parents do. The legal relationship that exists is between the two remarried adults. Even being a stepparent for several years gives no rights for custody.

2. *A stepparent and a stepchild owe courtesy and respect to one another.* That is the extent of their obligation. Neither owes the other love. If love develops in the course of interacting and maintaining a relationship, that is fortunate for the participants, but it should not be expected to emerge spontaneously and is not required in order to make a success of stepfamily living.

3. *Two significant myths that need to be debunked are those of "instant love" and "the wicked stepmother"* (Visher & Visher, 1979). A stepparent has not failed if he or she does not experience instant affection

for stepchildren or elicit instant love from the youngsters. The wicked stepmother myth probably stems from two sources. The first is from folklore and literature devolving from double standard, or sexist, attitudes that devalued women and blamed them for problems in family relationships. The second comes from the fact that in the past stepfamilies were formed following the death of a parent and that stepmothers frequently had their new spouse's children residing with them.

4. *Stepparents may perform a variety of roles, but there is no single right or wrong pattern.* Therapists should encourage stepparents to explore the possible roles open to them. Three models for the stepmother proposed by Draughon (1975) are "primary mother," "other mother," and "friend," for example. These roles can be generalized to both parents. Stepparents certainly should not try to compete with the biological parent, or to substitute unless the biological parent is clearly unavailable for the children and psychologically dead for them. The major issues in the various forms of stepparent relationships that have been gleaned from research have been summarized by Visher and Visher (1979).

5. *The nuclear family from which the participants in stepfamilies emerge does not provide guidelines or models that are workable for stepfamilies.* A considerable amount of confusion, frustration, conflict, and disappointment may result from the efforts of stepfamily members to apply what they have learned in their "basic training" in their family of origin or in their first-marriage nuclear family to stepfamily situations. Following the course of "doing what comes naturally" or "doing things the right way" (i.e., the way they were learned and done in the previous family) is an understandable inclination but a course that invites trouble.

The stepfamily at this juncture needs to understand not only that theirs is a different family form than the nuclear family but also that it is a new form that requires the development of new models of expectations and behaviors among its members. (A comprehensive and helpful listing of differences between the two kinds of family systems in terms of structure, purpose, tasks, nature of the bonding, factors influencing the children, and forces that impinge on the system itself has been provided by Sager and associates [1983].)

THERAPEUTIC INTERVENTIONS

Entering into a therapeutic relationship with the stepfamily system opens the way for the therapist to engage the members in careful exploration and clarification of various unresolved feelings including grief, anger, loss, and hope. It also helps the family to focus on the fact that there are a variety of ways in which stepfamilies can be organized other than the patterns learned in nuclear families. The therapist may provide illustrations and examples of how stepfamilies are different from nuclear families, including calling attention to the various patterns of remarriage and resultant relationship patterns mentioned earlier in this chapter.

Work with stepfamilies seems to be most effective when the therapist conducts it in an atmosphere of sympathetic understanding and with an explicit acknowledgment of the complexity of the family members' situation. Acknowledging the stress involved in understanding and dealing with multiple change situations, as well as recognizing the loyalty conflicts faced by various members, helps the family to settle down and begin to function more cooperatively and effectively. In order to be able to help, I need to comprehend clearly how the family members are involved in multiple life cycle changes and development in their individual, marital, and family life cycles in a complicated pattern of process and change.

Working with Remarried Families in the Formation Stage

Achieving stepfamily reorganization is seen as the goal of family therapy by the Vishers (1979). Certainly this is true in the early stages of stepfamily formation. There are some indications that the initial reorganization period, the time needed for stepfamilies to become integrated and to begin functioning as a family unit, lasts at least 2 years, and often much longer. The establishment of good marital bonding and freedom of movement for children between two different living situations typically are key elements in the achievement of stepfamily reorganization (Visher & Visher, 1979).

If the relationship between the two new marital partners is strong and can overcome efforts by children and others to weaken the alliance, the stepfamily is likely to function adequately. Both clinical observation and research indicate that the cohesiveness of the couple in the family is a very important dimension in emotionally healthy families (Lewis, Beavers, Gossett, & Phillips, 1976). Clinically, one seeks to determine the strength of the marital relationship and how it is affected by others, especially by the children. A key issue is often the length of time the new partners have had to secure bonding and integration.

Assessment

The complexity of the stepfamily makes it essential to begin with a careful assessment of the organization of the stepfamily system, including both subsystems and suprasystem (the system of extended family and the context of other systems in which the stepfamily functions and with which it links).

Such assessment starts even during the first telephone call, when some preliminary decisions are made about who is to be included in the assessment and treatment. In an original nuclear family, it is relatively simple to determine who is to be included in the therapy sessions. One usually includes the father, mother, dependent children, and anyone else living in the home, including, in a multigenerational approach, the grandparents.

Deciding whom to include for assessment with stepfamilies is more complicated. With families in which the children are living in a binuclear situation (living in two nuclear families), it is sometimes helpful to bring in all four adults, or three adults if one of the parents has not remarried, and, again, perhaps the grandparents. Decisions have to be made early about the potential assets and liabilities of trying to involve various groupings and individuals who compose the extended or suprafamily system in the assessment and treatment.

The constructs, and some of the therapeutic interventions, of structural family therapy (Minuchin, 1974; Colapinto, 1991) are particularly helpful in conceptualizing and dealing with remarried families. Organizationally, the stepfamily tends in some ways to resemble Aponte's (1976) urban poor family in that both are likely to be underorganized. This is particularly true in the early stages of stepfamily organization. Aponte dealt with family structure in terms of boundary, alignment, and force.

Boundaries

It is important to ask, "Who is to be included? What are the real boundaries of the family?" At the very outset, it may be necessary to spend some time getting the people settled down sufficiently to determine who is to be included inside the boundaries of the family. In strong contrast to the optimism that often goes with entry into a first marriage, there frequently is limited confidence and sometimes confusion about the second family.

The therapist has to keep in mind the fact that stepfamily members themselves may be quite uncertain as to who is in the family at a particular time. The construction of a genogram may disclose, for example, that "the family" is different for different members. Children in the family may be faced with the task of relating to at least four parental or quasiparental figures and with six or eight "grandparents" (i.e., the parents of the children's parents or stepparents).

The boundaries are not only permeable (Messinger, 1976), but they also may change suddenly. Members may move in and out of the family system with varying degrees of frequency. The shifting of boundaries may occur several years after a stepfamily has been formed and the boundaries ostensibly established. A child can abruptly leave one parent and move in with the other, for example, beginning to reside permanently in the stepfamily where he or she previously has been a weekend or vacation guest. Part of the immediate therapeutic task that accompanies integrating the youngster into the family's daily routines consists of examining whether there is any need for mourning on the part of any of the participants, whether there are significant loyalty conflicts on the child's part, and whether there are unrealistic expectations for "instant love" on the part of a stepparent or the child (Nichols, 1980).

Common boundary disputes that arise between adults include disagreements over the custody rights or privileges of custodial and noncustodial parents. The grandparents may be involved where there is change from past family holiday patterns and observance of rituals. When there is little contact between the various adults involved in situations and little clarity or agreement, the children have many opportunities to manipulate one system against the other (Visher & Visher, 1979).

Common complaints also arise from the fact that the children move back and forth between households that may have very different sets of standards and expectations. One household may embody strict behavioral expectations and the other may be much less restrictive and more permissive. One of the early therapeutic tasks may be that of helping the child to recognize the differences and to realize that one has to learn how to cope and adapt in the face of diverse expectations in different settings. Similarly, a parent may need reassurance that children can adapt to different patterns and rules if the expectations are presented to them clearly and firmly.

At the same time, for the sake of the child there may be an urgent need to help the formerly married persons diminish their continuing emotional ties and struggles with each other or to help a stepparent clarify his or her role so that the boundary issues become more clear. I have found it helpful to spend a considerable amount of time trying to establish a solid working relationship with these conflicted adults. Understandably, the more clearly I can demonstrate firmness and fairness in dealing with them, the greater the possibility that they may be able to accept my efforts to help them set clear boundaries. With some persons, any progress that one can make is helpful.

Family boundaries also may be assessed in terms of rules that determine the limits of the family system. What are the rules concerning how each of the formerly married persons deals with and relates to his or her children? How clear are they? How adequate are the rules? Are they flexible and adaptable enough to fit changing needs? Both an independent relationship between each parent and each child and a viable relationship of cooperation between the formerly married persons is required if a successful transition is to be made through divorce and into a workable stepfamily situation (Ahrons, 1980).

The remarried family has to negotiate four areas of boundary difficulty, according to Carter and McGoldrick (1988a). These areas, as adapted here, can be recalled through a mnemonic or memory device of M-A-S-T, which includes the following components:

Membership: Who are the "real" members of the family?
Authority: Who is in charge of decisions, discipline, money, and so forth?
Space: Where does one really belong and what space is theirs?
Time: Who gives how much to whom?

Alignment

The second construct used by Aponte (1976), "alignment," refers to the ways in which one member of the family may be united with or opposed to another with regard to conducting family operations. The term is being used here primarily to refer to the structuring of generational boundaries. One very important task in many families, for example, is the rebuilding of generational boundaries that have been weakened during the period between divorce and remarriage. During that time, a child may have become parentified into a surrogate spouse role. The remarriage of the parent can be used as the beginning of the liberation of the child who has been in a spousal role (confidant, companion to the single parent) or in a parental role (in relation to another child). However, this change may be seen by the youngster as a threat and potential loss. Often, this shift is experienced as rejection. Even after he or she has been replaced by the parent's new spouse following the parental remarriage, there may be a need and opportunity for the therapist to help the young person become a child again and to function at an age-appropriate level with the siblings.

Parent–child alignments in the stepfamily also may need to be strengthened. The biological parent and the child can be united around the task of taking responsibility for the child's behavior. Reinforcing the authority and disciplinary ties between them may prevent stepparent and stepchild conflict. Clashes arising from resentment on the part of the youngster at being disciplined by a stepparent, and role confusion on the part of the stepparent can be avoided by strengthening parent–child alignments. The uncertainty of stepparents, stemming largely from the lack of norms for stepfamilies, as well as from their frequent fears about security in either the marriage or the stepfamily, contribute significantly to alignment problems.

The alignment in a family may be too tight or too loose. In an underorganized family, it is not clear who can be depended on to carry out what tasks or responsibilities. In remarried families, the important issue for children and adults frequently is, "Who can be counted on to help with family-related tasks or functions?" If a significant number of things "fall between the cracks" in nuclear families, it is even more likely to be the case with stepfamilies. One biological parent, for example, may assume that a certain task is the responsibility of the other biological parent with whom he or she has limited communication and who simply may not be in a position to handle the task, or may be unwilling, resistant, or defiant. The alignments in a family system shift over time as different circumstances arise and as there is a need to fulfill different tasks.

Force and Power

"Force," the third ingredient in this approach to organization, refers to the distribution of power in the family system. Power may be assigned in a system on the basis of position or role. It also may be assumed by an individual. In an underorganized family, the force or power is not distributed in an orderly way (Aponte, 1976).

Difficulties may arise from various sources. Some members may not use the power assigned to their position; other members may assume power inappropriately and use it in ways that disrupt the family system. For example, in a stepfamily situation in which a widowed man and his teenage daughter joined a divorced woman and her younger daughter, the father abdicated the authority/disciplinary position almost entirely. Into the vacuum created by the father's failure to use his assigned power, his adolescent daughter moved to assume and exercise power out of proportion to her age. Although he was the legitimate possessor of power, the daughter was the one who put it into effect. The result was an ongoing conflict between his daughter and her stepmother. In another family composed of two parents who had brought their children together in one residence in an effort to create a genuinely blended family, the wife was both the possessor and the one who used power. She used not only power that was assigned to her because of her position as an adult and parent but also assumed additional power in the face of her husband's failure to use the power assigned to his position. This resulted in the kind of skewed system sometimes observed in original nuclear families.

The distribution of power varies as time passes in the life cycle (e.g., the child's dependency on the parents decreases and his or her own independence appropriately increases with age [Aponte, 1976]).

Clinical Example from the Formation Stage

One clinical example may help to tie together the present use of "boundary," "alignment," and "force" and some of the educational and therapeutic issues mentioned above. A major problem with the Jones family centered around the efforts to integrate John Jones into an ongoing family unit with his new wife and her three adolescent daughters. The alignment between Mrs. Jones and her daughters was so well established and powerful that Mr. Jones was excluded from effective participation in the stepfamily. During the first year of the new marriage, there had been conflict whenever Mr. Jones attempted to exert parental influence that he did not possess. When the marital partners dealt with each other separately from the adolescents, their relationship worked well.

The therapeutic interventions—which were all done directly with the marital partners—involved changing boundaries and alignments, and clarifying roles. Rather than starting with the problematic areas, the therapist initially concentrated on the marital relationship, attempting to build on available strengths. "How do you feel about each other?" "What do you want to do with the marriage?" "What attracted you to [the spouse]?" Discourse based on typical marital therapy exploratory questions indicated that there was genuine caring and desire to remain together between the partners.

Once the couple's commitment was established and it was clear that they wanted the same things in their relationship, it was possible to address the issues that stood in the way. Once again, the therapist sought clarity about what they desired and about their anxieties and concerns:

THERAPIST: John, we know that you are bothered by some of the girls' attitudes and the things that they do. But, putting it briefly, what is it that you want from them?

MR. JONES: I just want them to do right. To do what they should, to do some work around the house, to be respectful, and the older one and her boyfriend not to be climbing all over each other and pawing each other all the time. I want some peace and tranquility around the house.

Following some probing and additional clarification, the therapist asked Mrs. Jones, "What do you want from the girls?" Her responses indicated that, while more flexible and liberal in her expectations than her husband, she also wanted "some peace and tranquillity" in the home.

THERAPIST: You both want some of the same things, less arguing, less conflict, and more cooperation and harmony. Do you have any ideas about how you might achieve some of those things, and be able to enjoy your marriage and each other more?

Later, Mr. Jones was asked, "Do you really want the job of telling the girls what to do and trying to keep them in line?"

MR. JONES: Godsakes no!

MRS. JONES: Then stay out of it and let me handle things. It just gets worse when you try to step in and tell them what to do, or yell at them.

MR. JONES: If you would make them do right, I would. I would be glad to.

MRS. JONES: You have to let me do it my way. You can't expect me to do things the way you would. You have to loosen up and not expect them to do everything just the way you want it.

During the ensuing discussion, Mr. Jones appeared to gain some awareness that his attempts to be the disciplinarian were the source of much of the "disrespect" from the girls. The therapist explained how his efforts to act as a parent and to do what he thought he should might be producing loyalty conflicts for the girls as well as undesired outcomes for him. Explanations of the possible roles stepparents could appropriately play other than that of "parent" provided Mr. Jones with some viable alternatives. All of this opened the door for him to consider the possibility that he could "loosen up" and "back off" from his current approach to his stepchildren.

Some exploration of family-of-origin patterns for both partners illuminated their definitions of what was "right" and desirable in childrearing. This led to some negotiation and compromise. Mr. Jones decided that he could tolerate some things that made him uncomfortable if he had assurance that his wife would support his desires regarding other behaviors on the part of the adolescents. At least, he was "willing to give it a try. Anything is better than what we have now."

By agreement, the mother was given primary responsibility for guidance and discipline. The excessively strong ties between Mrs. Jones and her daughters that had developed during the years that she was single gradually diffused and the marital bonds and spousal subsystem simultaneously strengthened as the partners became more dependent on each other for companionship and for assistance with decision making. Also, Mr. Jones was helped to cope with problems of sexual attraction and defenses against his impulses so that he could relate to the adolescent females more comfortably. As this change occurred and his position was made more secure in the marriage and the stepfamily, he decreased his tendencies to exert force inflexibly. Over a period of time as the subsystems in the stepfamily were clearly differentiated and the generational boundaries firmly established, the teenagers moved back into appropriate places in their developmental cycles and began moving toward adulthood in a more timely and orderly fashion.

Working with Established Remarried Families

A majority of the literature on remarried families appears to be focused on the early stages of stepfamily formation. There are both different and similar issues between the remarried family in the process of formation, sometimes called the "reconstituting stepfamily," and the remarried family that has moved past the formation or reconstituting stage. Remarried families that have existed for 10 or more years are well past the initial reorganization stage, for example, but some still may be coping with "ghost" issues.

The developmental phases of the family in the process of formation have been described as recovering from loss and entering the new relationship, conceptualization and planning of the new marriage, and reconstitution of the family (Ransome, Schlesinger, & Derdeyn, 1979). To date, developmental tasks for stepfamilies have not been set for stages that go much beyond the formation period. There are some guidelines for therapeutic intervention, however. Sager and associates (Sager et al., 1983) have provided some excellent material on adolescents in stepfamilies that are related to developmental task schema for stepfamilies. Some assessment and intervention strategies for use with established remarried families can be adapted and evolved from the developmental schema presented in preceding chapters with regard to the particular life cycle stage of the family system and its members.

"Normal" Family Issues

Some remarried families eventually begin to function much like original nuclear families. Treatment in such cases primarily is concerned with the same kinds of issues that arise in nuclear families. Mr. and Mrs. Smith asked for help with their children some 3 years after forming a stepfamily. Each had two children from a former marriage. Mr. Smith's children had come to live with him and his new wife when their mother had been killed in an accident a few weeks after the remarriage. Mrs. Smith's children spent 1 or 2 weeks a year with their biological father. Otherwise, the six persons in the Smith family functioned essentially as a nuclear family. An assessment of the situation with Mr. and Mrs. Smith disclosed that their concerns about their children were basically normal childrearing concerns related to a variety of common problems such as curfews and limits, which fit with the children's developmental stages.

It was apparent that the more pressing concerns of the Smiths pertained to their marital relationship. Marital therapy became the treatment of choice. The presenting problems about the children were handled by the couple without the necessity of the children attending therapy sessions. The Smith family was notable in that it had worked through the early developmental issues of mourning and the establishment of relationships so that the youngsters had been permitted to get back on their appropriate individual life cycle paths. The boundaries were clear and the subsystems adequately separated and delineated.

Shifts in Boundaries

As a remarried family evolves over time and begins to become an established unit, there may be shifts in the attitudes and allegiances of the new family that require particular attention. For example, in one new family involving a wife/mother, her 8-year-old daughter from a previous marriage, and the husband/stepfather, things began to change after approximately two years. The child's biological father remarried and had an 11-year-old stepdaughter who served as a kind of sibling for the younger child. Things went reasonably well in the binuclear arrangement until the biological father, a substance abuser, created a wild physical scene in which he fought with his second wife and virtually wrecked the house during a weekend in which the 8-year-old was present. As a result, the child's mother decided to allow only daytime visits in the future, but to forbid overnight visits, something that was within her scope of power under the custody arrangements. In response, the biological father cut off contact with his daughter.

The mother worked in an appropriate manner to help the child recognize that the father was a seriously disturbed individual. Even though she wished to maintain contact with her stepsister, the child began to diminish her investment in the biological father and his family as she started to realize that the man had become very disturbed emotionally and that he did not love her. It took only a limited amount of probing with the youngster to discover that she was far more disturbed by the loss of contact with the stepsister than by the cutoff from her father. The only sibling that she had would no longer be available.

The child began to regard her stepfather, a warm and caring person, even more as a father figure. Eventually he began to function as a genuine parent. The binuclear situation withered and the stepfamily in which she resided became essentially the family of the child. This does not appear to be an unusual outcome of binuclear family living after a period of years.

Unresolved Tasks

Failure to resolve early tasks may create problems later or contribute to perennial difficulties in remarriage and stepfamily living. After nearly 20 years of marriage, Mr. and Mrs. Williams still had not succeeded in obtaining a remarried family organization that would have enabled them to function without large amounts of friction. A widower with three young children, Mr. Williams had remarried a single woman 13 years younger than he. During the early days, she struggled with her mother-in-law over control of the children, trying to take over the mothering role that the older woman had assumed during her son's days as a widower. The young woman's continuing conflicts with her stepchildren were a textbook example of "instant love" and "wicked stepmother" problems. The harder she tried to be a good mother to the three children, to make up to them for their losses, the more they resisted, and the more she became labeled a bad stepmother throughout the extended family system.

When Mr. and Mrs. Williams sought professional help, it was for the purpose of resolving marital problems. Working first with conflict over continuing relations with Mr. Williams's by then grown children, the therapist spent some time in clarifying current and original expectations on the part of both partners as to stepmother–stepchildren relations. A considerable amount of support and interpretation resulted in the diminishing of bewilderment and hurt on Mrs. Williams's part and resentments on the part of both partners. Understanding how things had gone off the track in the early days and had continued because of unclear and incompatible expectations aided them to lower tensions. As this occurred, it was possible to deal with other more specifically marital issues including temperamental differences between the mates. Mrs. Williams also was able to alter her current dealings and relationships with her stepchildren so that tensions there were lowered as well. She recognized that they probably would never be close to her, but a workable degree of amiable relating was obtained.

SUMMARY

Assessment and intervention with the stepfamily system are concerned with the current organization and functioning of the various individuals in the system, with the remarriage, with the family system itself, and with the system as part of a larger intergenerational network. What are the strengths of the remarried family and its members? What are the strengths of the remarriage? What are the problems of the individuals, of the remarriage, and of the remarried family?

Although it is axiomatic in a family therapy orientation that issues are examined and understood in terms of their systemic context, that point needs to be doubly emphasized where remarried family assessment and treatment are concerned. Working with remarried families may stir the clinician's emotional reactivity more readily than most other therapeutic challenges. Not only the emotional reactions but also the clinician's lack of knowledge about and experience with remarried families may contribute to his or her difficulty in comprehending what is being presented. Even veteran clinicians can become confused by the behavior of stepfamily members, unless they are acquainted with the significant differences between the cultures of original nuclear families and remarried families.

Sager and associates (Sager et al., 1983) have noted that the intensity of responses that they found, particularly among children who were reacting to parental separation and remarriage, often led them to regard stepfamily members as being very disturbed. When reexamined more carefully, the behaviors were seen as appropriate responses to disturbing and chaotic stepfamily situations. They found that more than four-fifths of the children in their clinical population were involved in a dysfunctional relationship with parents or stepparents. Not all required treatment. Many of those children and adults could be helped through educational channels.

CONCLUDING THOUGHTS

We have focused probably too much on therapeutic approach and
not enough on the skill of the therapist
—SOL GARFIELD,
Clinical Psychology: Science and Practice

Those words are from one of the foremost psychologists endeavoring to study and advance integration and eclecticism in psychotherapy. They reflect an attitude that has guided the writing of this book. I hope that it has been clear that, while I consider techniques important in psychotherapy, I regard them as secondary to the skill of the individual using them.

It has long been noted that there is nothing so practical as a good theory. This book embodies an attempt to emphasize that we deal with individuals in context. Hence, the theoretical approach offered here is one that emphasizes both the "inside" and the "outside" dimensions of the client. This holds whether the client is one person or many. One deals best with the system in its setting; with its dynamic, interactive relationship with larger systems; and with the internal dynamics of the system.

Understanding the developmental nature of clients as human beings, family members, married persons is also crucial in effective therapy. The more we can know about what our clients face in their attempts to wend their way through their various life cycles, the better we can understand them and work with them. This I regard as a truism whether we are trying to comprehend their narratives, restructure their family, help them to detriangulate, design strategic interventions, interpret their systemic functioning, or modify faulty cognitions. This book offers a developmental framework that can be helpful in comprehending what clients face and in intervening with them.

Understanding ourselves should not be overlooked in the therapist's continuing preparation for working with clients. There is much truth in a statement made a colleague long ago that "the person of the therapist sharpened and matured is the best tool that we have" for working with people. The therapist as tool refers not merely to the knowledge we possess or the verbal facility we exhibit, but, also to the ability to be empathic and, most importantly, to the kindness that we can deliver to our clients.

We need to give renewed and serious attention to what the therapist knows and is, not simply to what he or she does. Bringing a balance among those three to the therapeutic arena may be the most useful contribution that we can make to our clients. The therapist's own personal triangle consists of what we are, know, and do.

REFERENCES

Ackerman, N. W. (1958). *The psychodynamics of family life*. New York: Basic Books.

Ackerman, N. W. (1964). Prejudicial scapegoating and neutralizing forces in the family group. *International Journal of Social Psychiatry, 2*, 90–94. (Reprinted in Bloch, D. A. & Simons, R. [Eds.] [1982]. *The strength of family therapy: Selected papers of Nathan W. Ackerman* [pp. 195–200]. New York: Brunner/Mazel.)

Ackerman, N. W. (1966). *Treating the troubled family*. New York: Basic Books.

Ahrons, C. R. (1980). Redefining the divorced family: A conceptual framework for post-divorce family system reorganization. *Social Work, 25*, 437–441.

Ahrons, C. R. (1981). The continuing coparental relationship between divorced spouses. *American Journal of Orthopsychiatry, 51*, 315–328.

Ahrons, C. R. (1994). *The good divorce*. New York: HarperCollins.

Ahrons, C. R., & Rodgers, R. H. (1987). *Divorced families: A multidisciplinary developmental view*. New York: Norton.

Allport, G. W. (1955). *Becoming: Basic considerations for a psychology of personality*. New Haven: Yale University Press.

Allport, G. W. (1961). *Pattern and growth in personality*. New York: Holt, Rinehart & Winston.

Amato, P. R. (1993). Children's adjustment to divorce: Theories, hypotheses, and empirical support. *Journal of Marriage and the Family, 55*, 23–28.

Ambert, A. M. (1988). Relationships with former in-laws after divorce: A research note. *Journal of Marriage and the Family, 50*, 679–686.

American Association for Marriage and Family Therapy. (1992). *Family therapy glossary*. Washington, DC: Author.

American Psychiatric Association. (1987). *Diagnostic and statistical manual of mental disorders* (3rd ed., rev.). Washington, DC: Author.

American Psychiatric Association (1994). *Diagnostic and statistical manual of mental disorders* (4th ed.). Washington, DC: Author.

Andersen, T. (1993). Comfortable interventions. In T. S. Nelson & T. S. Trepper (Eds.), *101 interventions in family therapy* (pp. 418–420). New York: Haworth Press.

Anderson, C. M., Reiss, D. J., & Cahalane, J. F. (1986). Marital therapy with schizophrenic patients. In N. S. Jacobson & A. S. Gurman (Eds.), *Clinical handbook of marital therapy* (pp. 537–556). New York: Guilford Press.

Anderson, C. M., Reiss, D. J., & Hogarty, G. E. (1986). *Schizophrenia and the family*. New York: Guilford Press.

Anderson, C. M., & Stewart, S. (1983). *Mastering resistance: A practical guide to family therapy*. New York: Guilford Press.

Aponte, H. J. (1976). Underorganization in the poor family. In P. J. Guerin (Ed.), *Family therapy: Theory and practice* (pp. 432–448). New York: Gardner Press.

Arbarbanel, A. (1979). Shared parenting after separation and divorce: A study of joint custody. *American Journal of Orthopsychiatry, 49,* 320–329.

Ashby, W. R. (1952). *Design for a brain*. New York: Wiley.

Association of Marital and Family Therapy Regulatory Boards. (1989). *Information for candidates: Examination in marital and family therapy*. New York: Professional Examination Service.

Baber, K. M., & Allen, K. R. (1992). *Women and families: Feminist reconstructions*. New York: Guilford Press.

Baker, F. M. (1984). Group psychotherapy with patients over fifty: An adult developmental approach. *Journal of Geriatric Psychiatry, 17,* 79–108.

Bank, S. P., & Kahn, M. D. (1982). *The sibling bond*. New York: Basic Books.

Barnhill, L., & Longo, D. (1978). Fixation and regression in the family life cycle. *Family Process, 17,* 469–478.

Bateson, G. (1972). *Steps to an ecology of mind*. New York: Ballantine.

Bateson, G. (1979). *Mind and nature*. New York: Bantam Books.

Baucom, D. H., & Epstein, N. (1990). *Cognitive-behavioral marital therapy*. New York: Brunner/Mazel.

Beavers, W. R. (1977). *Psychotherapy and growth: A family systems perspective*. New York: Brunner/Mazel.

Beavers, W. R., & Hampson, R. B. (1990). *Successful families: Assessment and intervention*. New York: Norton.

Beavers, W. R., & Voeller, M. N. (1983). Family models: Comparing and contrasting the Olson circumplex model with the Beavers systems model. *Family Process, 22,* 85–97.

Beels, C. C., & Ferber, A. (1969). Family therapy. *Family Process, 9,* 280–318.

Beels, C. C., & Ferber, A. (1972). What family therapists do. In A. Ferber, M. Mendelsohn, & A. Napier (Eds.), *The book of family therapy* (pp. 168–232). New York: Science House.

Bell, J. E. (1975). *Family therapy*. New York: Jason Aronson.

Belsky, J., & Rovine, M. (1990). Patterns of marital change across the transition to parenthood: Pregnancy to three years postpartum. *Journal of Marriage and the Family, 52,* 5–19.

Berg, B., & Kelly, B. (1979). The measured self-esteem of children from broken, rejected, and accepted families. *Journal of Divorce, 2,* 363–369.

Berg, B., & Rosenblum, N. (1977). Fathers in family therapy: A survey of family therapists. *Journal of Marriage and Family Counseling, 3*(2), 85–91.

Bergler, E. (1948). *Divorce won't help.* New York: Hart.

Berman, E. M. (1982). The individual interview as a treatment technique in conjoint therapy. *American Journal of Family Therapy, 10,* 27–37.

Berman, E. M., & Lief, H. I. (1975). Marital therapy from a psychiatric perspective. *American Journal of Psychiatry, 132,* 583–592.

Berman, E. M., Miller, W. R., Vines, N., & Lief, H. I. (1977). The age 30 and the 7-year itch. *Journal of Marital and Sex Therapy, 3,* 197–204.

Bernard, J. (1972). *The future of marriage.* New York: World.

Bernard, J. M. (1989). School interventions. In M. Textor (Ed.), *The divorce and divorce therapy handbook* (pp. 267–284). Northvale, NJ: Jason Aronson.

Beutler, L. E., & Consoli, A. J. (1992). Systematic eclectic psychotherapy. In J. C. Norcross & M. R. Goldfried (Eds.), *Handbook of psychotherapy integration* (pp. 264–299). New York: Basic Books.

Blanck, R., & Blanck, G. (1968). *Marriage and personal development.* New York: Columbia University Press.

Bloom, B. L., White, S. W., & Asher, S. J. (1979). Marital disruption as a stressful life event. In G. Levinger & O. C. Moles (Eds.), *Divorce and separation* (pp. 184–200). New York: Basic Books.

Bohannon, P. (Ed.). (1970). *Divorce and after.* Garden City, NY: Doubleday.

Bordin, E. S. (1979). The generalizability of the psychoanalytic concept of the working alliance. *Psychotherapy: Theory, Research and Practice, 16,* 252–260.

Boszormenyi-Nagy, I. (1966). From family therapy to a psychology of relationships: Fictions of the individual and fictions of the family. *Comprehensive Psychiatry, 7,* 408–423.

Boszormenyi-Nagy, I. (1967). Relational modes and meaning. In G. H. Zuk & I. Boszormenyi-Nagy (Eds.), *Family therapy and disturbed families* (pp. 58–73). Palo Alto, CA: Science & Behavior Books.

Boszormenyi-Nagy, I., & Krasner, B. R. (1986). *Between give and take: A clinical guide to contextual therapy.* New York: Brunner/Mazel.

Boszormenyi-Nagy, I., & Spark, G. M. (1973). *Invisible loyalties.* New York: Harper & Row.

Boszormenyi-Nagy, I., & Ulrich, D. N. (1981). Contextual family therapy. In A. S. Gurman & D. P. Kniskern (Eds.), *Handbook of family therapy* (pp. 159–186). New York: Brunner/Mazel.

Bowen, M. (1966). The use of theory in family therapy. *Comprehensive Psychiatry, 7,* 345–374.

Bowen, M. (1978). *Family therapy in clinical practice.* New York: Jason Aronson.

Bowlby, J. (1969). *Attachment and loss.* New York: Basic Books.

Bradt, J. O. (1988). Becoming parents: Families with young children. In B. Carter

& M. McGoldrick (Eds.), *The changing family life cycle: A framework for family therapy* (2nd ed., pp. 237–254). New York: Gardner Press.

Breunlin, D. C. (1988). Oscillation theory and family development. In C. J. Falicov (Ed.), *Family transitions: Continuity and change over the life cycle* (pp. 133–155). New York: Guilford Press.

Breunlin, D. C., Schwartz, R. C., & MacKune-Karrer, B. (1992). *Metaframeworks: Transcending the models of family therapy.* San Francisco: Jossey-Bass.

Broden, A. R. (1970). Reaction to loss in the aged. In B. Schoenberg, A. C. Carr, D. Peretz, & A. H. Kutscher (Eds.), *Loss and grief: Psychological management in medical practice* (pp. 199–217). New York: Columbia University Press.

Broderick, C. B., & Schrader, S. S. (1991). The history of professional marriage and family therapy. In A. S. Gurman & D. P. Kniskern (Eds.), *Handbook of family therapy* (pp. 5–35). New York: Brunner/Mazel.

Broderick, C. B., & Schrader, S. S. (1981). The history of professional marriage and family therapy. In A. S. Gurman & D. P. Kniskern (Eds.), *Handbook of family therapy* (Vol. II, pp. 3–40). New York: Brunner/Mazel.

Bugen, L. A. (1977). Human grief: A model for prediction and intervention. *American Journal of Orthopsychiatry, 47,* 196–206.

Burgess, A. W. (1975). Family reactions to homicide. *American Journal of Orthopsychiatry, 45,* 391–398.

Butler, R. N., & Lewis, M. T. (1977). *Aging and mental health.* St. Louis: C. V. Mosby.

Campbell, A. (1975, May). The American way of mating: Marriage, si, children only maybe. *Psychology Today,* 37–43.

Capra, F. (1983). *The turning point.* New York: Bantam Books.

Carni, E. (1989). To deal or not to deal with death: Family therapy with three older couples. *Family Therapy, 16,* 59–68.

Carter, B., & McGoldrick, M. (Eds.). (1980). *The family life cycle: A framework for family therapy.* New York: Gardner Press.

Carter, B., & McGoldrick, M. (Eds.). (1988a). *The changing family life cycle: A framework for family therapy* (2nd ed.). New York: Gardner Press.

Carter, B., & McGoldrick, M. (1988b). Overview: The changing family life cycle. In B. Carter & M. McGoldrick (Eds.), *The changing family life cycle: A framework for family therapy* (2nd ed., pp. 3–28). New York: Gardner Press.

Christ, J. (1976). Treatment of marital disorders. In H. Grunebaum & J. Christ (Eds.), *Contemporary marriage: Structure, dynamics, and therapy* (pp. 371–399). Boston: Little, Brown.

Colapinto, J. (1988). Teaching the structural way. In H. A. Liddle, D. C. Breunlin, & R. C. Schwartz (Eds.), *Handbook of family therapy training and supervision* (pp. 17–37). New York: Guilford Press.

Colapinto, J. (1991). Structural family therapy. In A. S. Gurman & D. P. Kniskern (Eds.), *Handbook of family therapy* (Vol. II, pp. 417–443). New York: Brunner/Mazel.

Colarusso, C. A., & Nemiroff, R. A. (1987). Clinical implications of adult developmental theory. *American Journal of Psychiatry, 144,* 1263–1270.

Cooney, T. M., Smyer, M. A., Hagestad, C. O., & Klock, R. (1986). Parental divorce in young adulthood: Some preliminary findings. *American Journal of Orthopsychiatry, 56,* 470–477.

Coyne, J. C. (1986). Marital therapy for depression. In N. S. Jacobson & A. S. Gurman (Eds.), *Clinical handbook of marital therapy* (pp. 495–511). New York: Guilford Press.

Coyne, J. C. (1988). Strategic therapy. In J. F. Clarkin, G. L. Haas, & I. D. Glick (Eds.), *Affective disorders and the family: Assessment and treatment* (pp. 89–113). New York: Guilford Press.

Cuber, J. F., & Harroff, P. (1966). *Sex and the significant Americans.* Baltimore: Penguin Books.

Daniels, P., & Weingarten, K. (1982). *Sooner or later: The timing of parenthood in adult lives.* New York: Norton.

Davatz, U. (1981). Establishing a therapeutic alliance in family systems therapy. In A. S. Gurman (Ed.), *Questions and answers in the practice of family therapy* (pp. 46–48). New York: Brunner/Mazel.

Dell, P. F. (1982). Beyond homeostasis: Toward a concept of coherence. *Family Process, 21,* 21–44.

Dell, P. F. (1986). In defense of linear causality. *Family Process, 25,* 513–521.

Denton, W. (1990). A family system analyis of DSM-III-R. *Journal of Marital and Family Therapy, 16,* 113–125.

Derdeyn, A. P., & Scott, E. (1984). Joint cutody: A critical analysis and appraisal. *American Journal of Orthopsychiatry, 54,* 199–209.

de Shazer, S. (1982). Diagnosis = researching + doing therapy. In B. P. Keeney (Ed.), *Diagnosis and assessment in family therapy* (pp. 125–132). Rockville, MD: Aspen.

Dicks, H. V. (1963). Object relations theory and marital studies. *British Journal of Medical Psychology, 36,* 125–129.

Dicks, H. V. (1967). *Marital tensions.* New York: Basic Books.

DiCocco, B. E. (1986). A guide to family/school intervention for the family therapist. *Contemporary Family Therapy, 8,* 50–61.

Dobson, K. S., Jacobson, N. S., & Victor, J. (1988). Integration of cognitive therapy and behavioral marital therapy. In J. F. Clarkin, G. L. Haas, & I. D. Glick (Eds.), *Affective disorders and the family: Assessment and treatment* (pp. 53–88). New York: Guilford Press.

Donnelly, D., & Finkelhor, D. (1992). Does equality in custody arrangements improve the quality of the parent–child relationship? *Journal of Marriage and the Family, 54,* 837–845.

Downey, D. B., & Powell, B. (1993). Do children in single-parent households fare better living with same-sex parents? *Journal of Marriage and the Family, 55,* 55–71.

Draughon, M. (1975). Stepmother's model of identification in relation to mourning in the child. *Psychological Reports, 9*(1), 183–189.

Duhl, B. S., & Duhl, F. J. (1981). Integrative family therapy. In A. S. Gurman & D. P. Kniskern (Eds.), *Handbook of family therapy* (pp. 483–513). New York: Brunner/Mazel.

Duvall, E. M. (1957). *Family development.* Philadelphia: Lippincott.

Duvall, E. M. (1971). *Family development* (4th ed.). Philadelphia: Lippincott.

Duvall, E. M. (1977). *Marriage and family development* (5th ed.). Philadelphia: Lippincott.

Epstein, N. B., Baldwin, L. M., & Bishop, D. S. (1983). The McMaster family assessment device. *Journal of Marital and Family Therapy, 9,* 171–180.

Eagle, M. (1984). Theoretical and clinical shifts in psychoanalysis. *American Journal of Orthopsychiatry, 57,* 175–185.

Erikson, E. H. (1950). *Childhood and society.* New York: Norton.

Everett, C. A., Halperin, S., Volgy, S., & Wissler, A. (1989). *Treating the borderline family: A systemic approach.* San Deigo: Psychological Corporation.

Everett, C. A., & Volgy, S. (1989). Mediating child custody disputes. In M. Textor (Ed.), *The divorce and divorce therapy handbook.* Northvale, NJ: Jason Aronson.

Everett, C. A., & Volgy, S. (1994). *The healthy divorce: A guide for parents and children.* San Francisco: Jossey-Bass.

Fairbairn, W. R. D. (1952). *Psychoanalytic studies of the personality.* London: Routledge & Kegan Paul.

Fairbairn, W. R. D. (1954). *An object relations theory of the personality.* New York: Basic Books.

Fairbairn, W. R. D. (1963). Synopsis of an object-relations theory of the personality. *International Journal of Psycho-Analysis, 44,* 224–225.

Falloon, I. R. H. (1988). Behavioural family therapy: Systems, structures, and strategies. In E. Smith & W. Dryden (Eds.), *Family therapy in Britain* (pp. 101–126). Philadelphia: Milton Keynes.

Farmer, S., & Galaris, D. (1993). Support groups for children of divorce. *American Journal of Family Therapy, 21,* 41–50.

Feldman, L. B. (1979). Marital conflict and marital intimacy: An integrative psychodynamic-behavioral-systemic model. *Family Process, 18,* 69–78.

Feldman, L. B. (1985). Integrative multi-level therapy: A comprehensive interpersonal and intrapsychic approach. *Journal of Marital and Family Therapy, 11,* 357–372.

Feldman, L. B. (1992). *Integrating individual and family therapy.* New York: Brunner/Mazel.

Feldman, L. B., & Pinsof, W. M. (1982). Problem maintenance in family systems: An integrative model. *Journal of Marital and Family Therapy, 8,* 295–308.

Fisch, R. (1983). Commentary. *Family Process, 22,* 438–441.

Fisher, E. O. (1974). *Divorce: The new freedom.* New York: Harper & Row.

Fisher, L. (1977). On the classification of families. *Archives of General Psychiatry, 34.* (Reprinted in Howells, J. G. [Ed.]. [1979]. *Advances in general psychiatry* [Vol. 1, pp. 27–52]. New York: International Universities Press.)

Foster, S. W. (1986). Marital treatment of eating disorders. In N. S. Jacobson & A. S. Gurman (Eds.), *Clinical handbook of marital therapy* (pp. 575–593). New York: Guilford Press.

Framo, J. L. (1965). Rationale and techniques of intensive family therapy. In I.

Boszormenyi-Nagy & J. L. Framo (Eds.), *Intensive family therapy: Theoretical and practical aspects* (pp. 143–212). New York: Hoeber–Harper & Row.

Framo, J. L. (1970). Symptoms from a family transactional viewpoint. In N. W. Ackerman (Ed.), Family therapy in transition. *International Psychiatric Clinics, 7*(4), 125–171.

Framo, J. L. (1976). Family of origin as a therapeutic resource for adults in marital and family therapy: You can and should go home again. *Family Process, 15*, 193–210.

Framo, J. L. (1980). Marriage and marriage therapy: Issues and initial interview techniques. In M. Andolfi & I. Zwerling (Eds.), *Dimensions of family therapy* (pp. 49–71). New York: Guilford Press.

Framo, J. L. (1992). *Family-of-origin therapy: An intergenerational approach.* New York: Brunner/Mazel.

Freud, S. (1959). On psychotherapy. In E. Jones (Ed.), J. Riviere (Trans.), *Collected papers* (Vol. 1). New York: Basic Books. (Original work published 1906)

Friedman, E. H. (1985). *Generation to generation: Family process in church and synagogue.* New York: Guilford Press.

Galper, M. (1978). *Co-parenting: Sharing your child equally.* Philadelphia: Running Press.

Gardner, R. A. (1976). *Psychotherapy with children of divorce.* New York: Jason Aronson.

Giovacchini, P. (1958). Mutual adaptation in various object relationships. *International Journal of Psycho-analysis, 34*, 1–8.

Glaser, B., & Strauss, A. (1968). *Time for dying.* Chicago: Aldine.

Glick, I. D., & Kessler, D. R. (1974). *Marital and family therapy.* New York: Grune & Stratton.

Glucksman, M. L. (1987). Introduction. In M. L. Glucksman & S. L. Warner (Eds.), *Dreams in new perspective: The royal road revisited* (pp. 11–21). New York: Human Sciences Press.

Goldner, V. (1985). Feminism and family therapy. *Family Process, 24*, 31–48.

Goode, W. J. (1956). *After divorce (Women in divorce).* New York: Free Press.

Goodrich, W. (1968). Toward a taxonomy of marriage. In J. Marmor (Ed.), *Contemporary psychoanalysis* (pp. 407–423). New York: Basic Books.

Gray, W., & Rizzo, N. R. (1969). History and development of general system theory. In W. Gray, F. J. Duhl, & N. J. Rizzo (Eds.), *General systems theory and psychiatry* (pp. 7–31). Boston: Little, Brown.

Green, S. L., & Hansen, J. C. (1989). Ethical dilemmas faced by family therapists. *Journal of Marital and Family Therapy, 15*, 149–158.

Greenberg, J. R., & Mitchell, S. A. (1983). *Object relations in psychoanalytic theory.* Cambridge, MA: Harvard University Press.

Greene, B. L. (1970). *A clinical approach to marital problems: Evaluation and management.* Springfield, IL: Charles C. Thomas.

Greene, B. L., Lee, R. R., & Lustig, N. (1975). Treatment of marital disharmony where one spouse has a primary affective disorder (manic–depressive illness): I. General overview—100 couples. *Journal of Marriage and Family Counseling, 1*, 39–50.

Greif, J. B. (1979). Fathers, children, and joint custody. *American Journal of Orthopsychiatry, 49*, 311–319.

Grunebaum, H., & Christ, J. (Eds.). (1976). *Contemporary marriage: Structure, dynamics, and therapy*. Boston: Little, Brown.

Guntrip, H. (1969). *Schizoid phenomena, object relations, and the self*. New York: International Universities Press.

Gurman, A. S. (1980). Behavioral marriage therapy in the 1980s: The challenge of integration. *American Journal of Family Therapy, 8*(2), 86–96.

Gurman, A. S. (1981). Integrative marital therapy: Toward the development of an interpersonal approach. In S. Budman (Ed.), *Forms of brief therapy* (pp. 415–457). New York: Guilford Press.

Gurman, A. S. (1982). Creating a therapeutic alliance in marital therapy. In A. S. Gurman (Ed.), *Questions and answers in the practice of family therapy* (Vol. II). New York: Brunner/Mazel.

Gurman, A. S., & Kniskern, D. P. (1978). Research on marital and family therapy: Progress, perspective, and prospect. In S. L. Garfield & A. E. Bergin (Eds.), *Handbook of psychotherapy and behavior change: An empirical analysis* (2nd ed., pp. 817–901). New York: Wiley.

Gurman, A. S., & Kniskern, D. P. (Eds.). (1981). *Handbook of family therapy*. New York: Brunner/Mazel.

Gurman, A. S., & Kniskern, D. P. (Eds.). (1991). *Handbook of family therapy* (Vol. II). New York: Brunner/Mazel.

Gurman, A. S., Kniskern, D. P., & Pinsof, W. N. (1986). Research on the process and outcome of family therapy. In S. L. Garfield & A. E. Bergin (Eds.), *Handbook of psychotherapy and behavior change* (3rd ed., pp. 525–623). New York: Wiley.

Guttman, H. A. (1991). Systems theory, cybernetics, and epistemology. In A. S. Gurman & D. P. Kniskern (Eds.), *Handbook of family therapy* (Vol II, pp. 41–62). New York: Brunner/Mazel.

Hafner, R. J. (1986). Marital therapy for agoraphobia. In N. S. Jacobson & A. S. Gurman (Eds.), *Clinical handbook of marital therapy* (pp. 471–493). New York: Guilford Press.

Haley, J. (1963). Marriage therapy. *Archives of General Psychiatry, 8*, 213–234.

Haley, J. (1973). *Uncommon therapy: The psychiatric techniques of Milton H. Erickson, M.D.* New York: Norton.

Haley, J. (1976). *Problem solving therapy: New strategies for effective family therapy*. San Francisco: Jossey-Bass.

Haley, J. (1986). Behavior modification and a family view of children. In H. C. Fishman & B. L. Rosman (Eds.), *Evolving models for family change: A volume in honor of Salvador Minuchin* (pp. 44–61). New York: Guilford Press.

Hardy, K. V., & Laszloffy, T. A. (1992). Training racially sensitive family therapists: Context, content, and contact. *Families in Society: The Journal of Contemporary Human Services, 73*, 364–370.

Havighurst, R. J. (1953). *Human development and education*. New York: Longmans, Green.

Hawkins, A. J., Christensen, S. L., Sargent, K. P., & Hill, E. J. (1993). Rethinking fathers' involvement in child care: A developmental perspective. *Journal of Family Issues, 14,* 531–549.

Hetherington, E. M., Stanley-Hagan, M., & Anderson, E. R. (1989). Marital transitions: A child's perspective. *American Psychologist, 44,* 302–312.

Hill, R. (1949). *Families under stress.* New York: Harper & Row.

Hill, R. (1958). Generic features of families under stress. *Social Casework, 49,* 139–150.

Hill, R. (1970). *Family development in three generations.* Cambridge, MA: Schenkman.

Hill, R. (1971). Modern social science and the family. *Social Science Information,* pp. 7–26. (Reprinted in Sussman, M. B. [Ed.]. [1974]. *Sourcebook in marriage and the family* [4th ed., pp. 302–313]. Boston: Houghton Mifflin.)

Hill, R., & Rodgers, R. H. (1964). The developmental approach. In H. T. Christensen (Ed.), *Handbook of marriage and the family* (pp. 171–211). Chicago: Rand McNally.

Hinsie, L. E., & Campbell, R. J. (1960). *Psychiatric dictionary* (3rd. ed.). New York: Oxford University Press.

Hobbs, D. F., & Cole, S. P. (1976). Transition to parenthood: A decade replication. *Journal of Marriage and the Family, 38,* 723–731.

Hoffman, L. (1975). Enmeshment and the too richly cross-joined system. *Family Process, 14,* 457–468.

Hoffman, L. (1981). *Foundations of family therapy.* New York: Basic Books.

Hoffman, L. (1985). Beyond power and control: Toward a "second order" family systems medicine. *Family Systems Medicine, 3,* 381–396.

Hollingshead, A. B. (1950). Cultural factors in the selection of marriage mates. *American Sociological Review, 15,* 619–627.

Howells, J. G. (1975). *Principles of family psychiatry.* New York: Brunner/Mazel.

Imber-Black, E. (1988). *Families and larger systems: A family therapist's guide through the labyrinth.* New York: Guilford Press.

Imber-Black, E. (1991). A family–larger-system perspective. In A. S. Gurman & D. P. Kniskern (Eds.), *Handbook of family therapy* (Vol. II, pp. 583–605). New York: Brunner/Mazel.

Isaacs, M., Montalvo, B., & Abelsohn, D. (1986). *The difficult divorce: Therapy for children and families.* New York: Basic Books.

Jacobson, N. S., & Gurman, A. S. (Eds.). (1986). *Clinical handbook of marital therapy.* New York: Guilford Press.

Jacobson, N. S., & Margolin, G. (1979). *Marital therapy.* New York: Brunner/Mazel.

Jacobson, N. S., & Martin, B. (1976). Behavioral marriage therapy: Current status. *Psychological Bulletin, 83,* 540–556.

James, K., & McIntyre, D. (1983). The reproduction of families: The social role of family therapy? *Journal of Marital and Family Therapy, 15,* 133–138.

Johnson, C. F. (1993). Detriangulation and conflict management in parent–adolescent relationships: A model. *Contemporary Family Therapy, 15,* 185–195.

Johnson, P., Wilkinson, W. K., & McNeil, K. (1995). The impact of parental divorce on the attainment of the developmental tasks of young adulthood. *Contemporary Family Therapy, 17,* 249–264.

Johnston, J. R., Kline, M., & Tschann, J. M. (1989). Ongoing postdivorce conflict: Effects on children of joint custody and frequent access. *American Journal of Orthopsychiatry, 59,* 576–592.

Jones, E. (1953). *The life and work of Sigmund Freud, Vol. 1: 1856–1900—The formative years and great discoveries.* New York: Basic Books.

Jourard, S. M. (1975). Marriage is for life. *Journal of Marriage and Family Counseling, 1,* 199–208.

Kalter, N. (1984). Conjoint mother–daughter treatment: A beginning phase of psychotherapy with adolescent daughters of divorce. *American Journal of Orthopsychiatry, 54,* 490–497.

Kalter, N. (1987). Long-term effects of divorce on children: A developmental vulnerability model. *American Journal of Orthopsychiatry, 57,* 587–600.

Kalter, N., Pickar, J., & Lesowitz, M. (1984). School-based developmental facilitation groups for children of divorce: A preventive intervention. *American Journal of Orthopsychiatry, 54,* 613–623.

Kaplan, H. S. (1974). *The new sex therapy: Active treatment of sexual dysfunction.* New York: Brunner/Mazel.

Kaplan, H. S. (1979). *The new sex therapy: Volume II. Disorders of sexual desire and other new concepts and techniques in sex therapy.* New York: Brunner/Mazel.

Kaplan, H. S. (1987). *Sexual aversion, sexual phobias, and panic disorder.* New York: Brunner/Mazel.

Karpel, M. A. (1980). Family secrets: I. Conceptual and ethical issues in the relational context. II. Ethical and practical considerations in therapeutic management. *Family Process, 19,* 295–306.

Karpel, M. A., & Strauss, E. A. (1983). *Family evaluation.* New York: Gardner Press.

Kaslow, F. W. (1981). Divorce and divorce therapy. In A. S. Gurman & D. P. Kniskern (Eds.), *Handbook of family therapy* (pp. 662–296). New York: Brunner/Mazel.

Kaslow, F. W., & Schwartz, L. L. (1987). *The dynamics of divorce: A life cycle perspective.* New York: Brunner/Mazel.

Kaufman, E., & Kaufmann, P. N. (Eds.). (1979). *Family therapy of drug and alcohol abuse.* New York: Gardner Press.

Kazak, A. E., Jarmas, A., & Snitzer, L. (1988). The assessment of marital satisfaction: An evaluation of the dyadic adjustment scale. *Journal of Family Psychology, 2,* 82–91.

Keith, V. M., & Finlay, B. (1988). The impact of parental divorce on children's educational attainment, marital timing, and probability of divorce. *Journal of Marriage and the Family, 50,* 797–809.

Kelly, J. B. (1993). Current research on children's postdivorce adjustment: No simple answers. *Family and Conciliation Courts Review, 31,* 29–49.

King, P. H. (1980). The life cycle as indicated by the transference in the psychoanalysis of the middle-aged and elderly. *International Journal of Psycho-Analysis, 61*, 153–160.

Kinney, P., Ravich, R., Ford, P., & Vos, B. (1987, Summer). A typology of families: An interview with the Typology Task Force. *AFTA Newsletter, 28*, 21–27.

Kirschner, D. A., & Kirschner, S. (1986). *Comprehensive family therapy: An integration of systemic and psychodynamic treatment models.* New York: Brunner/Mazel.

Kitchener, K. S. (1984). Intuition, critical evaluation, and ethical principles: The foundation for ethical decisions in counseling psychology, *Counseling Psychology, 12*, 43–55.

Klein, H. A. (1974). Behavior modification as therapeutic paradox. *American Journal of Orthopsychiatry, 44*, 353–361.

Klein, M. (1932). *The psycho-analysis of children.* London: Hogarth Press.

Klein, M. (1948). *Contributions to psycho-analysis.* London: Hogarth Press.

Kluckhohn, C., & Murray, H. A. (1956). Personality formation: The determinants. In C. Kluckhohn, H. A. Murrray, & D. M. Schneider (Eds.), *Personality in nature, society, and culture* (2nd ed., pp. 53–67). New York: Knopf.

Koeske, G. F., & Koeske, R. D. (1990). The buffering effect of social support on parental stress. *American Journal of Orthopsychiatry, 60*, 440–451.

Kohut, H. (1971). *The analysis of the self.* New York: International Universities Press.

Kohut, H. (1977). *The restoration of the self.* New York: International Universities Press.

Korchin, S. K. (1976). *Modern clinical psychology.* New York: Basic Books.

Kovacs, L. (1988). Couple therapy: An integrated developmental and family system model. *Family Therapy, 15*, 133–156.

Krantzler, M. (1974). *Creative divorce.* New York: Evans.

Kris, E. (1934). *Psychoanalytic explorations in art.* New York: International Universities Press.

Kubie, L. S. (1956). Psychoanalysis and marriage. In V. Eisenstein (Ed.), *Neurotic interaction in marriage* (pp. 10–43). New York: Basic Books.

Kübler-Ross, E. (1969). *On death and dying.* New York: Macmillan.

L'Abate, L. (1975). Pathogenic role rigidity in fathers: Some observations. *Journal of Marriage and Family Counseling, 1*, 69–79.

L'Abate, L., & Bagarozzi, D. A. (1993). *Sourcebook of marriage and family evaluation.* New York: Brunner/Mazel.

L'Abate, L., & McHenry, S. (1983). *Handbook of marital interventions.* New York: Grune & Stratton.

Lane, A. R., Wilcoxson, S. A., & Cecil, J. H. (1988). Family-of-origin experiences and the transition to parenthood: Considerations for marriage and family therapists. *Family Therapy, 15*, 23–30.

Lansky, M. R. (1985). *Family approaches to major psychiatric disorders.* Washington, DC: American Psychiatric Press.

Lansky, M. R. (1986). Marital therapy for narcissistic disorders. In N. S. Jacobson & A. S. Gurman (Eds.), *Clinical handbook of marital therapy* (pp. 537–556). New York: Guilford Press.

Lederer, W. J., & Jackson, D. D. (1968). *The mirages of marriage.* New York: Norton.

LeMasters, E. E. (1957). Parenthood as crisis. *Marriage and Family Living, 19,* 352–355.

Levinson, D. J., Darrow, C. N., Klein, E. B., Levinson, M. H., & McKee, B. (1974). The psychological development of men in early adulthood and the mid-life transition. In D. F. Ricks, A. Thomas, & M. Roff (Eds.), *Life history in psychopathology* (pp. 243–258). Minneapolis: University of Minnesota Press.

Levinson, D. J., Darrow, C. N., Klein, E. B., Levinson, M. H., & McKee, B. (1978). *The seasons of a man's life.* New York: Alfred A. Knopf.

Lewis, J., Beavers, W. R., Gossett, J. P., & Phillips, V. (1976). *No single thread.* New York: Brunner/Mazel.

Lewis, M., & Rosenblum, L. A. (Eds.). (1990). *The effects of the infant on its care giver.* New York: Wiley.

Liberman, R. P. (1970). Behavioral approaches to family and couple therapy. *American Journal of Orthopsychiatry, 40,* 106–118.

Lidz, T. (1963). *The family and human adaptation.* New York: International Universities Press.

Lopata, H. Z. (1973). *Widowhood in an American city.* Cambridge, MA: Schenkman.

Maccoby, E. E., Depner, C. E., & Mnookin, R. H. (1990). Coparenting in the second year after divorce. *Journal of Marriage and the Family, 52,* 141–155.

Madanes, C. (1984). *Behind the one-way mirror: Advances in the practice of strategic therapy.* San Francisco: Jossey-Bass.

Mallouk, T. (1982). The interpersonal context of object relations: Implications for family therapy. *Journal of Marital and Family Therapy, 8,* 429–441.

Martin, P. A. (1976). *A marital therapy manual.* New York: Brunner/Mazel.

Marziali, E., & Alexander, L. (1991). The power of the therapeutic relationship. *American Journal of Orthopsychiatry, 6,* 383–391.

Maturana, H. R. (1978). Biology of language: The epistemology of reality. In G. A. Miller (Ed.), *Psychology and biology of language and thought: Essays in honor of Eric Lenneberg* (pp. 27–63). New York: Academic Press.

McCollum, E. E. (1993). Beyond intervention. In T. S. Nelson & T. S. Trepper (Eds.), *101 interventions in family therapy* (pp. 414–417). New York: Haworth Press.

McCubbin, M. A., & McCubbin, H. I. (1989). Theoretical orientations to family stress and coping. In C. R. Figley (Ed.), *Treating stress in families* (pp. 3–43). New York: Brunner/Mazel.

Lindemann, E. (1944). Symptomatology and management of acute grief. *American Journal of Psychiatry, 101,* 141–148.

London, P. (1986). *The models and morals of psychotherapy* (2nd ed.). New York: Hemisphere.

McFarlane, W. R. (Ed.). (1983). *Family therapy in schizophrenia.* New York: Guilford Press.

McFarlane, W. R. (1991). Family psychoeducational treatment. In A. S. Gurman

& D. P. Kniskern (Eds.), *Handbook of family therapy* (Vol. II, pp. 363–395). New York: Brunner/Mazel.

McGoldrick, M. (1980). The joining of family through marriage: The new couple. In E. A. Carter & M. McGoldrick (Eds.), *The family life cycle: A framework for family therapy* (pp. 93–119). New York: Gardner Press.

McGoldrick, M., & Gerson, R. (1985). *Genograms in family assessment.* New York: Norton.

McGoldrick, M., Pearce, J. K., & Giordano, J. (Eds.). (1982). *Ethnicity and family therapy.* New York: Guilford Press.

McGoldrick, M., & Walsh, F. (1991). A time to mourn: Death and the family life cycle. In F. Walsh & M. McGoldrick (Eds.), *Living beyond loss: Death in the family* (pp. 30–49). New York: Norton.

McLanahan, S., & Bumpass, L. (1988). Intergenerational consequences of family disruption. *American Journal of Sociology, 94,* 130–152.

Meissner, W. W. (1980). A note on projective identification. *Journal of the American Psychoanalytic Association, 28,* 43–67.

Messinger, L. (1976). Remarriage between divorced people with children from previous marriages: A proposal for remarriage. *Journal of Marriage and Family Counseling, 2,* 193–200.

Miller, I. W., Kabacoff, R. I., Epstein, N. B., Bishop, D. S., Keitner, G. I., Baldwin, L. M., & van der Spuy, H. I. J. (1994). The development of a clinical rating scale of the McMaster Model of Family Functioning. *Family Process, 33,* 53–69.

Miller, J. G. (1969). Living systems: Basic concepts. In W. Gray, F. J. Duhl, & N. J. Rizzo (Eds.), *General systems theory and psychiatry* (pp. 51–133). Boston: Little, Brown.

Miller, J. G., & Miller, J. I. (1980). The family as a system. In C. K. Hofling & J. M. Lewis (Eds.), *The family: Evaluation and treatment* (pp. 141–184). New York: Brunner/Mazel.

Miller, S., Wackman, D., Nunnally, E., & Saline, C. (1982). *Straight talk.* New York: New American Library.

Minuchin, P. (1985). Families and individual development: Provocations from the field of family development. *Child Development, 56,* 289–302.

Minuchin, S. (1974). *Families and family therapy.* Cambridge, MA: Harvard University Press.

Minuchin, S. (1982). Reflections on boundaries. *American Journal of Orthopsychiatry, 52,* 655–663.

Minuchin, S., & Fishman, H. C. (1981). *Family therapy techniques.* Cambridge, MA: Harvard University Press.

Minuchin, S., Montalvo, B., Guerney, B., Rosman, B., & Schumer, F. (1967). *Families in the slums.* New York: Basic Books.

Mishne, J. M. (1993). *The evolution and application of clinical theory: Perspectives from four psychologies.* New York: Free Press.

Moss, D. M., & Lee, R. R. (1976). Homogamous and heterogamous marriages. *International Journal of Psychoanalytic Psychotherapy, 5,* 395–412.

Mullahy, P. (1955). *Oedipus: Myth and complex.* New York: Grove Press.

Multicultural practice [Special issue]. (1992). *Families in Society: The Journal of Contemporary Human Services, 73.*

Murstein, B. I. (1961). The complementary needs hypothesis in newlyweds and middle-aged married couples. *Journal of Abnormal and Social Psychology, 63,* 194–197.

Napier, A. Y. (1971). The marriage of families: Cross-generational complementarity. *Family Process, 9,* 373–393.

Napier, A. Y. (1976). Beginning struggles with families. *Journal of Marriage and Family Counseling, 2,* 3–12.

Napier, A. Y. (1978). The rejection–intrusion pattern: A central family dynamic. *Journal of Marriage and Family Counseling, 4,* 5–12.

Napier, A. Y., & Whitaker, C. A. (1978). *The family crucible.* New York: Harper & Row.

National Center for Health Statistics. (1993). Annual summary of births, marriages, divorces, and death: United States, 1992. *Monthly Vital Statistics Report, 41*(3). Hyattsville, MD: U.S. Public Health Service.

Neill, J., & Kniskern, D. P. (Eds.). (1982). *From psyche to system: The evolving therapy of Carl Whitaker.* New York: Guilford Press.

Nelson, T. S., & Trepper, T. S. (Eds.). (1993). *101 interventions in family therapy.* New York: Haworth Press.

Nerin, W. F. (1986). *Family reconstruction: Long day's journey into light.* New York: Norton.

Nichols, W. C. (1977). Divorce and remarriage education. *Journal of Divorce, 1,* 153–161.

Nichols, W. C. (1978). The marriage relationship. *Family Coordinator, 27,* 185–191.

Nichols, W. C. (1980). Stepfamilies: A growing family therapy challenge. In L. R. Wolberg & M. L. Aronson (Eds.), *Group and family therapy 1980* (pp. 335–344). New York: Brunner/Mazel.

Nichols, W. C. (1984). Therapeutic needs of children in family system reorganization. *Journal of Divorce, 7*(4), 23–34.

Nichols, W. C. (1985a). A differentiating couple: Some transgenerational issues in marital therapy. In A. S. Gurman (Ed.), *Casebook of marital therapy* (pp. 199–228). New York: Guilford Press.

Nichols, W. C. (1985b). Family therapy with children of divorce. *Journal of Psychotherapy and the Family, 1*(2), 55–68.

Nichols, W. C. (1986). Sibling subsystem therapy in family system reorganization. *Journal of Divorce, 9*(3), 13–31.

Nichols, W. C. (1988). *Marital therapy: An integrative approach.* New York: Guilford Press.

Nichols, W. C. (1989). Problems and needs of children. In M. Textor (Ed.), *The divorce and divorce therapy handbook* (pp. 61–76). Northvale, NJ: Jason Aronson.

Nichols, W. C. (1992). *Treating adult survivors of childhood sexual abuse.* Sarasota, FL: Professional Resource Press.

Nichols, W. C., & Everett, C. A. (1986). *Systemic family therapy: An integrative approach*. New York: Guilford Press.

Nichols, W. C., & Pace-Nichols, M. A. (1993). Developmental perspectives and family therapy: The marital life cycle. *Contemporary Family Therapy, 15*, 299–315.

Norcross, J. C. (1991). Prescriptive matching in psychotherapy: Psychoanalysis for simple phobias? *Psychotherapy, 28*, 439–443.

Norcross, J. C., & Napolitano, G. (1986). Defining our journal and ourselves. *International Journal of Eclectic Psychotherapy, 5*, 249–255.

Norcross, J. C., & Newman, C. F. (1992). Psychotherapy integration: Setting the context. In J. C. Norcross & M. R. Goldfried (Eds.), *Handbook of psychotherapy integration* (pp. 3–45). New York: Basic Books.

Oates, W. E. (1955). *Anxiety in Christian experience*. Philadelphia: Westminster Press.

O'Farrell, T. J. (1986). Marital therapy in the treatment of alcoholism. In N. S. Jacobson & A. S. Gurman (Eds.), *Clinical handbook of marital therapy* (pp. 513–535). New York: Guilford Press.

O'Leary, K. D., & Turkewitz, H. (1978). The treatment of marriage and marriage disorders from a behavioral perspective. In T. J. Paolino & B. S. McCrady (Eds.), *Marriage and marital therapy* (pp. 240–297). New York: Brunner/Mazel.

Olson, D. H. (1988). Capturing family change: Multi-system level assessment. In L. C. Wynne (Ed.), *The state of the art in family therapy research: Controversies and recommendations* (pp. 75–80). New York: Family Process Press.

Orgun, I. M. (1973). Playroom setting for diagnostic family interviews. *American Journal of Psychiatry, 130*, 540–542.

Palazzoli, M. S., Boscolo, L., Cecchin, G., & Prata, G. (1978). *Paradox and counterparadox*. New York: Jason Aronson.

Paolino, T. J., & McCrady, B. S. (Eds.). (1978). *Marriage and marital therapy*. New York: Brunner/Mazel.

Papajohn, J., & Spiegel, J. (1975). *Transactions in families*. San Francisco: Jossey-Bass.

Papp, P. (1980). The Greek chorus and other techniques of paradoxical therapy. *Family Process, 19*, 45–57.

Papp, P. (1981). Paradoxical strategies and countertransference. In A. S. Gurman (Ed.), *Questions and answers in the practice of family therapy* (pp. 201–203). New York: Brunner/Mazel.

Papp, P. (1983). *The process of change*. New York: Guilford Press.

Parkes, C. M. (1973). *Bereavement*. New York: International Universities Press.

Parloff, M. B. (1986). Frank's "common elements" in psychotherapy: Nonspecific factors and placebos. *American Journal of Orthopsychiatry, 56*, 521–530.

Parsons, T., & Bales, R. F. (1955). *The family, socialization and interaction process*. Glencoe, IL: Free Press.

Patterson, G. R. (1974). Retraining of aggressive boys by their parents: Review of recent literature and followup evaluation. *Canadian Psychiatric Association Journal, 19*, 142–161.

Patterson, G. R. (1982). A social learning approach to family intervention. Vol. 3. Coercive family process. Eugene, OR: Castalia.

Patterson, G. R., & Reid, J. B. (1970). Reciprocity and coercion: Two facets of social systems. In C. Neuringer & J. L. White (Eds.), Behavior modification in clinical psychology (pp. 137–177). New York: Appleton-Century-Crofts.

Paul, N. L., & Paul, B. B. (1975). A marital puzzle: Transgenerational analysis in marriage counseling. New York: Norton.

Pearson, J., & Thonennes, N. (1990). Custody after divorce: Demographic and attitudinal patterns. American Journal of Orthopsychiatry, 60, 233–249.

Peck, E. (1971). The baby trap. New York: Geis.

Peck, J. S., & Manocherian, J. (1988). Divorce in the changing family life cycle. In B. Carter & M. McGoldrick (Eds.), The changing family life cycle: A framework for family therapy (2nd ed., pp. 335–369). New York: Gardner Press.

Pedro-Carroll, J. L., & Cowen, E. L. (1987). The children of divorce intervention program: An investigation of the efficacy of a school-based prevention program. Journal of Consulting and Clinical Psychology, 53, 603–611.

Peretz, D. (1970a). Development, object-relationships, and loss. In B. Schoenberg, A. C. Carr, D. Peretz, & A. H. Kutscher (Eds.), Loss and grief: Psychological management in medical practice (pp. 3–19). New York: Columbia University Press.

Peretz, D. (1970b). Reaction to loss. In B. Schoenberg, A. C. Carr, D. Peretz, & A. H. Kutscher (Eds.), Loss and grief: Psychological management in medical practice (pp. 20–35). New York: Columbia University Press.

Peterson, M. A. (1992). At personal risk: Boundary violations in professional–client relationships. New York: Norton.

Piercy, F. P., Sprenkle, D. H., & Associates. (1986). Family therapy sourcebook. New York: Guilford Press.

Pincus, L., & Dare, C. (1978). Secrets in the family. New York: Pantheon Books.

Pinsof, W. M. (1983). Integrative problem-centered therapy: Toward the synthesis of family and individual psychotherapies. Journal of Marital and Family Therapy, 9, 19–35.

Pinsof, W. M. (1990, November). What's wrong with family therapy. Paper presented at the annual meeting of the American Association for Marriage and Family Therapy, Washington, DC.

Pinsof, W. M., & Catherall, D. R. (1986). The integrative psychotherapy alliance: Family, couple, and individual therapy scales. Journal of Marital and Family Therapy, 12, 137–151.

Prochaska, J. O., & DiClemente, C. C. (1992). The transtheoretical approach. In J. C. Norcross & M. R. Goldfried (Eds.), Handbook of psychotherapy integration (pp. 300–334). New York: Basic Books.

Ransom, J. W., Schlesinger, S., & Derdeyn, A. P. (1979). A stepfamily in formation. American Journal of Orthopsychiatry, 49, 36–43.

Rapoport, A. (1968). Foreword. In W. Buckley (Ed.), Modern systems research for the behavioral scientist (pp. xiii–xxii). Chicago: Aldine.

Rapoport, R., & Rapoport, R. N. (1964). New light on the honeymoon. *Human Relations, 17*(1), 33–56.

Reiss, D. (1980). Pathways to assessing the family: Some choice points and a sample route. In C. K. Hofling & J. M. Lewis (Eds.), *The family: Evaluation and treatment* (pp. 86–121). New York: Brunner/Mazel.

Rice, J. K., & Rice, D. G. (1986). *Living through divorce: A developmental approach to divorce therapy.* New York: Guilford Press.

Rodgers, R. H. (1973). *Family interaction and transaction: A transactional approach.* Englewood Cliffs, NJ: Prentice-Hall.

Rollins, B. C., & Feldman, H. (1970). Marital satisfaction over the family life cycle. *Journal of Marriage and the Family, 32,* 20–28.

Roman, M., & Haddad, W. (1974). *The disposable parent: The case for joint custody.* New York: Penguin.

Roos, P. A. (1985). *Gender and work: A comparative analysis of industrial societies.* Albany: State University of New York Press.

Rosenberg, E. B. (1980). Therapy with siblings in reorganizing families. *International Journal of Family Therapy, 2,* 139–150.

Rosenberg, E. B. (1992). *The adoption life cycle: The children and their families through the years.* New York: Free Press.

Rosman, B. L. (1986). Developmental perspectives in family therapy with children. In C. H. Fishman & B. L. Rosman (Eds.), *Evolving models for family change: A volume in honor of Salvador Minuchin* (pp. 227–233). New York: Guilford Press.

Rossi, A. (1968). Transition to parenthood. *Journal of Marriage and the Family, 30,* 26–39.

Rossiter, A. B. (1988). A model for group intervention with preschool children experiencing separation and divorce. *American Journal of Orthopsychiatry, 58,* 387–396.

Rutledge, A. L. (1963). Should the marriage counselor ever recommend divorce? *Marriage and Family Living, 25,* 319–324.

Ryder, R., & Hepworth, J. (1990). AAMFT ethical code: "Dual relationships." *Journal of Marital and Family Therapy, 16,* 127–132.

Sager, C. J. (1966). The treatment of marital couples. In S. Arieti (Ed.), *American handbook of psychiatry* (Vol. 3, pp. 213–224). New York: Basic Books.

Sager, C. J. (1976). *Marriage contracts and couples therapy.* New York: Brunner/Mazel.

Sager, C. J. (1981). Couples therapy and marriage contracts. In A. S. Gurman & D. P. Kniskern (Eds.), *Handbook of family therapy* (pp. 85–130). New York: Brunner/Mazel.

Sager, C. J., Brown, H. S., Crohn, H., Engel, T., Rodstein, E., & Walker, L. (1983). *Treating the remarried family.* New York: Brunner/Mazel.

Sander, F. M. (1979). *Individual and family therapy: Toward an integration.* New York: Jason Aronson.

Satir, V. (1964). *Conjoint family therapy.* Palo Alto, CA: Science & Behavior Books.

Sawyer, M. C., Baghurst, P. A., Cross, D. G., & Kalucy, R. S. (1988). Family

Assessment Device: Reports from mothers, fathers, and adolescents in community and clinic families. *Journal of Marital and Family Therapy,* 4, 287–296.

Scharff, D. E., & Scharff, J. S. (1987). *Object relations family therapy.* Northvale, NJ: Jason Aronson.

Scharff, D. E., & Scharff, J. S. (1991). *Object relations couples therapy.* Northvale, NJ: Jason Aronson.

Scharff, J. S. (Ed.). (1989). *Foundations of object relations family therapy.* Northvale, NJ: Jason Aronson.

Scherz, F. H. (1971). Maturational crises and parent–child interaction. *Social Casework,* 52, 362–369.

Schibuk, M. (1989). Treating the sibling subsystem: An adjunct of divorce therapy. *American Journal of Orthopsychiatry,* 59, 226–237.

Schnarch, D. M. (1991). *Constructing the sexual crucible: An integration of sexual and marital therapy.* New York: Norton.

Schoenberg, B., & Senescu, R. A. (1970). The patient's reaction to fatal illness. In B. Schoenberg, A. C. Carr, D. Peretz, & A. H. Kutscher (Eds.), *Loss and grief: Psychological management in medical practice* (pp. 221–237). New York: Columbia University Press.

Schupack, D. (July 7, 1994). Young love, brief marriage, early divorce. *The New York Times,* pp. B2, B5.

Seagraves, R. T. (1982). *Marital therapy: A combined psychodynamic-behavioral approach.* New York: Plenum Press.

Segal, H. (1964). *Introduction to the work of Melanie Klein.* New York: Basic Books.

Seligman, M. (1975). *Helplessness: On depression, development, and death.* San Francisco: Freeman.

Shapiro, R. J., & Budman, S. H. (1973). Separation, termination, and continuation in family and individual therapy. *Family Process,* 12, 55–67.

Sholevar, G. P., & Sonne, J. C. (1979). *A family based intervention with children of marital disruption.* Unpublished manuscript, Jefferson Medical College, Philadelphia. (Cited in Sholevar, G. P. [Ed.]. [1981]. *The handbook of marriage and marital therapy.* New York: SP Medical and Scientific Books.)

Skinner, B. F. (1953). *Science and human behavior.* New York: Macmillan.

Skynner, A. C. R. (1981). An open-systems, group-analytic approach to family therapy. In A. S. Gurman & D. P. Kniskern (Eds.), *Handbook of family therapy* (pp. 39–84). New York: Brunner/Mazel.

Slipp, S. (1984). *Object relations: A dynamic bridge between individual and family treatment.* New York: Jason Aronson.

Slipp, S. (1988). *The technique and practice of object relations family therapy.* Northvale, NJ: Jason Aronson.

Slipp, S., Ellis, S., & Kressel, K. (1974). Factors associated with engagement in family therapy. *Family Process,* 13, 413–427.

Sluzki, C. (1975). The coalitionary process in initiating family therapy. *Family Process,* 14, 67–77.

Solomon, A. (1992). Clinical diagnosis among diverse populations: A multicultural perspective. *Families in Society: The Journal of Contemporary Human Services, 73*, 371–377.

Solomon, M. A. (1973). A developmental, conceptual framework for family therapy. *Family Process, 12*, 179–188.

Solomon, M. A. (1977). The staging of family treatment: An approach to developing the therapeutic alliance. *Journal of Marriage and Family Counseling, 3*, 59–66.

Somers, M. (1993). A comparison of voluntarily childfree adults and parents. *Journal of Marriage and the Family, 55*, 643–650.

Spanier, G. B., & Casto, R. F. (1979). Adjustment to separation and divorce: A qualitative analysis. In G. Levinger & O. C. Moles (Eds.), *Divorce and separation* (pp. 201–227). New York: Basic Books.

Spanier, G. B., & Glick, P. C. (1980). Paths to remarriage. *Journal of Divorce, 3*, 283–298

Spanier, G. B., & Thompson, L. (1984). *Parting: The aftermath of separation and divorce.* Beverly Hills, CA: Sage.

Steinglass, P. (1978). The conceptualization of marriage from a systems theory perspective. In T. J. Paolino & B. S. McCrady (Eds.), *Marriage and marital therapy* (pp. 298–365). New York: Brunner/Mazel.

Steinglass, P., Bennett, L. A., Wolin, S. J., & Reiss, D. (1987). *The alcoholic family.* New York: Basic Books.

Steinman, S. (1981). The experience of children in a joint-custody arrangement: A report of a study. *American Journal of Orthopsychiatry, 51*, 403–414.

Stewart, R. H., Peters, T. C., Marsh, S., & Peters, M. J. (1975). An object-relations approach to psychotherapy with marital couples, families, and children. *Family Process, 14*, 161–178.

Stierlin, H. (1974). *Separating parents and adolescents.* New York: Quadrangle.

Stierlin, H. (1977). *Psychoanalysis and family therapy.* New York: Jason Aronson.

Stierlin, H. (1981). *Separating parents and adolescents.* New York: Jason Aronson.

Stuart, R. B. (1980). *Helping couples change: A social learning approach to marital therapy.* Guilford Press.

Sullivan, H. S. (1953a). *Conceptions of modern psychiatry.* New York: Norton.

Sullivan, H. S. (1953b). *The interpersonal theory of psychiatry.* New York: Norton.

Sullivan, H. S. (1954). *The psychiatric interview.* New York: Norton.

Sullivan, H. S. (1962). *Schizophrenia as a human process.* New York: Norton.

Sullivan, H. S. (1964). *The fusion of psychiatry and social science.* New York: Norton.

Teismann, M. W. (1980). Convening strategies in family therapy. *Family Process, 19*, 393–400.

Tmychuk, A. J. (1979). *Parents and family therapy.* New York: SP Medical and Scientific Books.

Thibaut, J. W., & Kelley, H. H. (1959). *The social psychology of groups.* New York: Wiley.

Thomas, E. J. (1977). *Marital communication and decision making.* New York: Wiley.

Toman, W. (1993). *Family constellation: Its effect on personality and social behavior* (4th ed.). New York: Springer.

Touliatos, J., Perlmutter, B. F., & Straus, M. A. (Eds.). (1990). *Handbook of family measurement techniques*. Newbury Park, CA: Sage.

Trad, P. V. (1990). *Infant previewing: Predicting and sharing interpersonal outcome*. New York: Springer-Verlag.

Trad, P. V. (1992). *Interventions with parents: The theory and practice of previewing*. New York: Wiley.

Trad, P. V. (1993). Menarche: A crossroads that previews developmental change. *Contemporary Family Therapy, 15,* 223–246.

Unger, R. K., & Crawford, M. (1993). Commentary: Sex and gender: The troubled relationship between terms and concepts. *Psychological Science, 4,* 122–124.

Veevers, J. E. (1973). Voluntary childlessness: A neglected area of family study. *Family Coordinator, 22,* 199–205.

Veevers, J. E. (1974). Voluntary childlessness and social policy: An alternative view. *Family Coordinator, 23,* 397–406.

Veevers, J. E. (1975). The moral careers of voluntarily childless wives: Notes on the defense of a variant world view. *Family Coordinator, 24,* 473–487.

Vincent, C. E. (1972). An open letter to the "caught generation." *Family Coordinator, 21,* 143–150.

Vincent, J. P. (Ed.). (1980). *Advances in family intervention, assessment, and theory*. Greenwich, CT: JAI Press.

Visher, E. B., & Visher, J. S. (1979). *Stepfamilies*. New York: Brunner/Mazel.

Visher, E. B., & Visher, J. S. (1990). Dynamics of successful stepfamilies. *Journal of Divorce and Remarriage, 14*(1), 3–12.

Vogel, E., & Bell, N. W. (1960). The emotionally disturbed child as a family scapegoat. In N. W. Bell & E. Vogel (Eds.), *The family* (pp. 382–397). Glencoe, IL: Free Press.

von Bertalanffy, L. (1968). *General system theory*. New York: Braziller.

Wachtel, E. F., & Wachtel, P. L. (1986). *Family dynamics in individual psychotherapy: A guide to clinical strategies*. New York: Guilford Press.

Wachtel, P. L. (1977). *Psychoanalysis and behavior therapy: Toward an integration*. New York: Basic Books.

Wachtel, P. L. (1987). *Action and insight*. New York: Guilford Press.

Wachtel, P. L., & McKinney, M. K. (1992). Cyclical psychodynamics and integrative psychodynamic therapy. In J. C. Norcross & M. R. Goldfried (Eds.), *Handbook of psychotherapy integration* (pp. 335–370). New York: Basic Books.

Wahlroos, S. (1974). *Family communication*. New York: New American Library.

Wallace, P. M., & Gotlieb, I. H. (1990). Marital adjustment during the transition to parenthood: Stability and predictors of change. *Journal of Marriage and the Family, 52,* 21–29.

Wallerstein, J. S. (1983). Children of divorce: The psychological tasks of the child. *American Journal of Orthopsychiatry, 53,* 230–243.

Wallerstein, J. S. (1991). Tailoring the intervention to the child in the separating and divorced family. *Family and Conciliation Courts Review, 29,* 448–459.

Walsh, F., & McGoldrick, M. (Eds.) (1991). *Living beyond loss: Death in the family.* New York: Norton.

Watzlawick, P., Beavin, J., & Jackson, D. D. (1967). *Pragmatics of human communication: A study on interactional patterns, pathologies and paradoxes.* New York: Norton.

Watzlawick, P., Weakland, J. H., & Fisch, R. (1974). *Change: Principles of problem formation and problem solution.* New York: Norton.

Weiner-Davis, M. (1992). *Divorce busting: A revolutionary and rapid program for "staying together."* New York: Summit Books.

Weiss, R. L. (1978). The conceptualization of marriage and marriage disorders from a behavioral perspective. In T. J. Paolino & B. S. McCrady (Eds.), *Marriage and marital therapy* (pp. 165–239). New York: Brunner/Mazel.

Weiss, R. L., Hops, H., & Patterson, G. R. (1973). A framework for conceptualizing marital conflict: A technology for altering it, some data for evaluating it. In L. A. Hammerlynck, L. C. Handy, & E. J. Mash (Eds.), *Behavior change: Methodology, concepts, and practice* (pp. 309–342). Champaign, IL: Research Press.

Weiss, R. S. (1975). *Marital separation.* New York: Basic Books.

Westley, W. A., & Epstein, N. B. (1969). *The silent majority.* San Francisco: Jossey-Bass.

Whitaker, C. A. (1958a). *Psychotherapy of chronic schizophrenic patients.* Boston: Little, Brown.

Whitaker, C. A. (1958b). Psychotherapy with couples. *American Journal of Psychotherapy, 12,* 18–23.

Whitaker, C. A., & Bumberry, W. M. (1988). *Dancing with the family: A symbolic–experiential approach.* New York: Brunner/Mazel.

Whitaker, C. A., & Keith, D. V. (1981). Symbolic–experiential family therapy. In A. S. Gurman & D. P. Kniskern (Eds.), *Handbook of family therapy* (pp. 187–225). New York: Brunner/Mazel.

Wile, D. B. (1981). *Couples therapy.* New York: Wiley.

Wilkinson, I. (1993). *Family assessment.* New York: Gardner Press.

Willi, J. G. (1982). *Couples in collusion.* New York: Jason Aronson.

Willi, J. G. (1984). *Dynamics of couples therapy.* New York: Jason Aronson.

Willi, J. G. (1992). *Growing together, staying together.* Los Angeles: Jeremy P. Tarcher.

Williamson, D. S. (1991). *The intimacy paradox: Personal authority in the family system.* New York: Guilford Press.

Wills, T. A., Weiss, R. L., & Patterson, G. R. (1974). A behavioral analysis of the determinants of marital satisfaction. *Journal of Consulting and Clinical Psychology, 42,* 802–811.

Wilson, G. T., & Evans, I. (1977). The patient–therapist relationship in behavior therapy. In A. S. Gurman & A. M. Razin (Eds.), *Effective psychotherapy: A handbook of research.* New York: Pergamon.

Winch, R. F. (1958). *Mate selection.* New York: Harper & Row.

Wolpe, J. (1958). *Psychotherapy by reciprocal inhibition.* Stanford, CA: Stanford University Press.

Woody, J. D. (1990). Resolving ethical issues in clinical practice: Toward a pragmatic model. *Journal of Marital and Family Therapy, 16,* 133–150.

World Health Organization. (1979). *The international classification of diseases* (9th rev.). *Clinical modification (ICD-9-CM)* (Vol 2). Los Angeles: Practice Management Information Corporation (PMIC).

Wynne, L. C. (1965). Some indications and contraindications for exploratory family therapy. In I. Boszormenyi-Nagy & J. L. Framo (Eds.), *Intensive family therapy: Theoretical and practical aspects* (pp. 289–322). New York: Hoeber–Harper & Row.

Wynne, L. C. (1983). Family research and family therapy: A reunion. *Journal of Marital and Family Therapy, 9,* 113–117.

Wynne, L. C. (1986). Structure and lineality in family therapy. In H. C. Fishman & B. L. Rosman (Eds.), *Evolving models for family change: A volume in honor of Salvador Minuchin* (pp. 251–260). New York: Guilford Press.

Wynne, L. C. (Ed.). (1988). *The state of the art in family therapy research: Controversies and recommendations.* New York: Family Process Press.

Wynne, L. C., McDaniel, S. H., & Weber, T. T. (Eds.). (1986). *Systems consultation: A new perspective for family therapy.* New York: Guilford Press.

Young, D. M. (1989). Group intervention for children of divorced families. In M. Textor (Ed.), *The divorce and divorce therapy handbook* (pp. 267–284). Northvale, NJ: Jason Aronson.

Zemon-Gass, G., & Nichols, W. C. (1981). *Changing marital developmental tasks: Continuing family therapy issues.* Unpublished manuscript.

Zemon-Gass, G., & Nichols, W. C. (1988). Gaslighting: A marital syndrome. *Contemporary Family Therapy, 10,* 3–16.

Zilbach, J. J., Bergel, E., & Gass, C. (1972). The role of the young child in family therapy. In C. J. Sager & H. S. Kaplan (Eds.), *Progress in group and family therapy* (pp. 385–399). New York: Brunner/Mazel.

Zinner, J. (1976). The implications of projective identification for marital interaction. In H. Grunebaum & J. Christ (Eds.), *Contemporary marriage: Structure, dynamics, and therapy* (pp. 293–308). Boston: Little, Brown.

Zinner, J., & Shapiro, R. L. (1989). The family group as a single psychic entity: Implications for acting out in adolescence. In J. S. Scharff (Ed.), *Foundations of object relations therapy* (pp. 187–202). Northvale, NJ: Jason Aronson.

Zuk, G. H. (1967). Family therapy. *Archives of General Psychiatry, 16,* 71–79.

Zuk, G. H. (1969). Triadic-based family therapy. *International Journal of Psychiatry, 8,* 539–548.

Zuk, G. H. (1976). Family therapy: Clinical hodgepodge or clinical science? *Journal of Marriage and Family Counseling, 2,* 299–303.

Zuk, G. H. (1986). *Process and practice in family therapy* (2nd ed.). New York: Human Sciences Press.

Zygmond, M. J., & Boorhem, H. (1989). Ethical decision making in family therapy. *Family Process, 28,* 269–280.

INDEX